Optics of the Human Eye

Optics of the Human Eye

David A. Atchison
BScOptom MScOptom PhD GradCertEd FAAO

School of Optometry, Queensland University of Technology

George Smith
BSc MSc PhD

Department of Optometry and Vision Sciences, University of Melbourne

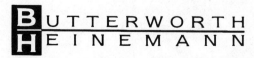

OXFORD   AUCKLAND   BOSTON   JOHANNESBURG   MELBOURNE   NEW DELHI

Butterworth-Heinemann
An imprint of Elsevier Science Limited
Robert Stevenson House
1–3 Baxter's Place
Leith Walk
Edinburgh EH1 3AF

First published 2000
Reprinted 2002

British Library Cataloguing in Publication Data
A catalogue record for this book is available from the British Library

Library of Congress Cataloging in Publication Data
A catalog record for this book is available from the Library of Congress

ISBN 0 7506 3775 7

your source for books,
journals and multimedia
in the health sciences
www.elsevierhealth.com

Typeset by E & M Graphics, Midsomer Norton, Bath
Printed and bound in Great Britain by The Bath Press, Somerset

Contents

Acknowledgements

Several colleagues have commented on drafts or provided references and advice. In particular, we thank Brian Brown, Niall Strang and Tom Raasch, who read substantial sections of drafts. Others include Ray Applegate, Pablo Artal, Harold Bedell, Arthur Bradley, Neil Charman, Nicolas Chateau, Michael Doughty, Dave Elliot, Richard Guy, Douglas Horner, Tony Joblin, Phil Kruger, Barbara Pierscionek, Katrina Schmid, Lawrence Stark, Peter Swann, Christopher Tyler, Barry Winn, Joanne Wood and Russell Woods.

We are grateful to Pablo Artal, Michael Cox, Larry Thibos and Barry Winn for providing data for some figures; these are also acknowledged at the appropriate figure captions. We thank the American Academy of Optometry, the Optical Society of America, Elsevier Press and the Association for Research in Vision and Ophthalmology for permission to use previously published data; again, these are acknowledged at the appropriate figure captions.

Finally, we thank our wives, Janette and Yolette, for their support.

Sign convention and symbols

When we examine image formation and ray-tracing, we need a sign convention. Although the choice of a sign convention is arbitrary, it must be consistent. In this book we use the standard cartesian and trigonometric sign conventions. Distances to the left of a surface or other reference position or below the optical axis are negative, and those to the right or above are positive. Angles due to anticlockwise rotations of the ray from the optical axis are positive, and those due to clockwise rotations are negative.

Distance notation and sign

Points are denoted by Roman letters in bold. Distances are denoted by either a single lower case letter such as l, or by two upper case letters such as **PF**. In this example, **P** and **F** are both points and **PF** denotes the distance from **P** to **F**. If **F** is to the right of **P**, this distance is positive, and if **F** is to the left of **P**, this distance is negative.

Greek alphabet

Greek letters are used extensively throughout the book.

αA	alpha	βB	beta	γΓ	gamma
δΔ	delta	εE	epsilon	ζZ	zeta
ηH	eta	θΘ	theta	ιI	iota
κK	kappa	λΛ	lambda	μM	mu
νN	nu	ξΞ	xi	oO	omicron
πΠ	pi	ρP	rho	σΣ	sigma
τT	tau	υY	upsilon	φΦ	phi
χX	chi	ψΨ	psi	ωΩ	omega

Units and their abbreviations

metre	m
centimetre	cm
millimetre	mm
micrometre	μm
nanometre	nm
dioptre	D
prism dioptre	Δ
Joule	J
Watt	W
candela	cd
lumens	lm
steradian	st
second	s
Hertz	Hz
Kelvin	K
radian	rad
degree	°, deg
minutes of arc	min. arc

Introduction

The purpose of this book is to describe the optical structure and optical properties of the human eye. It will be useful to those who have an interest in vision, such as optometrists, ophthalmologists, vision scientists, optical physicists, and students of visual optics. An understanding of the optics of the human eye is particularly important to designers of ophthalmic diagnostic equipment and visual optical systems such as telescopes.

Most animals have some sort of eye structure or sophisticated light sense. Like humans, some rely heavily on vision, including predatory birds and insects such as honeybees and dragonflies. However, many animals rely much more on other senses, particularly hearing and smell, than on vision. The visual sense is very complex and is able to process huge amounts of information very rapidly. How this is done is not fully understood; it requires greater knowledge of how the neural components of vision (retina, visual cortex, and other brain centres) process the retinal image. However, the first stage in this complex process is the formation of the retinal image. In this text, we investigate how the image is formed and discuss factors that affect its quality.

The majority of animal eyes can be divided into two groups: compound eyes (as possessed by most insects), and vertebrate eyes (such as the human eye). Compared with vertebrate eyes, there is considerable variation in the compound eyes. Compound eyes contain a large number of optical elements (ommatidia), each with its own aperture to the external world. Vertebrate eyes have a single aperture to the external world, which is used by all the detectors. A number of other animals have simple eyes, which can be described as less developed versions of the vertebrate eye. All eyes, of whatever type, involve compromises between the need for detection (sensitivity), particularly at low light levels, and spatial resolving capability in terms of the direction or form of an object.

Although this book is about the optics of the human eye we do not wish to consider the optics in complete isolation from the neural components, as otherwise we cannot appreciate what influence changes in the retinal image will have on vision performance. As an example, altering the optics has considerable influence on resolution of objects for central vision but not for peripheral vision. This is because the retina's neural structure is fine enough at its centre, but not in the periphery, for large changes in optical quality to be of importance (Chapter 18). Thus, the neural components of the visual system, particularly the retinal detector, rate some mention in the book. The neural structures of the retina themselves produce optical effects. As an example, the photoreceptors exhibit waveguide properties that make light arriving from some directions more efficient at stimulating vision than light arriving from other directions. Another example is that the regular arrangement of the nerve fibre layers produces polarization effects.

While image formation in the eye is similar to that in man-made optical systems such as cameras and must obey the conventional optical laws, there are some interesting differences because of the eye's biological basis. Perhaps the greatest difference is that, as a living organ, the eye responds to its environment, often in an attempt to give the best image under different circumstances. Also, it grows, ages and suffers disease. Unlike most man-made optical systems, the eye is not rotationally symmetrical about a single axis, and different axes must be used to define image formation.

There are many interesting and important optical effects associated with ocular diseases such as keratoconus (conical cornea) and cataract. Furthermore, the balance between optical and neural contributions to overall vision performance changes with diseases of the retina and beyond. Although there are some passing references to cataract, we have concentrated on the healthy human eye. We give some prominence to age-related changes in the optics of the eye throughout the book, and devote Chapter 20 to this topic.

To make the book easy to read it is divided into a number of short chapters, with each chapter dedicated to a single theme. The most commonly useful topics are at the beginning, and topics with narrower appeal (such as ocular aberrations) are placed towards the end. Section 1 covers the basic optical structure of the human eye, including the refracting components, the pupil, axes and simple models of the eye. Section 2 is about image formation and refraction of the eye. This includes the refractive errors of the eye, their measurement and correction, and paraxial treatments of focused and defocused image sizes and positions. Section 3 deals with the interactions between light and the eye, considering transmission, reflection and scatter in the media of the eye and at the fundus. Section 4 deals with aberrations and retinal image quality. As well as considering these for real eyes, it covers the modelling of eyes and the performance of a range of schematic eyes of different levels of sophistication. Section 5 considers the topics of depth-of-field and age-related changes in the optics of the eye. While depth-of-field effects could possibly have been placed earlier in the book, understanding them well requires some knowledge about aberration and diffraction. The book concludes with 4 appendices, three of which (Appendices 1, 2 and 4) cover some mathematics relating to paraxial optics, aberrations theory and image quality criteria. Appendix 3 lists construction data, optical parameters and the aberrations of a number of schematic eyes.

Section 1:

Basic optical structure of the human eye

1

The human eye: an overview

Introduction

This chapter is a short overview of the optical structure and function of the human eye. It mentions briefly some important aspects such as the cornea, the lens and ocular axes, which are covered in more detail in later chapters. Other important topics, such as the passage of light, aberrations and retinal image quality, are also discussed in later chapters.

The structure of the human eye is shown in Figure 1.1. The outer layer is in two parts: the anterior **cornea** and the posterior **sclera**. The cornea is transparent and approximately spherical with a radius of curvature of about 8 mm. The sclera is a dense, white, opaque, fibrous tissue that is mainly protective in function and is approximately spherical with a radius of curvature of about 12 mm. The centres of curvature of the sclera and cornea

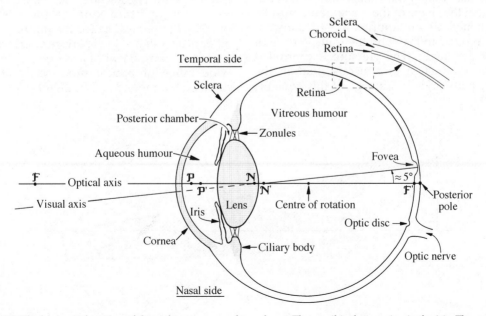

Figure 1.1. The horizontal section of the right eye as seen from above. The pupil is the opening in the iris. The cardinal points (**F**, **F'**, **P**, **P'**, **N** and **N'**) are for the relaxed eye.

are separated by about 5 mm. More accurate measures of shapes are given in subsequent chapters.

The middle layer of the eye is the uveal tract. It is composed of the **iris** anteriorly, the **choroid** posteriorly, and the intermediate **ciliary body**. The iris plays an important optical function through the size of its aperture, the ciliary body is important to the process of **accommodation**, and both the ciliary body and choroid support important vegetative processes.

The inner layer of the eye is the **retina**, which is an extension of the central nervous system and is connected to the brain by the optic nerve.

The inside of the eye is divided into three compartments:

1. The **anterior chamber**, between the cornea and iris, which contains the aqueous fluid.
2. The **posterior chamber**, between the iris, the ciliary body and the lens, which contains the aqueous fluid.
3. The **vitreous chamber**, between the lens and the retina, which contains a transparent colourless and gelatinous mass called the vitreous humour or vitreous body.

The internal pressure of the eye must be higher than that of the atmosphere in order to maintain the shape of the cornea, and must be maintained at an approximately constant level in order to maintain the transparency of the ocular media. The pressure is controlled by the production of aqueous fluid in the ciliary body and by drainage of this aqueous fluid from the eye. This drainage is through the angle of the anterior chamber (between the cornea and the iris) to the canal of Schlemm (not shown in Figure 1.1) and, finally, to the venous drainage of the eye.

The eye rotates in its socket by the action of six extra-ocular muscles.

More detailed anatomical descriptions of the human eye can be found in books such as those by Hogan *et al.* (1971) and Snell and Lemp (1997).

Optical structure and image formation

The principles of image formation by the eye are the same as for man-made optical systems such as the camera lens. Image-forming light enters the eye through the cornea, and is refracted by the cornea and the lens to be focused at the retina. Of the two refracting elements, the cornea has the greater power. However, whereas the corneal power is constant, the power of the lens can be changed when the eye needs to focus at different distances. This process is called **accommodation**, and occurs because of an alteration in the lens shape. It is discussed further in Chapter 20. The diameter of the incoming beam of light is controlled by the iris, which forms the **aperture stop** of the eye. The opening in the iris is called the **pupil**. As with all optical systems, the aperture stop is a very important component of a system, affecting a wide range of optical processes, and it is discussed in more detail in Chapter 3.

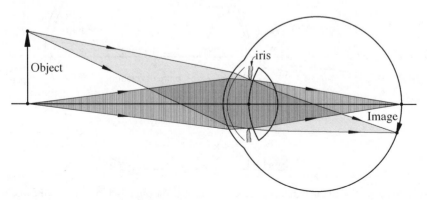

Figure 1.2. Image formation of the human eye.

Figure 1.2 shows two light beams from object points forming images on the retina. The image is inverted, as it is for a camera. We discuss this image formation in more detail in Chapter 6.

The retina

The light-sensitive tissue of the eye is the **retina**. It is shown in Figure 1.3, and consists of a number of cellular and pigmented layers and a nerve fibre layer. These layers have varying degrees of optical significance, with the amount of incoming light specularly reflected and scattered by each layer being of particular importance. This aspect is dis-cussed in greater depth in Chapter 14. The thickness of the retina varies from 50 μm (0.05 mm) at the foveal centre to about 600 μm (0.6 mm) near the optic disc.

There is a layer of light-sensitive cells at the back of the retina, and the light must pass through the other layers to reach these cells. These receptor cells are of two types, known as **rods** and **cones**. The names refer to their shapes, but considerable variations in shape occur with location, and it is not always possible to distinguish between the two types on this basis. Figure 1.4 shows their distribution along the horizontal temporal section of the retina. There are about 100 million rods in the retina, and they reach their maximum density at about 20° from the fovea.

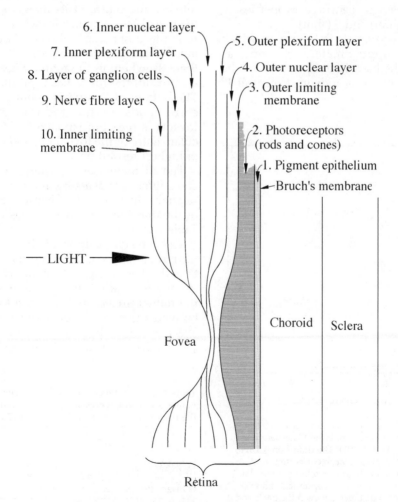

Figure 1.3. The layers at the back of the human eye (based on Polyak, 1941).

There are approximately 5 million cones in the retina.

In general, rods are longer and narrower than cones. Rods are sometimes described as highly sensitive low-level light detectors in comparison with cones. However, much of this is due to the neural wiring that occurs rather than differences between the receptors. The retinal neural network of rods is such that the output of about 100 rods can combine on the way to the brain, so that the rod system has very high sensitivity to light but poor spatial resolution. In contrast, the output of fewer cones is combined, so the cone system functions at higher light levels and is capable of higher spatial resolution. Cones recover from exposure to light more quickly than rods. The first stage in colour vision is the existence of three types of cones, each with different wavelength sensitive properties: L (long), M (medium) and S (short) cones.

The cones predominate in the **fovea**, which is 1.5 mm or approximately 5° wide as subtended at the back nodal point **N'** of the eye. The fovea is free of rods in its central 1°

field. At high light levels the best resolution is attained by the cones in the fovea, which occupies only about 1/1000th of the total retinal area. Despite the predominance of cones at the fovea, it contains only a small proportion (1 per cent) of the total cones (Tyler, 1996), and an even smaller proportion (0.05 %) of cones is found in the high-resolution **foveola**. Therefore, the vast majority of cones are distributed throughout the peripheral retina. At low light levels the cones at the fovea do not operate; thus the centre of the fovea is 'night blind', and it is necessary to look eccentrically to see objects using the rods. At very low light levels, maximum visual acuity and detection ability occur about 10–15° away from the fovea.

The location of the fovea is shown in Figure 1.1. When the eye fixates on an object of interest, the centre of its image is formed on the foveal centre, which is inclined at about 5° from the 'best fit' optical axis. At the fovea, the layers overlying the receptor cells are thinner than elsewhere in the retina (Figure 1.3) and, as a result, the fovea has a pit-like structure. The bottom of this pit is about 1° wide, and corresponds to the rod-free region. The foveola is the approximately 0.5°-wide avascular centre of the foveal pit, and is the region of highest resolution.

The diameters and packing of the foveal cones affect visual acuity, and we examine this relationship briefly in Chapter 18. Estimates of the diameters of foveal cones are given in Table 1.1.

The off-axis position of the fovea is most intriguing since aberration theory predicts that the best image of an optical system is usually formed on the optical axis. Therefore the retinal image quality at the fovea should be worse than at the posterior pole. The off-axis position of the fovea has some interesting visual effects which we discuss in **Chapter 17**.

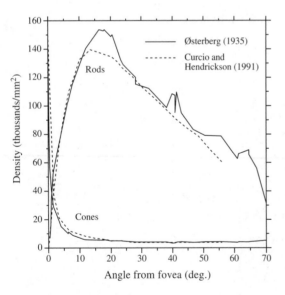

Figure 1.4. The density of cones and rods across the retina in the temporal direction. From Østerberg (1935), Curcio and Hendrickson (1991). The data from Curcio and Hendrickson (1991) have been converted from distances along the retina to angles relative to the back nodal point of the eye, assuming a spherical retina of diameter 12 mm and a distance between the back nodal point and retina of 17.054 mm.

Table 1.1. Diameters of foveal cones. The angular values are calculated assuming the distance between the back nodal point and the fovea is 17 mm.

	μm	min. arc	
Polyak (1941)	1.0–1.5	0.2–0.3	central fovea
	3.5–4.0	0.7–0.8	outer fovea
O'Brien (1951)*	2.3	0.46	

*Actually centre-to-centre spacing between cones.

The fovea is the central part of the **macula**, whose peripheral limits are where the cells of the outer nuclear layer are reduced to a single row (Hogan *et al.*, 1971). The macular diameter is 5.5 mm (19°).

The optic disc and blind spot

The vascular supply to the outer layers of the retina is carried in the choroid, which lies between the retina and the sclera. The vascular supply to the inner retina enters the eye at the optic disc, whose location is shown in Figure 1.1. There are no cones or rods here, and hence this region is blind. The name given to the corresponding region in the **visual field** is the '**blind spot**'. The optic disc is approximately 5° wide horizontally and 7° vertically, and its centre is approximately 15° nasally and 1.5° upwards relative to the fovea. Correspondingly, the blind spot is 15° temporally and 1.5° downwards relative to the point of fixation. Figure 1.5 provides a demonstration of the blind spot.

The cardinal points

Every centred optical system that has some equivalent power (i.e. is not afocal) has six cardinal points that lie on the optical axis. These are in three pairs. Two are focal points which we denote by the symbols **F** and **F′**, two are principal points denoted by the symbols **P** and **P′**, and two are nodal points denoted by the symbols **N** and **N′**. The positions of these cardinal points in an eye depend upon its structure and the level of accommodation. For an eye focused at infinity, the approximate positions of these cardinal points are shown in Figure 1.1. More precise positions are given in Chapter 5, where we discuss schematic eyes

Figure 1.5. Demonstration of the blind spot. Look steadily at the cross with your right eye (left eye closed) from a distance of about 20 cm. Vary this distance until you find a position for which the spot disappears.

and their properties. These cardinal points are as follows:

1. *Focal points* (**F** and **F′**). Light leaving the front (also first and anterior) focal point **F** passes into the eye, and would be imaged at infinity after final refraction by the lens if the retina were not in the way. Light parallel to the axis and coming into the eye from an infinite distance is imaged at the back (also second and posterior) focal point **F′**. Thus, for the eye focused at infinity, the retina coincides with the back focal point.
2. *Principal points* (**P** and **P′**). These are images of (or conjugate to) each other, such that their transverse magnification is +1. That is, if an object were placed at one of these points, an erect image of the same size would be formed at the other point.
3. *Nodal points* (**N** and **N′**). These are also images or conjugates of each other, but have a special property such that a ray from an off-axis point passing towards **N** appears to pass through **N′** on the image side of the system, while inclined at the same angle to the axis on each side of the system. Such a ray is called the **nodal ray**, and when the off-axis point is the point of fixation, the ray is called the **visual axis**.

We make use of these cardinal points frequently in the following chapters.

The equivalent power and focal lengths

One of the important properties of any optical system is its **equivalent power**. This is a measure of the ability of the system to bend or deviate rays of light. The higher the power, the greater is the ability to deviate rays. We denote the equivalent power of an optical system by the symbol F. The equivalent power of the eye is related to the distances between the focal and principal points by the equation

$$F = -\frac{1}{\mathbf{PF}} = \frac{n'}{\mathbf{P'F'}} \tag{1.1}$$

where n' is the refractive index in the vitreous chamber. The average power of the eye for adults is about 60 m^{-1} or 60 D, but the value varies greatly from eye to eye. Using this power and the commonly accepted refractive index n' of the vitreous chamber (1.336), the focal lengths of the eye are

$$\textbf{PF} = -16.7 \text{ mm and } \textbf{P}'\textbf{F}' = +22.3 \text{ mm} \qquad (1.2)$$

While the equivalent power of the eye is a very important property of the eye, it is not easy to measure directly. Its value is usually inferred from the other measurable quantities such as surface radii of curvature, surface separations and eye length, and assumed refractive indices of the ocular media.

However, more important than equivalent power is **refractive error**. The refractive error can be regarded as an error in the equivalent power due to a mismatch between the equivalent power and the eye length. For example, if the equivalent power is too high for a certain eye length, the image is formed in front of the retina and this results in a **myopic** refractive error. If the power is too low, the image is formed behind the retina and results in a **hypermetropic** refractive error. Refractive errors are discussed in Chapter 7.

Axes of the eye

The eye has a number of axes. Figure 1.1 shows two of these: the **optical axis** and the **visual axis**. The optical axis is usually defined as the line joining the centres of curvatures of the refracting surfaces. However, the eye is not perfectly rotationally symmetric, and therefore even if the four refracting surfaces were each perfectly rotationally symmetric, the four centres of curvatures would not be co-linear. Thus in the case of the eye, we define the optical axis as the line of best fit through these non co-linear points. The visual axis is defined as the line joining the object of interest and the fovea, and which passes through the nodal points. These and the other axes are discussed in greater detail in Chapter 4.

Centre-of-rotation

The eye rotates in its socket under the action of the six extra-ocular muscles. Because of the way these muscles are positioned and operate, there is no unique centre-of-rotation;

however, we can nominate a mean position for this point. The rotation of the eye in the horizontal plane was studied by Fry and Hill (1962), who found that the mean centre-of-rotation for 31 subjects was about 15 mm behind the cornea. Often it is assumed to lie along the optical axis.

Field-of-vision

Examination of the pupil from different angles shows that the pupil can still be seen at angles greater than 90° in the temporal field. Light is able to enter the pupil from about 105° to the side, as shown in Figure 1.6. While this suggests that the radius of the field-of-view may be as great as 105°, the real extent of the field-of-vision depends upon the extent of retina in the extreme directions. On the nasal side, vision is cut-off at about 60° because of the combination of the nose and the limited extent of the temporal retina.

Binocular vision and binocular overlap

The use of two eyes provides better perception of the external world than one eye

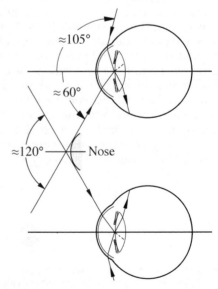

Figure 1.6. The horizontal field of view in monocular and binocular vision.

alone. Binocular vision improves contrast sensitivity and visual acuity slightly over those obtained with monocular vision (Campbell and Green, 1965; Home, 1978). Two laterally displaced eyes give the potential for a three-dimensional view of the world, which includes the perception of depth known as **stereopsis**. The degree of stereopsis depends partly upon the distance between the two eyes, which is called the **interpupillary distance**. Stereopsis can be improved considerably by optical devices such as rangefinders, which increase the effective interpupillary distance.

Interpupillary distance

The interpupillary distance, or **PD**, is usually measured by the distance between the centres of the two pupils of the eyes. The **distance PD** is measured for the eyes looking straight ahead; that is, the visual axes are parallel. When the eyes focus on nearby objects, the eyes rotate inwards and hence there is a corresponding decrease in interpupillary distance. The **near PD** can then be measured or determined from the distance PD using simple trigonometry.

Harvey (1982) provided distance PDs for various armed services. Means ranged from 61 to 65 mm, with standard deviations of 3–4 mm. These values were mainly for men.

Binocular overlap

As shown in Figure 1.6, the total field-of-view in the horizontal plane is about 210° with a 120° binocular overlap.

Typical dimensions

All dimensions of the eye vary greatly between individuals. Some depend upon accommodation and age. Representative data are shown in Figure 1.7. Average values have been used to construct representative or schematic eyes, which we discuss in Chapter 5. More detailed data are presented in later chapters.

Summary of main symbols

F equivalent power of the eye
n' refractive index of vitreous humour (usually taken as 1.336)
R radius of curvature in millimetres
F, F' front and back focal points
N, N' front and back nodal points
P, P' front and back principal points

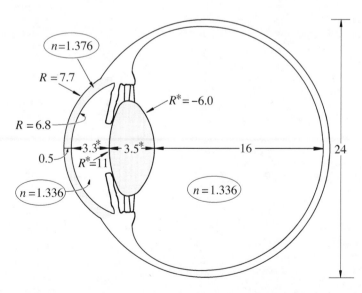

Figure 1.7. Representative dimensions (millimetres) and refractive indices of the (relaxed) eye. The starred values depend upon accommodation.

References

Campbell, F. W. and Green, D. G. (1965). Monocular versus binocular visual acuity. *Nature*, **208**, 191–2.

Curcio, C. A. and Hendrickson, A. E. (1991). Organization and development of the primate photoreceptor mosaic. *Prog. Retinal Res.*, **10**, 89–120.

Fry, G. A. and Hill, W. W. (1962). The center of rotation of the eye. *Am. J. Optom. Arch. Am. Acad. Optom.*, **39**, 581–95.

Harvey, R. S. (1982). Some statistics of interpupillary distance. *Optician*, **184** (4766), 29.

Hogan, M. J., Alvarado, J. A. and Weddell, J. E. (1971). *Histology of the Human Eye*. W. B. Saunders and Co.

Home, R. (1978). Binocular summation: A study of contrast sensitivity, visual acuity and recognition. *Vision Res.*, **18**, 579–85.

O'Brien, B. (1951). Vision and resolution in the central retina. *J. Opt. Soc. Am.*, **41**, 882–94.

Østerberg, G. (1935). Topography of the layers of rods and cones in the human retina. *Acta Ophthal.* (Suppl.), **6**, 1–103.

Polyak, S. L. (1941). *The Retina*, p. 201. University of Chicago Press.

Snell, R. S. and Lemp, M. A. (1997). *Clinical Anatomy of the Eye*, 2nd edn. Blackwell Scientific Publications.

Tyler, C. W. (1996). Analysis of human receptor density. In *Basic and Clinical Applications of Vision Science, The Professor Jay M. Enoch Festschrift Volume* (V. Lakshminarayanan, ed.), pp. 63–71. Kluwer Academic Publishers.

2

Refracting components: cornea and lens

Introduction

The refracting elements of the eye are the cornea and the lens. In order to provide a good quality retinal image, these elements must be transparent and have appropriate curvatures and refractive indices. Refraction takes place at four surfaces, the anterior and posterior interfaces of the cornea and the lens,

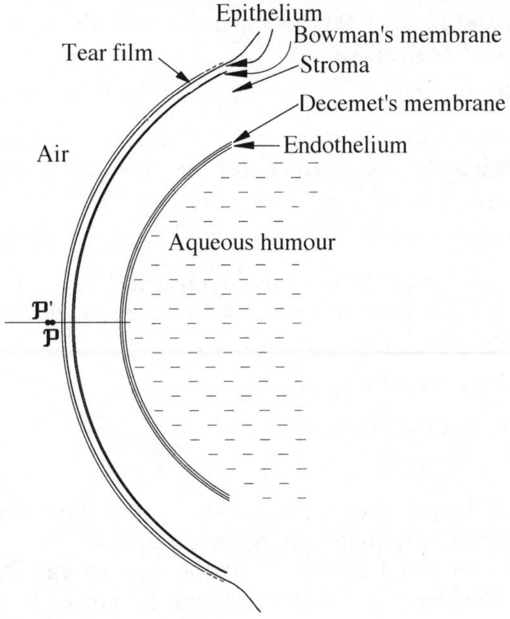

Figure 2.1. The structure of the cornea and the approximate positions of the principal points.

and there is also continuous refraction within the lens.

In this chapter we describe the optical structure of the normal cornea and lens, but we must be aware that in many eyes there are significant departures from these norms. Some of these are due to serious ocular defects or irregularities, which can have a major impact on vision. There are also changes with age, and any descriptions given in this section relate only to mean adult values. More detail on age dependencies is given in Chapter 20.

Cornea

The majority of the refracting power is provided by the **cornea**, the clear, curved 'window' at the front of the eye. It has about two-thirds of the total power for the relaxed eye, but this fraction decreases as the lens increases in power during accommodation.

Anatomical structure

The schematic cross-sectional structure of the cornea is shown in Figure 2.1. It has a **tear film** at its front surface, and several distinct parts. These are, in order from the outer surface of the eye, the **epithelium**, **Bowman's membrane**, the **stroma**, **Descemet's membrane** and the **endothelium**. Approximate thicknesses of these components are given in Table 2.1.

Table 2.1. Thicknesses (μm) of corneal layers (Hogan *et al.*, 1971).

Tear film	4–7
Epithelium	50
Bowman's membrane	8–14
Stroma*	500
Descemet's membrane	10–12
Endothelium	5
Total	~ 580

*The stroma thickens by at least an additional 150 μm from the centre to the edge of the cornea.

The tear film is 4–7 μm thick (Tomlinson, 1992). It is composed of oily, aqueous and mucous layers, with 98 per cent of the thickness being provided by the aqueous layer. The tear film is essential for clear vision because it moistens the cornea and smooths out the 'roughness' of the surface epithelial cells. The tear film does not contribute significant refractive power itself, since it is very thin and consists effectively of two very closely spaced surfaces of almost equal radii. However, the importance of this tear film is realized if it dries out. If this occurs, the transparency of the cornea decreases significantly.

The **epithelium** protects the rest of the cornea by providing a barrier against water, larger molecules and toxic substances. It consists of approximately six layers of cells, and only the innermost layer of these cells is able to divide. After cells are formed, they move gradually towards the surface as the superficial cells are shed.

Bowman's membrane is 8–14 μm thick, and consists mainly of randomly arranged collagen **fibrils**.

The **stroma** comprises 90 per cent of the corneal thickness, and consists mainly of 200 or more collagen lamellae. The collagen fibrils within each lamella run parallel to each other, and the successive lamellae run across the cornea at angles to each other. This arrangement maintains an ordered transparent structure while enhancing mechanical strength.

Descemet's membrane is the basement membrane of the endothelial cells.

The **endothelium** consists of a single layer of cells, which are hexagonal and fit together like a honeycomb. The endothelium regulates the fluid balance of the cornea in order to maintain the stroma at about 78 per cent hydration and thus retain transparency.

Refractive index

Each corneal layer has its own refractive index, but since the stroma is by far the thickest layer, its refractive index dominates. The mean value of refractive index is usually taken as 1.376.

Radii of curvature, vertex powers and total corneal power

Several studies have measured the anterior radius of curvature, but there have been far fewer investigations of the rear surface. Experimental distributions of the vertex radii (R) of curvature are given in Table 2.2. Similar results have been obtained by various investigators for the anterior cornea, but clearly there is a reasonable degree of variation between patients, and females have slightly steeper anterior corneas than males. There is a high linear correlation between the anterior and posterior radii of curvature (Lowe and Clark, 1973; Dunne *et al.*, 1992; Patel *et al.*, 1993) and a reasonable fit of this relationship is

$$R_2 = 0.81R_1 \qquad (2.1)$$

From these radii of curvature, we can calculate the surface powers (F) using the equation

$$F = (n' - n)/R \qquad (2.2)$$

where n and n' are the refractive indices on the incident and refracted side, respectively. At the anterior surface

$n = 1$ and $n' = 1.376$

and at the posterior surface

$n = 1.376$ and $n' = 1.336$

Surface power values, using these data and equations, are given in Table 2.2.

The total power F of the cornea can be calculated from the 'thick lens' equation:

$$F = F_1 + F_2 - F_1F_2d/\mu \qquad (2.3)$$

where F_1 is the anterior surface power, F_2 is

Table 2.2. Population distributions of corneal vertex radii of curvature *R* and corresponding powers calculated from equations (2.2) and (2.3), assuming corneal refractive index 1.376, aqueous refractive index 1.336 and a corneal thickness 0.5 mm. Where results were provided for more than one meridian, mean values have been used.

		Anterior		Posterior		Total
	S/N	R(mm)	F(D)	R(mm)	F(D)	F(D)
Donders (1864)						
females	38/-	7.80	48.2			
males	79/-	7.86	47.9			
Stenstrom (1948)	-/1000	7.86 ± 0.26	47.8			
Sorsby *et al.* (1957)	-/194	7.82 ± 0.29	48.1			
Lowe and Clark (1973)	46/92	7.65 ± 0.27	49.2	6.46 ± 0.26	−6.2	43.2
Kiely *et al.* (1982)	88/176	7.72 ± 0.27	48.7			
Edmund and Sjøntoft (1985)	40/80	7.76 ± 0.25	48.5			
Guillon *et al.* (1986)	110/220	7.78 ± 0.25	48.3			
Koretz *et al.* (1989)						
females	68/-	7.69 ± 0.23	48.9			
males	32/-	7.78 ± 0.24	48.3			
Dunne *et al.* (1992)						
females	40/40	7.93 ± 0.20	48.0	6.53 ± 0.20	−6.1	42.0
males	40/40	8.08 ± 0.16	47.1	6.65 ± 0.16	−6.0	41.2
Patel *et al.* (1993)	20/20	7.68 ± 0.40	49.0	5.81 ± 0.41	−6.9	42.2
Mean (unweighted)		7.83	48.0	6.34	−6.3	

S = number of subjects; N = number of eyes; - = number not provided.

the posterior surface power, *d* is the vertex corneal thickness and *μ* is the refractive index of the cornea (usually taken as 1.376). The power of the cornea can be estimated from the sum of the surface powers

$$F \approx F_1 + F_2 \qquad (2.3a)$$

This value is different from the exact value by an amount $F_1 F_2 d/\mu$. Using the data given by Patel *et al.* (1993) in Table 2.2, a corneal thickness of 0.5 mm and a refractive index of 1.376, the exact equation (2.3) gives a corneal power of 42.2 D and the approximate equation (2.3a) gives a slightly lower value of 42.1 D.

The above surface power values apply to the vertices of the cornea, and would apply to other parts of the corneal surfaces only if they were spherical. However, neither the anterior nor the posterior surfaces are perfectly spherical due to both toricity and asphericity. Therefore, the radii of curvature do not fully describe the shape of the cornea and its refracting properties.

Anterior surface shape

Toricity

Frequently the anterior corneal surface exhibits toricity, which produces astigmatism. In young eyes, the radius of curvature is generally greater in the horizontal than in the vertical meridian (referred as 'with the rule'), but this trend reverses with an increase in age.

Asphericity

In general, the radius of curvature increases with distance from the surface apex, so that the surface flattens away from the apex. Surfaces that are non-spherical in this sense are often described as **aspheric**.

The shape of the anterior corneal surface has been extensively studied, especially over the central 8 mm of its approximately 12 mm diameter. This central 'optical' zone is the maximum zone of the cornea through which light passes to form the foveal image. To investigate the shape over this zone, corneal surfaces are often represented by conicoids in three dimensions or conics in two dimensions. A conicoid can be expressed in the form

$$h^2 + (1+Q)Z^2 - 2ZR = 0 \qquad (2.4)$$

where

the *Z* axis is the optical axis
$h^2 = X^2 + Y^2$
R is the vertex radius of curvature and

Q is the surface asphericity, where
$Q < -1$ specifies a hyperboloid
$Q = -1$ specifies a paraboloid
$-1 < Q < 0$ specifies an ellipsoid, with the Z-axis being the major axis
$Q = 0$ specifies a sphere
$Q > 0$ specifies an ellipsoid with the major axis in the *X–Y* plane.

The effect of the value and sign of Q on the shape is shown in Figure 2.2. Sometimes asphericity is expressed in terms of a quantity p, which is related to Q by the equation

$$p = (1+Q) \tag{2.5}$$

The conicoid form described by equation (2.4) is not the only mathematical representation used in the literature to describe conic(oid)s. Many investigators have measured surface shapes separately in different sections, and fitted the data to ellipses, which can be described by the equation

$$\frac{(Z-a)^2}{a^2} + \frac{Y^2}{b^2} = 1 \tag{2.6}$$

where a and b are ellipse axes' semi-lengths. The shape of such ellipses is often described by the eccentricity e, which is related to a and

b by the equation

$$e^2 = 1 - b^2/a^2 \tag{2.7}$$

provided that the Z-axis is the major axis.

Equation (2.6) can be transformed easily into the form of equation (2.4). If we do this, we find that the vertex radius of curvature R is related to a and b by the equation

$$R = + b^2/a \tag{2.8}$$

and that the asphericity Q is given by the equation

$$Q = b^2/a^2 - 1 \tag{2.9}$$

It follows from equations (2.7) and (2.9), that the quantities e and Q are related by the equation

$$Q = -e^2 \tag{2.10}$$

Specifying asphericity using e is not completely satisfactory because e^2 may be negative, in which case e cannot have a value.

Other forms of representing corneal shape are described in Chapter 16. More complex forms are important to describe the shape of the cornea accurately, especially outside the optical zone.

Measured values of the anterior corneal

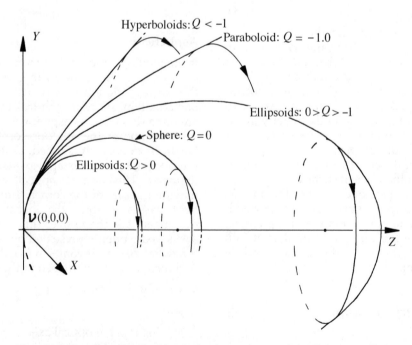

Figure 2.2. The effect of asphericity on the shape of a conicoid. All the curves have the same apex radius of curvature.

Table 2.3. Summary of asphericity data for the anterior surface of the cornea.

	No. of subjects/eyes	Q	s.d. or range
Lotmar (1971) (using Bonnet (1964)'s data)		–0.286	
El Hage and Berny (1973)	1/1	+0.16	
Mandell and St Helen (1971)	8/8	–0.23	–0.04 to –0.72
Kiely *et al.* (1982)	88/176	–0.26	0.18
Edmund and Sjøntoft (1985)	40/80	–0.28	0.13
Guillon *et al.* (1986)*	110/220	–0.18	0.15
Patel *et al.* (1993)	20/20	–0.01	0.25
Lam and Douthwaite (1997)	60/60	–0.30	0.13

*The mean of the steepest and shallowest meridians.

asphericity (Q) are given in Table 2.3. The values of Q are usually negative, indicating that the cornea flattens away from the vertex. Figure 2.3 shows the profiles of corneal surfaces, all with a radius of curvature of 7.8 mm but with different Q values.

Optical significance of corneal asphericity

There has been considerable speculation as to why the cornea flattens away from the centre. It has been argued that the cornea flattens in order to reduce spherical aberration, and certainly the flattening does lead to a lower spherical aberration, but the amount of asphericity in the average cornea is not sufficient to eliminate it. The value of Q

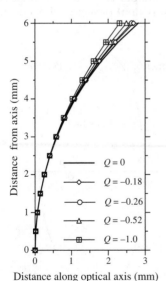

Figure 2.3. The anterior surface of a cornea with a vertex radius of curvature of 7.8 mm, with various values of the asphericity Q.

required to eliminate spherical aberration at the anterior surface is –0.528, given a corneal refractive index of 1.376. Perhaps an important reason for the flattening is the need for the cornea to make a smooth join with the main globe of the eye.

Off-axis radii of curvature

The radius of curvature at any point on a spherical surface and in any meridian is the same. However, for a conicoid surface, the radius of curvature at off-axis points depends not only upon the distance from the vertex, but also on the meridian at that point. There are two principal meridians: the tangential meridian, which lies along the radius line from the vertex, and the sagittal meridian, which is perpendicular to the tangential meridian. For conicoids, the corresponding equations for the sagittal radius of curvature (R_s) and the tangential radius of curvature (R_t) are

$$R_s = [R^2 - QY^2]^{1/2} \tag{2.11a}$$

and

$$R_t = [R^2 - QY^2]^{3/2}/R^2 = R_s^3/R^2 \tag{2.11b}$$

Figure 2.4 shows changes in R_t and R_s with distance Y from the corneal vertex for an asphericity Q value of –0.18 (Guillon *et al.*, 1986) and a vertex radius of curvature of 7.8 mm.

An alternative name for the tangential radius of curvature is the **instantaneous radius of curvature**, while the sagittal radius of curvature is also called the **axial radius of curvature**. Unfortunately, this last term may be readily confused with the vertex radius of curvature.

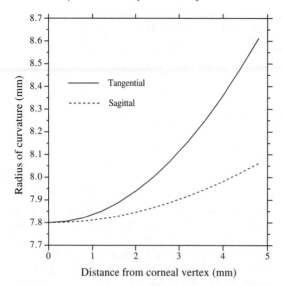

Figure 2.4. The radii of curvature in the sagittal and tangential directions of a cornea with a vertex radius of curvature of 7.8 mm and a corneal asphericity of $Q = -0.18$, from Guillon *et al.* (1986).

Posterior surface shape

This is difficult to measure because of the influence of anterior surface shape on any measurement. It is of lesser significance than the anterior surface shape because of the small refractive index difference across the posterior corneal boundary, but it is not of negligible significance.

Patel *et al.* (1993) estimated the shape of the posterior surface of 20 corneas from measured anterior surface shapes and peripheral values of corneal thickness. For the 20 subjects, they found a mean posterior vertex radius of 5.8 mm and a mean asphericity of $Q = -0.42$. However, Patel and co-workers used a mean anterior corneal shape that was almost spherical ($Q = -0.01$) and therefore much less aspheric than found in other studies. Lam and Douthwaite (1997) used a similar approach with a group of 60 young Chinese in Hong Kong, and obtained asphericity of $Q = -0.66 \pm 0.38$. In this case, the anterior surface asphericity was $Q = -0.31 \pm 0.13$.

Positions of the principal points

The positions of the principal points of the cornea depend upon the radii of curvatures of the anterior and posterior surfaces, the corneal thickness and the refractive indices. Representative positions are shown in Figure 2.1. Note that both principal points are in front of the cornea.

Lens

Figure 2.5 shows a cross-section of the lens. The lens bulk is a mass of cellular tissue of non-uniform gradient index, contained within an elastic **capsule**. We do not have an accurate measure of this index distribution. There is a layer of epithelial cells, extending from the anterior pole of the lens to the equator. The lens grows continually throughout life, with new epithelial cells forming at the equator. These cells elongate as fibres that wrap around the periphery of the lens, under the capsule and epithelium, to meet at sutures. The older fibres lose their nuclei and other intracellular organelles. Because of the continual growth of the lens throughout life, lenticular parameters are age-dependent.

The lens capsule plays an important role in the accommodation process. It is attached to the ciliary body via the zonules, as shown in a simplified fashion in Figure 2.6. Contraction of the ciliary muscle within the ciliary body leads to changes in zonular tension, which alter lens shape. This process causes a change in the equivalent power of the lens and hence

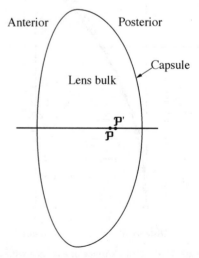

Figure 2.5. Cross-section of the lens showing the approximate positions of its principal points.

in the ocular equivalent power, and allows the eye to focus on objects at different distances. Note that contraction of the ciliary muscle *decreases* tension on the zonules and this allows the lens to take up a more curved form, appropriate for near vision.

Surface radii of curvature and shapes

Some values of the radii of curvature of the lens are given in Table 2.4. These values must be treated with caution for three reasons. First, the lens radii of curvature change with accommodation; second, the values are highly age-dependent; and third, any measurements of the lens *in vivo* (within the eye) depend upon knowing the value of all the optical parameters that precede the particular surface. This is a particular problem with the posterior surface because of the uncertainty of the refractive index distribution in any particular lens.

The most common method of determining the radii of curvature of the lenticular surfaces is by measurement of the Purkinje images,

Table 2.4. Population distributions of *in vivo* lens vertex radii of curvature (R).

	No. of subjects/ eyes	Anterior mm	Posterior mm
Lowe (1972)	46/92	10.29 ± 1.78	
Brown (1974)	100/-	12.4 ± 2.6	−8.1 ± 1.6

which are the images of an object formed through specular reflection at the ocular surfaces. Procedures for doing this are described by Tunnacliffe (1993), Smith and Garner (1996), Garner and Smith (1997) and Rabbetts (1998).

Howcroft and Parker (1977) provided shape data for *in vitro* lenses (outside the eye), but the lenses were in unknown accommodated states and probably did not represent the shape of lenses *in vivo*. Furthermore, the asphericity values were published as absolute values, thus losing the sign. Some attempts to extract asphericity Q values from the data are given in Table 2.5. There are some data for *in vivo* samples (Brown, 1974) that were analysed by Liou and Brennan (1997) to give Q values. From the results of Smith *et al.* (1991) it is clear that there is a wide variation in values, and this is probably due to a combination of the difficulty in accurate measurement of asphericity and inter-individual variations in asphericity values.

Thickness

The lens thickness is often taken to be about 3.6 mm in the relaxed state, but the lens thickens upon accommodation and with increasing age (for example, see Koretz *et al.*, 1989 and 1997). These changes in thickness are discussed further in Chapter 20.

Refractive index distribution

The refractive index within the lens is not constant, being greatest in the centre and least in the periphery (Nakao *et al.*, 1969; Pierscionek *et al.*, 1988; Pierscionek and Chan, 1989; Pierscionek, 1995). In the nuclear (central) region of the lens the index magnitude is almost constant, with the greatest variations occurring in the cortex

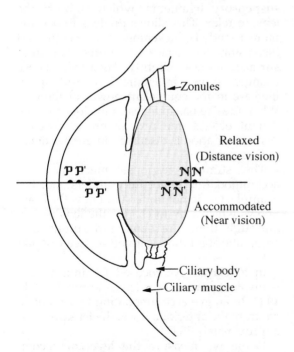

Figure 2.6. The effect of accommodation on the lens shape and lens position, and on the principal and nodal points of the eye.

Table 2.5. Population distributions of lens surface asphericities (*Q*).

	Sample size	Anterior	Posterior
In vitro values			
Kooijman (1983)[a]	–	–6.06	–1.19
Smith *et al.* (1991)[b]	59	–1.08 ± 9.41	–0.12 ± 1.74
In vivo values			
Liou and Brennan (1997)[c]	100	–0.94	+0.96

[a]The original values given by Kooijman in his paper were calculated from data published by Howcroft and Parker (1977) but were in error, and the above values are corrected values (private communication, 1985).
[b]Calculated from data on 59 eyes, supplied by Parker (private communication, 1985).
[c]Calculated from data of Brown (1974).

(periphery). This variation in index produces a progressive and continuous refraction of rays, and may improve the quality of the image by reducing spherical aberration.

Gullstrand (1909) gave an equation for the refractive index distribution within the lens. An equivalent form of his equation is

$$n(Y,Z) = 1.406 - 0.0062685(Z - Z_0)^2$$
$$+ 0.0003834(Z - Z_0)^3 - [0.00052375$$
$$+ 0.00005735(Z - Z_0) + 0.00027875$$
$$(Z - Z_0)^2]Y^2 - 0.000066717Y^4 \qquad (2.12)$$

This gives a maximum index of 1.406 at the nominal centre of the lens, which occurs at $Z = Z_0$, and an index of 1.386 at the edge of the lens. Gullstrand gave a value for Z_0 of 1.7 mm, and the total lens thickness as 3.6 mm.

Equivalent refractive index

If the real lens with its gradient index is replaced by one with the same thickness, same radii of curvature and a uniform refractive index, this index must be made higher than the maximum index. The equivalent refractive index is often taken as 1.42, compared with the maximum value of about 1.406.

Equatorial diameter

The equatorial diameter of the lens is between 8.5 and 10 mm (Pierscionek and Augusteyn, 1991).

Positions of principal points

The positions of the principal points of the lens depend upon the radii of curvature of the anterior and posterior lens surfaces, the lens thickness and its refractive index distribution. All of these depend upon the level of accommodation. The positions of the principal points depend also on the refractive indices of the surrounding media. Representative positions are shown in Figure 2.5.

Accommodation

During accommodation, when the eye needs to change focus from distant to closer objects, the ciliary muscle contracts and causes the suspensory ligaments, which support the lens, to relax. This allows the lens to become more rounded, thickening at the centre and increasing the surface curvatures. The front surface moves slightly forward. These changes (shown in Figure 2.6) result in an increase in the equivalent power of the eye. When the eye has to focus from close to more distant objects, the reverse process occurs. Accommodation is discussed in greater detail in Chapter 20.

The stimulus–response mechanism in accommodation is not fully understood. For example, we do not understand how the brain knows which way to change the lens power, although there are some indications that chromatic aberration is involved (see Chapter 17).

In a relaxed eye focused for infinity, the equivalent power of the lens is approximately 19 D. In an eye accommodating to a point 10 cm from the anterior cornea, the lens power is approximately 30 D.

While we measure the level of accommodation as the vergence of the 'in focus' object, this vergence should not be mistaken as the power of the eye. For the relaxed eye,

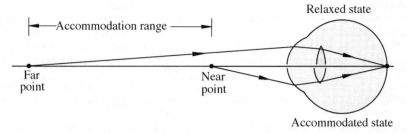

Figure 2.7. The near and far points of the eye. This is a myopic eye, because the far point is in front of it. For a hyperopic eye the far point would be behind the eye, and for the emmetropic eye the far point would be at infinity.

the accommodation level is zero, but the power of the eye is about 60 D. Although the accommodation level and increase in lens power are not the same, they are closely related.

There are physical limits to the range of lens shapes, and hence restrictions to changes in lens power and the range of clear vision. The furthest and closest object points along this range are called the **far** and **near points**, respectively, and are shown schematically in Figure 2.7. When the ciliary muscle is completely relaxed the eye is focused on the far point, which is conjugate to the retina. When the ciliary muscle is maximally contracted or the lens maximally relaxed, the eye has its greatest equivalent power and the near point is conjugate to the retina.

The distance between the far and near points is called the range of accommodation – for example, from infinity to 20 cm. The difference between the vergences of the far and near points is called the **amplitude of accommodation**.

Example 2.1: Calculate the amplitude of accommodation of an eye with a far point of 1.25 m and a near point of 10 cm.

Solution: The vergence of the far point is $1/1.25 = 0.8$ m^{-1} or 0.8 D. The vergence of the near point is $1/0.10 = 10.0$ m^{-1} or 10.0 D.
The difference is $10.0 - 0.8 = 9.2$ D.

The amplitude of accommodation is affected by age. It probably reaches a peak early in the second decade of life, and then gradually declines to become zero at approximately the middle of the sixth decade. This and other effects of age are discussed in Chapter 20.

As the two eyes accommodate to focus clearly on a close object, they also must rotate inwards to fixate on the object. This inward rotation is called convergence. Accommodation and convergence are controlled to some extent by the same nervous pathway from the brain, and there is an interaction between accommodation and convergence called a **synkinesis**. A stimulus to either accommodation or convergence can cause both to change. An example is that of placing an occluder in front of one eye and placing a negative-powered lens in front of the other eye. As well as the negative lens stimulating accommodation, the occluded eye turns inwards.

As the accommodation level increases, all the cardinal points of the eye move towards the anterior surface of the lens (Chapter 5).

Summary of main symbols

e eccentricity of an aspheric surface
n, n' refractive indices on incident and refraction sides of a surface
Q surface asphericity $(= -e^2)$
p surface asphericity $(= 1 + Q)$
R radius of curvature
Z optical axis
F equivalent power
X, Y distances perpendicular to optical axis

References

Bonnet, R. (1964). *La Topographie Cornéenne*. Desroches (cited by Lotmar, 1971).

Brown, N. (1974). The change in lens curvature with age. *Exp. Eye Res.*, **19**, 175–83.

Donders, F. C. (1864). *On the Anomalies of Accommodation and Refraction of the Eye* (translated by W. D. Moore), p. 89. The New Sydenham Society.

Dunne, M. C. M., Royston, J. M. and Barnes, D. A. (1992). Normal variations of the posterior corneal surface. *Acta Ophthal.*, **70**, 255–61.

Edmund, C. and Sjøntoft, E. (1985). The central–peripheral radius of the normal corneal curvature. *Acta Ophthal.*, **63**, 670–77.

El Hage, S. G. and Berny, F. (1973). Contribution of the crystalline lens to the spherical aberration of the eye. *J. Opt. Soc. Am.*, **63**, 205–11.

Garner, L. G. and Smith, G. (1997). Changes in equivalent and gradient refractive index of the crystalline lens with accommodation. *Optom. Vis. Sci.*, **74**, 114–19.

Guillon, M., Lydon, D. P. M. and Wilson, C. (1986). Corneal topography: a clinical model. *Ophthal. Physiol. Opt.*, **6**, 47–56.

Gullstrand, A. (1909). Appendix II: Procedure of the rays in the eye. Imagery – laws of first order. In *Helmholtz's Handbuch der Physiologischen Optik, Volume 1* (English translation edited by J. P. Southall, Optical Society of America, 1924).

Hogan, M. J., Alvarado, J. A. and Weddell, J. E. (1971). *Histology of the Human Eye*. W. B. Saunders and Co.

Howcroft, M. J. and Parker, J. A. (1977). Aspheric curvatures for the human lens. *Vision Res.*, **17**, 1217–23.

Kiely, P. M., Smith, G. and Carney, L. G. (1982). The mean shape of the human cornea. *Optica Acta*, **29**, 1027–40.

Kooijman, A. C. (1983). Light distribution on the retina of a wide-angle theoretical eye. *J. Opt. Soc. Am.*, **73**, 1544–50.

Koretz, J. F., Cook, C. A. and Kaufman, P. L. (1997). Accommodation and presbyopia in the human eye. Changes in the anterior segment and crystalline lens with focus. *Invest. Ophthal. Vis. Sci.*, **38**, 569–78.

Koretz, J. F., Kaufman, P. L., Neider, M. W. and Goeckner, P. A. (1989). Accommodation and presbyopia in the human eye – aging of the anterior segment. *Vision Res.*, **29**, 1685–92.

Lam, A. K. C. and Douthwaite, W. A. (1997). Measurement of posterior corneal asphericity on Hong Kong Chinese: a pilot study. *Ophthal. Physiol. Opt.*, **17**, 348–56.

Liou, H.-L. and Brennan, N. A. (1997). Anatomically accurate, finite model eye for optical modelling. *J. Opt. Soc. Am. A*, **14**, 1684–95.

Lotmar, W. (1971). Theoretical eye model with aspherics. *J. Opt. Soc. Am.*, **61**, 1522–9.

Lowe, R. F. (1972). Anterior lens curvature. Comparisons between normal eyes and those with primary angle-closure glaucoma. *Br. J. Ophthal.*, **56**, 409–13.

Lowe, R. F. and Clark, B. A. J. (1973). Posterior corneal curvature. Correlations in normal eyes and in eyes involved with primary angle-closure glaucoma. *Br. J. Ophthal.*, **57**, 464–70.

Mandell, R. B. and St Helen, R. (1971). Mathematical model of the corneal contour. *Br. J. Physiol. Opt.*, **26**, 183–97.

Nakao, S., Ono, T., Nagata, R. and Iwata, K. (1969). The distribution of refractive indices in the human crystalline lens. *Jpn. J. Clin. Ophthal.*, **23**, 903–6.

Patel, S., Marshall, J. and Fitzke, F. W. (1993). Shape and radius of posterior corneal surface. *Refract. Corn. Surg.*, **9**, 173–81.

Pierscionek, B. K. (1995). Variations in refractive index and absorbance of 670-nm light with age and cataract formation in human lens. *Exp. Eye Res.*, **60**, 407–14.

Pierscionek, B. K. and Augusteyn, R. C. (1991). Shapes and dimensions of *in vitro* human lenses. *Clin. Exp. Optom.*, **74**, 223–8.

Pierscionek, B. K. and Chan, D. Y. C. (1989). Refractive index gradient of human lenses. *Optom. Vis. Sci.*, **66**, 822–9.

Pierscionek, B. K., Chan, D. Y. C., Ennis, J. P. *et al.* (1988). Non-destructive method of constructing three-dimensional gradient index models for the crystalline lens: 1. Theory and Experiment. *Am. J. Optom. Physiol. Opt.*, **65**, 481–91.

Rabbetts, R. B. (1998). *Bennett and Rabbetts' Clinical Visual Optics*, 3rd edn. Butterworth-Heinemann.

Smith, G. and Garner, L. G. (1996). Determination of the radius of curvature of the anterior lens surface from the Purkinje images. *Ophthal. Physiol. Opt.*, **16**, 135–43.

Smith, G., Pierscionek, B. K. and Atchison, D. A. (1991). The optical modelling of the human lens. *Ophthal. Physiol. Opt.*, **11**, 359–69.

Sorsby, A., Benjamin, B., Davey, J. B. *et al.* (1957). *Emmetropia and its Aberrations. A Study in the Correlation of the Optical Components of the Eye*. Medical Research Council special report series no 293. HMSO.

Stenstrom, S. (1948). Investigations of the variation and correlation of the optical elements of the human eye. Part III, Chapter III (translated by D. Woolf) *Am. J. Optom. Arch. Am. Acad. Optom.*, **25**, 340–50.

Tomlinson, A. (1992). Tear film changes with contact lens wear. In *Complications of Contact Lens Wear* (A. Tomlinson, ed.), Ch. 8. Mosby Year Book.

Tunnacliffe, A. H. (1993). *Introduction to Visual Optics*, 4th edn. Association of British Dispensing Opticians.

3

The pupil

Introduction – the iris

The iris forms the **aperture stop** of the eye. Its aperture or opening is known as the **pupil**. The pupil size is determined by two antagonistic muscles, which are under autonomic (reflex) control:

1. The sphincter pupillae, which is a smooth muscle forming a ring around the pupillary margin of the iris. When it contracts, the pupil constricts. It is innervated by the parasympathetic fibres from the oculo-motor (3rd cranial) nerve by the way of the ciliary ganglion and the short ciliary nerves.
2. The dilator pupillae, which is more primitive and consists of myo-epithelial cells that extend radially from the sphincter into the ciliary body. It dilates the pupil and is innervated by sympathetic nerve fibres, which synapse in the superior cervical ganglion and enter the eye by way of the short and long ciliary nerves.

Iris colour varies markedly between different people, and depends upon the amount of pigmentation within the stroma and anterior limiting layer. Lightly pigmented irides appear blue, and the more pigment there is in the iris, the browner the eye appears.

In this chapter, we discuss the properties of the aperture stop/pupil, factors that affect pupil size and the effect of pupil size on the retinal image.

Entrance and exit pupils

In general optical systems, the opening in the aperture stop is not referred to as the pupil. The word 'pupil' is used for the images of the aperture stop. The image of the stop formed by the optical elements in front of it is the **entrance pupil** – in other words, the entrance pupil of an optical system is the image of the aperture stop formed in object space. The image of the aperture stop formed by the elements behind it is the **exit pupil**. Alternatively, we can say that the exit pupil is the image of the aperture stop formed in image space. When we look into an eye at the aperture stop, we see the image of the stop formed by the cornea (i.e. the entrance pupil). The exit pupil of the eye is the image of the aperture stop formed by the eye's lens.

With respect to the eye, and depending on the context, the term 'pupil' is generally used to refer to either the aperture stop opening – the 'real' or 'actual' pupil – or to the entrance pupil that we see. Compared with the entrance pupil, the exit pupil of the eye has little practical significance. In the rest of the chapter, when we refer to pupil size we are referring to the entrance pupil.

Given the ocular parameters of an eye (for example, as given for the schematic eyes in Appendix 3), paraxial optics can be used to determine the size and positions of the entrance and exit pupils. To determine the entrance pupil position and size, we need to trace a ray from the centre of the iris out of the

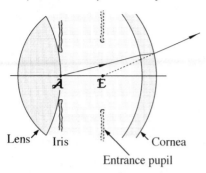

Figure 3.1. The formation of the entrance pupil.

eye. For the exit pupil, we trace a ray from the same point towards the retina. We show how this is done in Chapter 5. In such calculations, we assume that the actual pupil lies in the front vertex plane of the lens.

Figure 3.1 shows, in schematic form, a ray traced from the iris at **A** through the cornea and out of the eye. This ray appears to cross the axis at the point **E**, which locates the entrance pupil. This figure is not to scale, but shows correctly that the entrance pupil is forward to and larger than the aperture. The entrance pupil is actually only slightly forward to and larger than the aperture. In one schematic eye, the Gullstrand number 1 relaxed schematic eye, the aperture is 3.6 mm from the corneal vertex and the entrance pupil is 3.05 mm from the corneal vertex. The

entrance pupil is 13.3 per cent larger than the aperture. The exit pupil is 0.07 mm behind the aperture and 3.1 per cent larger. Figure 3.2 shows the positions and sizes of the aperture and entrance and exit pupils of this schematic eye.

Effect of aberrations

The above calculations are based upon paraxial optics, which ignore aberration effects. The predictions are valid only for small pupils observed along or close to the optical axis. Aberrations of the cornea have some effect for wide pupils and for oblique viewing. We discuss the effect of aberrations on pupil magnification in Chapter 15.

Accommodation

Upon accommodation, the anterior surface of the lens moves forward. Gullstrand's number 1 schematic eye has a highly accommodated version in which this movement and that of the aperture stop is 0.4 mm. The entrance and exit pupils move forward by similar amounts.

The paraxial marginal ray and paraxial pupil ray

If we wish to analyse the optical properties of the eye, two useful and special rays are the **paraxial marginal ray** and the **paraxial pupil ray** (also **paraxial chief ray**). These can be defined as follows:

- The paraxial marginal ray is the paraxial ray from an on-axis object point, which passes through the edges of the pupils and the aperture stop and to the image point (which also must be on axis).
- The paraxial pupil ray is the paraxial ray from an object point, at the edge of a nominated field-of-view, which passes through the centres of the pupils and the aperture stop.

The nominal paths of these two rays are shown in Figures 3.3a and 3.3b, with the actual paths for schematic eyes found by paraxial ray tracing (Appendix 1). These two rays are useful in various ways. For example,

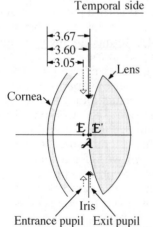

Figure 3.2. The iris and entrance and exit pupils of the Gullstrand number 1 relaxed schematic eye (unit is mm).

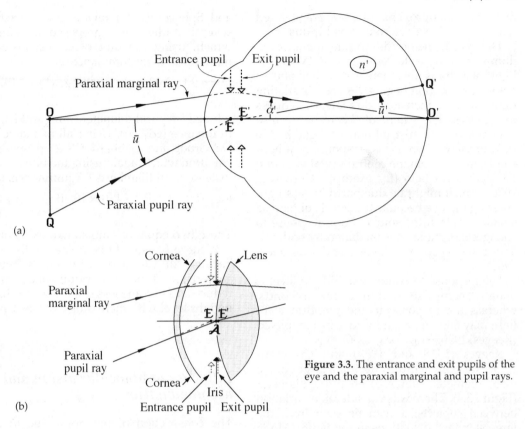

Entrance pupil Exit pupil

Paraxial marginal ray

n'

Paraxial pupil ray

(a)

Cornea Lens

Paraxial
marginal ray

Paraxial
pupil ray

Cornea

Iris

Entrance pupil Exit pupil

(b)

Figure 3.3. The entrance and exit pupils of the eye and the paraxial marginal and pupil rays.

the path of the paraxial marginal ray and the angle α' inside the eye are useful in determining retinal light level (Chapter 13). The paraxial pupil ray is useful in calculating the position of off-axis retinal images (see Chapters 6, 9 and 10), and both rays are useful in estimating the aberrations of the eye.

Pupil centration

In any rotationally symmetric optical system, the pupils are centred. However, the pupils of real eyes are usually decentred, often being displaced nasally by about 0.5 mm relative to the optical axis (Westheimer, 1970). The position of the (entrance) pupil controls the direction of the path of a beam passing into the eye, and therefore affects the amount and type of aberrations and hence retinal image quality.

The pupil centre may move with change in pupil diameter. Walsh (1988) found that in both naturally- and drug-induced pupil dilations, the pupil centre moved by up to 0.4 mm in some subjects. Wilson *et al.* (1992) confirmed Walsh's findings. Most subjects showed temporal movement of the pupil centre with increase in pupil size.

Pupil size

Some of the factors controlling or affecting pupil size are briefly discussed here. Loewenfeld (1993) gave a comprehensive review of these factors.

Level of illumination

This is the most important factor affecting pupil size. The diameter of the pupil may vary from about 2 mm at high illumination to about 8 mm in darkness, corresponding to approximately 16 times variation in area. At normal levels of photopic illumination, the pupil fluctuates in size at a temporal frequency of approximate 1.4 Hz, exaggerated cases of which are referred to as **hippus**.

The pupil responds to an increase in illumination by a decrease in size. When the light intensity is low, there is a latency of 0.5 s before constriction begins. As the stimulating light intensity increases, this latency reduces to 0.2–0.3 s. The extent of the response also depends on the distribution of light in the field-of-view. There is less response as a light source moves from the central visual field into the peripheral field (for example, Crawford, 1936), which might be due partly to less light entering the eye because the pupil subtends a smaller angle at the source. Pupil response to changes in light level is mediated by both rod and cone receptors (Alpern and Campbell, 1962).

The response to an increase in light level is usually complete within a few seconds, whereas the response to the withdrawal of light may take up to a minute to be completed (Reeves, 1920; Crawford, 1936).

Reeves (1918 and 1920) and Crawford (1936) investigated the effect of a large source ($\approx$55° diameter subtense) on pupil diameter (Figure 3.4). There was considerable variation between subjects, as can be seen from the large standard deviations in the figure. Moon and Spencer (1944) reviewed the results of several studies, and proposed an equation which, using the unit of cd/m² instead of millilamberts for luminance, is

$$D = 4.90 - 3.00 \tanh\{0.400[\log_{10}(L) + 1.0]\}$$
(3.1a)

where D is pupil diameter (mm) and L is field luminance (cd/m²). Using all available data, De Groot and Gebhard (1952) proposed an equation which, again using the unit of cd/m² instead of millilamberts for luminance, is

$$\log_{10}(D) = 0.8558 - 4.01 \times 10^{-4}[\log_{10}(L) + 8.6]^3$$
(3.1b)

These two equations are shown in Figure 3.4. The curve fits should be treated with caution because of the wide differences between subjects, and because pupil sizes tend to reduce and become less responsive to changes in light level with increasing age (see Chapter 20).

Influence of binocular vision and accommodation

The constriction of the pupil due to direct light stimulation is referred to as the **direct light reflex**. In a healthy visual system there is also a **consensual light reflex**, in which the pupils of both eyes respond equally to stimulation of only one eye. Pupil reactions are more extensive when both eyes of a person are stimulated than when only one eye is stimulated.

The pupil decreases in diameter when the eyes converge or accommodate. This is referred to as the **near reflex**.

Age

Pupil size decreases with increase in age, and pupils react less to changes in light level. This is considered further in Chapter 20.

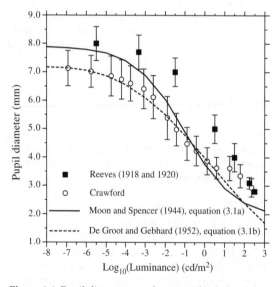

Figure 3.4. Pupil diameter as a function of light level for a uniformly extended field. Experimental data from Reeves (1918 and 1920) and Crawford (1936), and mathematical 'mean' curves of Moon and Spencer (1944) and De Groot and Gebhard (1952).

Drugs

Drugs that cause pupil dilation are called **mydriatics**. These can act by stimulating the sympathetic division of the autonomic nervous system (**sympathomimetics**) or by blocking its parasympathic division (**parasympatholytics**). Drugs that cause pupil constriction are called **miotics**, and can act by stimulating the parasympathic division (**parasympathomimetics**) or by blocking the sympathetic division (**sympatholytics**). Some drugs influence pupil size through their effects on the central nervous system.

Many drugs that affect pupil size also affect accommodation.

Psychological factors

Emotional states such as fear, joy and surprise cause the pupil to dilate. Hess (1965) found that pupil size was affected by mental activities. For example, pleasant, arousal-causing mental images increased pupil size, while unpleasant mental images decreased pupil size.

Shape of the obliquely viewed pupil

So far we have assumed that the pupil is circular, and we continue to make this assumption even though this is not true for some people. If we observe the pupil from increasingly oblique angles, the pupil becomes narrower in the direction of view (the **tangential section**) but remains approximately the same in the perpendicular section (the **sagittal section**), as shown in Figure 3.5. Thus, the apparent area of the pupil decreases as the oblique viewing angle is increased. The decrease in tangential diameter with viewing angle has important implications for (a) the oblique aberrations, and hence retinal image quality, and (b) the amount of light entering the eye from oblique angles, and hence the brightness of a peripheral retinal image (Sloan, 1950; Bedell and Katz, 1982).

We can estimate the apparent tangential diameter and area from simple geometry, as follows. In the simple geometrical model, a circle appears to be elliptical when viewed

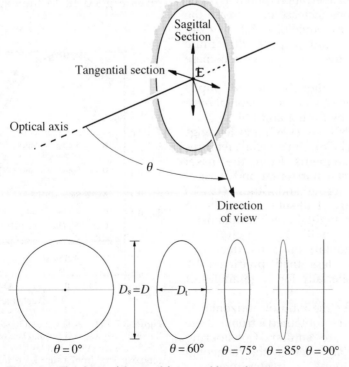

Figure 3.5. The shape of the pupil from an oblique direction.

obliquely. Thus, if we view an entrance pupil of diameter D from an oblique angle θ in any direction, the sagittal diameter D_s does not vary with the eccentricity but the tangential diameter D_t is given by the equation

$$D_t = D \cos(\theta) \tag{3.2}$$

which is shown in Figure 3.5. The projected or apparent area $A_p(\theta)$ is the area of an ellipse, and is given by the equation

$$A_p(\theta) = \pi D_s D_t / 4 \tag{3.3}$$

Alternatively, this area can be expressed in the form

$$A_p(\theta) = A(0)_p \cos(\theta) \tag{3.4}$$

where

$$A(0)_p = \pi D^2 / 4 \tag{3.4a}$$

Thus the apparent area decreases with $\cos(\theta)$, and the ratio of the apparent area at an angle θ to that for axial viewing is also $\cos(\theta)$.

This model assumes that the aperture stop (not the entrance pupil) is plane and does not suffer any aberration when imaged by the cornea. It assumes also that the iris rim has minimal thickness. Unless we resort to complex ray tracing, we cannot readily predict the effect of aberrations and determine whether aberrations increase or decrease the values predicted by equations (3.2) to (3.4). However, we would expect the finite thickness of the iris rim to decrease these values slightly.

Dimensions of obliquely viewed pupils when the direction of view is horizontal have been determined by Spring and Stiles (1948a and b), Sloan (1950), Jay (1962) and Jennings and Charman (1978), but facial features restricted measurements from the nasal direction. The mean horizontal and vertical diameters from Spring and Stiles' (1948b) photographic study of 13 subjects are shown in Figure 3.6. The sagittal (vertical) diameter varies very little with eccentricity. The tangential (horizontal) diameter decreases as expected, but less than predicted by equation (3.2), especially for large angles of eccentricity.

Figure 3.7 shows the ratio of horizontal to vertical diameters obtained from three studies. Results are similar. Considering Figures 3.6 and 3.7 together, the tangential diameter of the pupil is greater than that

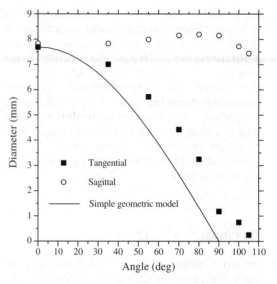

Figure 3.6. The vertical (sagittal) and horizontal (tangential) diameters of the obliquely viewed dilated pupil from the data of Spring and Stiles (1948b). The solid line is the ratio expected from a simple geometric model.

predicted by the simple geometric model. This is most likely to be due to pupil aberrations. A fourth-order equation that gives a good fit to the experimental results

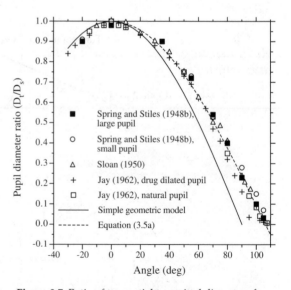

Figure 3.7. Ratio of tangential to sagittal diameters for the obliquely viewed pupil. Data of Spring and Stiles (1948a), Sloan (1950) and Jay (1962). The solid line is the ratio expected from a simple geometric model and the dotted line is the fit to the data given by equation (3.5a).

is

$$D_t = D_s(1 - 1.0947 \times 10^{-4}\ \theta^2 + 1.8698 \times 10^{-9}\ \theta^4)$$
(θ in degrees) (3.5a)

and this equation is shown on Figure 3.7. Assuming that D_s is the same as D, this equation can be converted into the apparent pupil area

$$A(\theta)_p = A(0)_p(1 - 1.0947 \times 10^{-4}\ \theta^2 + 1.8698 \times 10^{-9}\ \theta^4)$$
(3.5b)

Significance of pupil size

Pupil size has a number of effects on vision.

Depth-of-field

As with conventional optical systems, the diameter of the pupil affects the depth-of-field. The larger the pupil, the narrower is the depth-of-field. This is discussed in detail in Chapter 19.

Retinal light level

Obviously, pupil diameter affects retinal light level. A detailed analysis of the dependency is left until Chapter 13.

Retinal image quality and visual performance

For large pupil diameters, aberrations cause deterioration in retinal image quality. For small pupil diameters, diffraction limits image quality. There is an optimum pupil diameter range of 2–3 mm that gives the best balance between these two effects for the corrected eye. The effect of pupil diameter on retinal image quality is discussed in greater detail in Chapter 18.

Campbell and Gregory (1960) and Woodhouse (1975) found that the artificial pupil size that gives the optimum (corrected) visual acuity is close to the natural pupil size at various background lighting levels. The visual acuity of a defocused eye is strongly dependent upon pupil diameter. This is discussed further in Chapter 9.

Purpose of the pupillary light response

We may expect that pupil size varies in order to maintain a constant light level on the retina, but this is not so. The variation of pupil size with light level is not sufficient to ensure a constant retinal illuminance, because if the pupil size changes from 2 to 8 mm in diameter, the amount of light entering the pupil changes by a factor of only 16. By contrast, we operate comfortably over a 10^5 times luminance range, from full moonlight (≈ 0.01 cd/m^2) to bright daylight (≈ 1000 cd/m^2).

The work of Campbell and Gregory (1960) and Woodhouse (1975) suggests that pupil size variations optimize visual acuity for various light levels. This is only applicable for corrected eyes; uncorrected eyes require much smaller pupil sizes. Woodhouse and Campbell (1975) suggested that the purpose of pupil size changes with changes in light

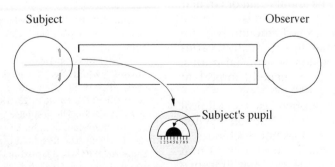

Figure 3.8. A simple pupillometer.

level is to reduce retinal illumination and thus help adaptation if there is a return to darkness.

Measurement of pupil size (pupillometry)

There are a number of experimental and clinical methods for measuring pupil diameter. These vary both in the level of intrusion to the subject and in accuracy. A simple clinical device has the construction shown in Figure 3.8. The inside surface of the end nearest the patient's eye contains a millimetre scale. Parallax is a source of error.

More accurate and less intrusive methods involve photography, either using standard photography or a video camera. A distinct advantage of a photographic method is that it can be done with infrared radiation in complete darkness, and therefore does not affect pupil size. The use of a video camera offers the further advantage that rapid changes in pupil diameter can be recorded and monitored.

Loewenfeld (1993) gave a comprehensive review of pupillometry.

Artificial pupils

Artificial pupils are often used to control the effective pupil size of the eye in visual experiments. The pupil of the eye must be dilated first. Artificial pupils can simply be apertures placed immediately in front of the eye, or they can be projected onto the plane of the actual pupil by a relay system. The artificial pupils may be annular, slit or circular pupils, and may be decentred relative to the actual pupil by a controlled amount. Because of aberrations, retinal image quality varies according to the position of artificial pupils, and careful centration is usually important (Walsh and Charman, 1988).

Artificial pupils are often used in clinical practice as an aid in refraction. When corrected visual acuity does not reach normal levels, placing a small pupil (e.g. 1 mm diameter) in front of the eye may improve visual acuity markedly if the refraction is not accurate, but a lack of improvement indicates a pathological basis for the poor vision. Medium-sized artificial pupils (e.g. 3–4 mm) may be used when the pupil has been previously dilated by drugs; the pupils reduce the influence of aberrations, which may make refraction difficult or inaccurate.

Summary of main symbols

$A_p(\theta)$ projected or apparent pupil area in the direction θ
D (entrance) pupil diameter
D_s pupil diameter in the sagittal section
D_t pupil diameter in the tangential section
L scene luminance (cd/m^2)
θ oblique angle

References

Alpern, M. and Campbell, F. W. (1962). The spectral sensitivity of the consensual light reflex. *J. Physiol.*, **164**, 478–507.

Bedell, H. E. and Katz, L. M. (1982). On the necessity of correcting peripheral target luminance for pupillary area. *Am. J. Optom. Physiol. Opt.*, **59**, 767–9.

Campbell, F.W. and Gregory, A. H. (1960). Effect of pupil size on visual acuity. *Nature*, **187**, 1121–3.

Crawford, B. H. (1936). The dependence of pupil size upon external light stimulus under static and variable conditions. *Proc. R. Soc. B.*, **121**, 376–95.

De Groot, S. G. and Gebhard, J. W. (1952). Pupil size as determined by adapting luminance. *J. Opt. Soc. Am.*, **42**, 492–5.

Hess, E. H. (1965). Attitude and pupil size. *Sci. Am.*, **212(4)**, 46–54.

Jay, B. S. (1962). The effective pupillary area at varying perimetric angles. *Vision Res.*, **1**, 418–28.

Jennings, J. A. M. and Charman, W. N. (1978). Optical quality in the peripheral retina. *Am. J. Optom. Physiol. Opt.*, **55**, 582–90.

Loewenfeld, I. E. (1993). *The Pupil. Anatomy, Physiology, and Clinical Applications*, vols. 1 and 2. Iowa State University Press.

Moon, P. and Spencer, D. E. (1944). On the Stiles–Crawford effect. *J. Opt. Soc. Am.*, 34, 319–29.

Reeves, P. (1918). Rate of pupillary dilation and contraction. *Psychol. Rev.*, **25**, 330–40.

Reeves, P. (1920). The response of the average pupil to various intensities of light. *J. Opt. Soc. Am.*, **4**, 35–43.

Sloan, L. (1950). The threshold gradients of the rods and cones: in the dark-adapted and in the partially light-adapted eye. *Am. J. Ophthal.*, **33**, 1077–89.

Spring, K. H. and Stiles, W. S. (1948a). Variation of pupil

size with change in the angle at which light strikes the retina. *Br. J. Ophthal.*, **32**, 340–46.

Spring, K. H. and Stiles, W. S. (1948b). Apparent shape and size of the pupil viewed obliquely. *Br. J. Ophthal.*, **32**, 347–54.

Walsh, G. (1988). The effect of mydriasis on pupillary centration of the human eye. *Ophthal. Physiol. Opt.*, **8**, 178–82.

Walsh, G. and Charman, W. N. (1988). The effect of pupil centration and diameter on ocular performance. *Vision Res.*, **28**, 659–65.

Westheimer, G. (1970). Image quality in the human eye. *Optica Acta.*, **17**, 641–58.

Wilson, M. A., Campbell, M. C. W. and Simonet, P. (1992). Change of pupil centration with change of illumination and pupil size. *Optom. Vis. Sci.*, **69**, 129–36.

Woodhouse, J. M. (1975). The effect of pupil size on grating detection at various contrast levels. *Vision Res.*, **15**, 645–8.

Woodhouse, J. M. and Campbell, F. W. (1975). The role of the pupil light reflex in aiding adaptation to the dark. *Vision Res.*, **15**, 649–53.

4

Axes of the eye

Introduction

Most man-made optical systems are rotationally symmetric about one line, the optical axis. If the reflecting and refracting surfaces are spherical, this is the line joining the centres of curvatures of these surfaces. Some systems contain astigmatic or toroidal components and have two planes of symmetry; the line of intersection of these two planes is the optical axis.

By contrast, to fully describe the optical properties of the eye, we need to introduce a number of axes. This is because of the lack of symmetry of the eye and because the fixation point and fovea are not along a best-fit axis of symmetry. The optical and visual axes were mentioned in Chapter 1. In this chapter we describe these and other axes, their significance, their applications, and how they may be determined.

The validity of some of these axes is dependent upon some idealized properties of the eye. For example, the visual axis requires the existence of the nodal points, which only exist if the eye is rotationally symmetric. A second example is the fixation axis, which requires the existence of a unique centre-of-rotation of the eye.

Some of the methods for determining the axes depend upon observing the images of a small light source formed by specular reflections from the refracting surfaces of the eye. These Purkinje images are discussed in greater depth in Chapter 12.

Direction of axes

These axes are meaningless without a means of determining their directions and where they enter the eye. The directions are defined relative to each other, and we often refer to the angles between the axes. Table 4.1 lists some axes, and the symbols used to denote the angles between them. Three of the axes pass through the centre of the pupil and, since the pupil centre can change with change in diameter (see Chapter 3), their directions depend upon pupil size.

Definitions and significance

Martin (1942) gave an early account of the angles and axes which highlighted the confusing array of terms that have been used in this area. The definitions of optical axis, line of sight, visual axis, pupillary axis and fixation axis given below are similar to those provided in dictionaries of visual science (Cline *et al.*, 1989; Millodot, 1993).

Optical axis

This is the line passing through the centres of curvatures of the refracting and reflecting surfaces of a centred system. The optical axis is not of particular importance by itself, but it is a useful reference for some of the other axes of the eye.

Table 4.1. Some different axes used for the eye and the symbols used to denote the angles between them.

	Optical axis	*Visual axis*	*Line of sight*	*Achromatic axis*
Visual axis	α	–	–	ψ
Pupillary axis	–	κ	λ	–
Fixation axis	γ	–	–	–

In a conventional centred optical system, the centres of curvatures of each refracting or reflecting surface lie on one line (i.e. they are co-linear). This line is the optical axis. The eye is not a centred system, and does not contain a true optical axis. The concept of optical axis can be applied to the eye by defining the optical axis as the line of 'best fit' through the centres of curvature of the 'best fit' spheres to each surface.

Line of sight

This is the line joining the fixation point and the centre of the entrance pupil.

The line of sight is the most important axis from the point of view of visual function, including refraction procedures, as it defines the centre of the beam of light entering the eye. As mentioned in the previous section, it is unfortunately not fixed because the pupil centre may alter with fluctuations in pupil size.

The fovea is usually on the temporal side of the optical axis (Chapter 1). Therefore, the point in object space conjugate to the fovea is also off axis, but on the nasal side of the optical axis. The line of sight is the central ray of the beam from the fixation point **T** as shown in Figure 4.1. In paraxial optics, the line of sight is called the paraxial pupil ray, which was defined in the previous chapter (see *Entrance and exit pupils*). The position at which it intercepts the cornea is called the **corneal sighting centre** (Mandell, 1995) or **visual centre of the cornea** (Cline *et al.*, 1989).

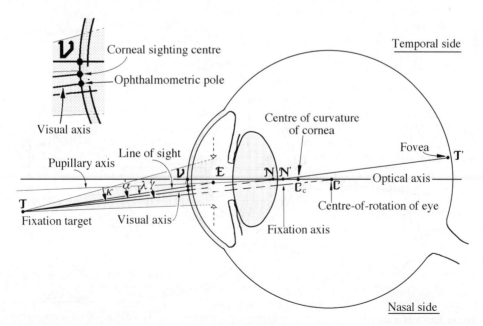

Figure 4.1. Most of the axes and angles referred to in this chapter. The object has been shown extremely close to the eye, thus exaggerating angular differences between visual axis, line of sight and fixation axis.

Visual axis

This is the line joining the fixation point and the foveal image by way of the nodal points.

The visual axis is a convenient reference axis for visual functions, particularly as it does not depend on pupil size. It is usually close to the line of sight at the cornea and entrance pupil (see following section, *Locating some axes*).

The visual axis is the line segments **TN** and **N'T'** shown in Figure 4.1. This is not a single straight line, since the nodal points are not coincident. Allowing for the exaggeration in Figure 4.1, this shows the proximity of the visual axis to the line of sight.

The **foveal achromatic axis** is closely related to the visual axis, and can be defined as the path from the fixation point to the fovea such that the ray does not suffer from any transverse chromatic aberration. Ignoring the small change in the nodal points that occurs with change in wavelength, this axis is the same as the visual axis and its definition can be used as a basis for locating the visual axis. Ivanoff (1953) referred to this axis as simply the **achromatic axis**. However, Thibos *et al.* (1990) redefined this term to refer to the **pupil nodal ray**, which is the ray passing through

the centre of the pupil and which has no transverse chromatic aberration. It is similar to the optical axis but, unlike the optical axis, it is dependent on pupil position. Where Ivanoff used the term achromatic axis, we use the term foveal achromatic axis, and we have adopted Thibos and co-workers' use of achromatic axis (Figure 4.2).

Rabbetts (1998) criticized the use of the term 'visual axis' for the ray passing through the nodal points, on the grounds that such a ray is not representative of the beam passing into the eye from a fixation target. He preferred to call it the 'nodal axis', and reserved the term 'visual axis' for the axis we have defined as the line of sight.

Le Grand and El Hage (1980) referred to the intersection of the visual axis with the cornea as the **ophthalmometric pole** (Figure 4.1).

Pupillary axis

This is the line passing through the centre of the entrance pupil, and which is normal to the cornea.

The pupillary axis is used as an objective measure to judge the amount of **eccentric fixation**, the condition in which a retinal point

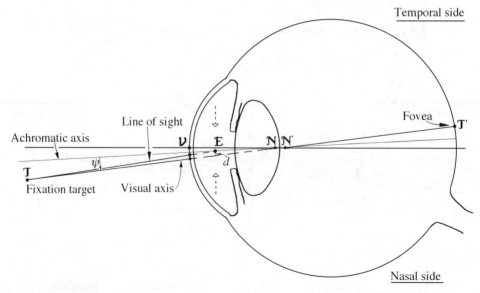

Figure 4.2. Ocular axes:
a. The optical axis, line of sight, visual axis and achromatic axis.
b. The angle ψ between the visual axis and the achromatic axis.
c. The distance d between the visual axis and line of sight at the entrance pupil.

other than the centre of the fovea is used for fixation. Eccentric fixation is an adaptation to **heterotropia** (squint or turned eye). We discuss the measurement of eccentric fixation and heterophoria further in the following section (*Locating some axes*).

If the eye was a centred system and the pupil was also centred, the pupillary axis would lie along the optical axis. However, the pupil is often not centred relative to the cornea and, furthermore, the cornea may not be a regular shape. Both these factors cause the pupil axis to lie in some other direction, and in general it does not pass through the fixation point **T** as shown in Figure 4.1.

Fixation axis

This is the line passing through the fixation point and the centre-of-rotation of the eye.

The fixation axis is the reference for measuring eye movements.

This axis is shown in Figure 4.1. There is no unique centre-of-rotation, and estimates of it depend on the direction of rotation of the eye (Alpern, 1969). Accordingly, the idea of a fixation axis is just an approximation, and estimates of it depend also upon the direction of rotation.

Keratometric axis

This is the axis of a keratometer or video-keratographic instrument, and it contains the centre of curvature of the anterior cornea.

This axis is used for alignment in corneal topography measurements. In the standard operation of a corneal topographic instrument, the axis intercepts the line of sight at the fixation target (Figure 4.3a), although the fixation target may be moved deliberately so that this is not the case (Figure 4.3b). According to Mandell (1994), in standard use a small but negligible variation occurs in this axis between different instruments, because of differences in the distance of the fixation point.

When a videokeratographic instrument is used in standard operation, the keratometric axis is neither the line of sight nor does it pass through the apex of the cornea (the point with the smallest radius of curvature (Mandell and St Helen, 1969)). The point at which the axis intercepts the cornea is sometimes called the vertex normal (Maloney, 1990), and is the centre of videokeratographs showing corneal contour. If the vertex normal is sufficiently decentred from the corneal apex, the videokeratograph gives a false representation of surface curvature across the cornea (Mandell and Horner, 1995).

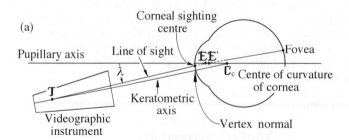

(a)

Corneal sighting centre

Pupillary axis Line of sight Fovea

E E'

C_c Centre of curvature of cornea

Keratometric axis

Videographic instrument

Vertex normal

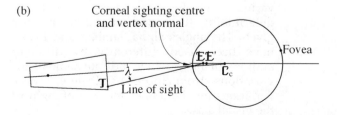

(b)

Corneal sighting centre and vertex normal

E E' Fovea

C_c

T Line of sight

Figure 4.3. The keratometric axis and the line of sight of a videokeratographic instrument.
a. Standard operation. The line of sight and the keratometric axis intersect at the fixation point.
b. The alignment has been altered so that the line of sight and the keratometric axis intersect at the cornea (corneal sighting centre). Based on Mandell *et al.* (1995).

Locating some axes

The line of sight

Many automated instruments have a video display showing the front of the eye. To achieve alignment while a patient is fixating a reference target, either the patient or the instrument is moved vertically and horizontally until the pupil is correctly centred. Thus the line of sight is made to coincide with the optical axis of the instrument. Sometimes this is aided by imaging a centred annulus as well as the eye.

The visual axis

The intercept of the visual axis at the cornea (ophthalmometric pole) can be determined by having the subject view a vernier target, half of which is blue and half of which is red. Two possible targets are shown in Figure 4.4. The subject views the vernier target through a small artificial pupil, say 1 mm diameter. If the artificial pupil is not centred on the visual axis, there is a break in the alignment of the blue and red halves of the target. The position of the subject's eye is adjusted until alignment is obtained. The reliability of the method should improve as the wavelength bands of the target are narrowed.

Thibos *et al.* (1990) indicated a simple way of estimating the separation of the visual axis from the line of sight at the entrance pupil (the distance *d* in Figure 4.2). The small artificial pupil, referred to in the previous paragraph, can be scanned across the eye both vertically and horizontally to find the real pupil limits at which the vernier target disappears. The mean of these positions corresponds to the corneal sighting centre (on the line of sight). This position is then compared with the ophthalmometric pole (visual axis intercept at the cornea). Thibos and co-workers measured five subjects with drug-induced pupil dilation, considering only the horizontal meridian. They obtained values of *d* between –0.1 mm and 0.4 mm, with a mean of +0.14 mm (a positive sign indicating that the visual axis is nasal to the line of sight in object space).

Simonet and Campbell (1990) used a videomonitor to determine the difference in horizontal position of the visual axis (which they referred to as the achromatic axis) and the line of sight. For natural (although generally large) pupils, the differences for eight eyes of five subjects were between –0.08 mm and +0.51 mm, with a mean of +0.11 mm.

Keratometric axis

Mandell *et al.* (1995) described methods of determining the location of the keratometric axis relative to the corneal sighting centre and the corneal apex. Using a videokeratographic instrument in its standard operation and 20 normal subjects, they found a mean difference between the keratometric axis and the corneal sighting centre of 0.38 ± 0.10 mm, with the majority of subjects having the keratometric axis below and nasal to the corneal sighting centre. The mean difference between the keratometric axis and the corneal apex was 0.62 ± 0.23 mm, with the majority of subjects having the keratometric axis above the corneal apex.

Angles between axes

Here we define some of the angles between various axes. In some cases, methods for determining these and measurements are given. The angles alpha, lambda and kappa have been used differently by different authors. In Table 4.2 we indicate some of the variations from those used here. These variations involve either the line of sight or the visual axis.

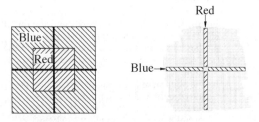

Figure 4.4. Two targets for locating the visual axis.

Table 4.2. Different terms used for angles.

Term used here	Millodot (1993)	Le Grand and El Hage (1980)	Cline et al. (1989)
α	α	α	α
–	κ^*	–	–
λ	–	κ	–
κ	–	–	–

*between line of sight and optical axis.

Visual axis and optical axis: the angle alpha (α)

Most authors use the term 'angle alpha' to refer to the angle between the optical and visual axes (Le Grand and El Hage, 1980; Cline *et al.*, 1989; Millodot, 1989). We have retained this use but, as the technique of measuring this angle involves the subject fixating on a target, it may be considered that the line of sight (i.e. centre of entrance pupil) is involved rather than the visual axis (i.e. nodal points). The distinction is of no practical importance.

In optical laboratories, a frequent need is to locate the optical axis of an optical system. One method of locating this axis is to shine a distant point source into the system and observe the images of this source of light reflected from each surface inside the system. In a centred optical system, if the source of light falls on the optical axis, it and the reflected images are co-linear.

Since the eye has four reflecting surfaces, there are four main reflected (Purkinje) images. However, as the eye is not a centred system, there is no position or direction of the light source that enables the Purkinje images to be aligned. All that can be done is to

minimize the spread of these images, and the corresponding direction of the source identifies the direction of the optical axis.

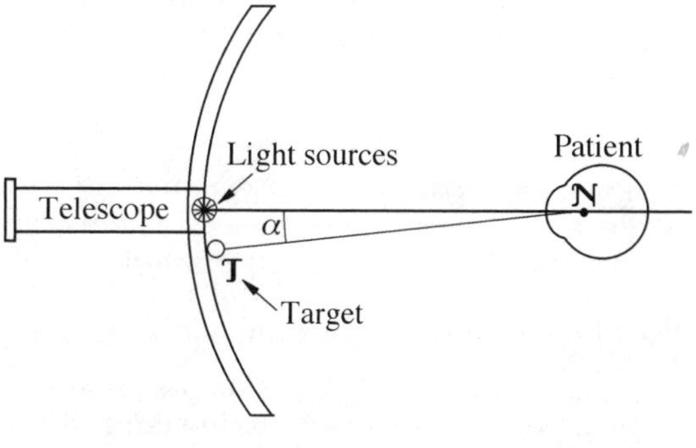

Clinically, the angle α is determined with the ophthalmophakometer (Figure 4.5). This instrument contains a graduated arc, with an observing telescope mounted centrally in the arc. The patient's eye is at the centre of curvature of the arc. Two small light sources are placed on the arc near the telescope, with one slightly above and one slightly below it. This gives pairs of Purkinje images. A small fixation object **T** is moved along the arc until the observer looking through the telescope judges that the Purkinje images are in the best possible alignment. At this point, the optical axis of the eye corresponds with the axis of the instrument. The angle α is given by the scale reading at the position of the fixation target. The instrument can be rotated through 90 degrees to obtain a value in the vertical direction. The distance between the eye and the arc is relatively large (typically 86 cm) so that discrepancies between the front nodal point and the centre of curvature of the arc are not critical.

The angle between the visual axis and the optical axis is considered to be positive if the visual axis is on the nasal side of the optical axis in object space. The mean value of angle α is often taken to be about +5° horizontally, but is usually in the range +3 to +5°, and is rarely negative. The visual axis is also downwards relative to the optical axis by 2–3° (Tscherning, 1990).

Pupillary axis and line of sight: angle lambda (λ)

This angle is one of the easiest to determine. It can be determined using the opthalmophakometer just described, but it is determined easily with simpler equipment (Figure 4.6).

Figure 4.5. The ophthalmophakometer.

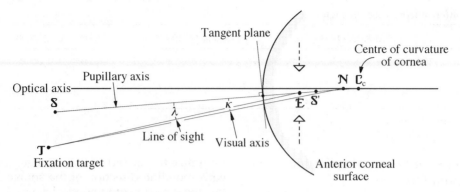

Figure 4.6. The pupillary axis and the line of sight.

The subject fixates on some suitable target **T**, and an observer watches the anterior corneal reflection (Purkinje image P_1) of a small source of light **S** close to the observer's eye. The position of the light is changed, and the observer's eye is maintained next to the light source, until the reflected image **S'** is seen in the centre of the pupil **E** (Figure 4.6). The observation axis is now the pupillary axis. The angle between the line of sight and the pupillary axis at the eye is the angle λ.

For most patients, the pupillary axis is temporal to the line of sight in object space. This is taken as a positive angle. Loper (1959) obtained angles of $1.4 \pm 1.6°$, and Franceschetti and Burian (1971) obtained angles of $2.6 \pm 1.7°$. Furthermore, the angles should be similar between the two eyes.

The angle λ is important for diagnosis of eccentric fixation and heterotropia. In testing for the presence of eccentric fixation, angle λ is determined monocularly (with the other eye occluded). A large angle indicates the likely presence of eccentric fixation. The line of sight as we have defined it is not being used, because the patient has rotated the eye to align a retinal point eccentric to the fovea with the fixation point. Angle λ is estimated binocularly (with both eyes open) to test for direction and amount of heterotropia in the **Hirschberg test**. In the presence of heterotropia, a large angle λ is observed because one eye rotates so that its fovea is not being used to align the fixation target. Either the fovea is being suppressed or another retinal point is being used for fixation (anomalous correspondence), or both are occurring. Again, we are not strictly measuring angle λ because of

the change in reference axis away from the line of sight.

The usual application of these tests involves the clinician shining a penlight at the patient's eye or eyes. The penlight is just in front of the clinician's face, and the patient is instructed to look at it. The clinician observes the position of the corneal reflection (or reflex) in the pupil (Figure 4.7). Usually the reflex is about half a millimetre nasal to the centre of the pupil (Figure 4.7a). Each millimetre change in reflex position away from this corresponds to approximately 22 prism dioptres ($13°$) of eye rotation (Grosvenor, 1996). Care must be taken in the monocular test, as some patients may have normal fixation but unusual angles. Results from the two eyes should be compared. Similarly, in the Hirschberg test it is important to compare the difference in reflex positions between the two eyes.

Pupillary axis and the visual axis: angle κ

In practical terms, this is the same as angle λ. It is shown in Figures 4.1 and 4.6.

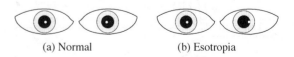

(a) Normal   (b) Esotropia

Figure 4.7. The Hirschberg test for measuring the angle of heterotropia.
a. Appearance of corneal reflexes for no heterotropia.
b. Appearance of reflexes for left esotropia (left eye turned in).

Visual axis and achromatic axis: angle psi (ψ)

Thibos *et al.* (1990) estimated this angle from the equation

$$\sin(\psi) = d/\mathbf{EN} \tag{4.1}$$

where d is the distance between the visual axis and line of sight at the entrance pupil and $\mathbf{EN}$ is the estimate of the distance between the entrance pupil and the nodal point (Figure 4.2). Based on either the Gullstrand No. 1 or No. 2 eyes, the distance $\mathbf{EN}$ is 4.0 mm. An approximate, but sufficiently accurate, method for determining d was given earlier in this chapter. Using five subjects, Thibos and co-workers determined a range of angles from $-1.2°$ to $+5.3°$, with a mean of $+2.1°$ (positive angles indicate the visual axis is inclined nasally to the achromatic axis in object space).

Fixation axis and optical axis: angle gamma (γ)

Figure 4.8 shows the relationship between angles γ and α. In this figure, y is the distance between the optical axis and the fixation target **T**, **N** is the front nodal point, **C** is the centre-of-rotation of the eye, and w is the distance from the projection of **T**, onto the optical axis, to the cornea at **V**. We have the equations

$$\tan(\alpha) = y/(w + \mathbf{VN}) \tag{4.2}$$

and

$$\tan(\gamma) = y/(w + \mathbf{VC}) \tag{4.3}$$

which, combined, give

$$\tan(\gamma) = \tan(\alpha)(w + \mathbf{VN})/(w + \mathbf{VC}) \tag{4.4}$$

Angle γ is within 1 per cent of angle α for object distances greater than 50 cm.

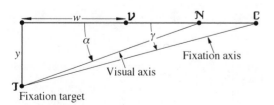

Figure 4.8. Determination of the angle γ.

Summary of main symbols

C	centre-of-rotation of the eye
C_c	centre of curvature of the anterior corneal surface
E, E′	centres of entrance and exit pupils
N, N′	front and back nodal points
T	fixation target
T′	conjugate of **T** on the retina, i.e. the fovea
S, S′	source of light and its image, used to find the pupillary axis
V	intersection of the optical axis with the cornea
d	distance between visual axis and line of sight at the entrance pupil
α	angle between visual axis and optical axis
γ	angle between fixation axis and optical axis
κ	angle between pupillary axis and visual axis
λ	angle between pupillary axis and line of sight
ψ	angle between visual axis and achromatic axis

References

Alpern, M. (1969). Specification of the direction of regard. In *Muscular Mechanisms*, Ch. 2. Vol. 3 of *The Eye*, 2nd edn (H. Davson, ed.), pp. 5–12. Academic Press.

Cline, D., Hofstetter, H. W. and Griffin, J. R. (1989). *Dictionary of Visual Science*, 4th edn. Chilton Trade Book Publishing.

Franceschetti, A. T. and Burian, H. M. (1971). L'angle kappa. *Bull. Mem. Soc. Fr. Ophtalmol.*, **84**, 209–14.

Grosvenor, T. P. (1996). *Primary Care Optometry*, 3rd edn, Ch. 6. Butterworth-Heinemann.

Ivanoff, A. (1953). Les aberrations de l'oeil. Leur role dans l'accommodation. Éditions de la *Revue d'Optique Théorique et Instrumentale*. Masson and Cie.

Le Grand, Y. and El Hage, S. G. (1980). *Physiological Optics* (translation and update of Le Grand, Y. (1968). La dioptrique de l'oeil et sa correction. In *Optique Physiologique*, vol. 1), pp. 71–4. Springer-Verlag.

Loper, L. R. (1959). The relationship between angle lambda and the residual astigmatism of the eye. *Am. J. Optom. Arch. Am. Acad. Optom.*, **36**, 365–77.

Maloney, R. K. (1990). Corneal topography and optical zone location in photorefractive keratectomy. *Refract. Corneal Surg.*, **6**, 363–71.

Mandell, R. B. (1994). Apparent pupil displacement in videokeratography. *CLAO J.*, **20**, 123–7.

Mandell, R. B. (1995). Location of the corneal sighting

centre in videokeratography. *J. Refract. Corneal Surg.*, **11**, 253–8.

Mandell, R. B. and Horner, D. (1995). Alignment of videokeratographs. In *Corneal Topography: The State of the Art* (J. P. Gills, D. R. Sanders, S. P. Thornton *et al.* eds.), Ch. 2. Slack Incorporated.

Mandell, R. B., Chiang, C. S. and Klein, S. A. (1995). Location of the major corneal reference points. *Optom. Vis. Sci.*, **72**, 776–84.

Mandell, R. B. and St Helen, R. (1969). Position and curvature of the corneal apex. *Am. J. Optom. Arch. Am. Acad. Optom.*, **46**, 25–9.

Martin, F. E. (1942). The importance and measurement of angle alpha. *Br. J. Ophthal.*, **3**, 27–45.

Millodot, M. (1993). *Dictionary of Optometry*, 3rd edn. Butterworth-Heinemann.

Rabbetts, R. B. (1998). *Bennett and Rabbetts' Clinical Visual Optics*, 3rd edn., Ch.12. Butterworths.

Simonet, P. and Campbell, M. C. W. (1990). The optical transverse chromatic aberration of the fovea of the human eye. *Vision Res.*, **30**, 187–206.

Thibos, L. N., Bradley, A., Still, D. L. *et al.* (1990). Theory and measurement of ocular chromatic aberration. *Vision Res.*, **30**, 33–49.

Tscherning, M. (1990). *Physiologic Optics*, 1st edn. (translated from the original French edition by C. Weiland). The Keystone.

5

Paraxial schematic eyes

Introduction

We can construct model eyes using population mean values for relevant ocular parameters. This can be done at different levels of sophistication. If we assume that the refractive surfaces are spherical and centred on a common optical axis, and that the refractive indices are constant within each medium, this gives a simple family of models referred to as **paraxial** schematic eyes.

Paraxial schematic eyes are only accurate within the paraxial region. They do not accurately predict aberrations and retinal image formation for large pupils or for angles at more than a few degrees from the optical axis. The paraxial region is defined in geometrical optics as the region in which the replacement of sines of angles by the angles leads to no appreciable error. If we limit the errors to less than 0.01 per cent, this limits object field angles to less than 2° and the entrance pupil diameter to less than 0.5 mm.

Paraxial schematic eyes serve as a framework for examining a range of optical properties. The location of the paraxial image plane or calculation of the paraxial image height has many useful applications. Information can be obtained from schematic eyes concerning magnification, retinal illumination, surface reflections (e.g. Purkinje images), entrance and exit pupils, and effects of refractive errors. A study of cardinal points of

the systems can also have practical applications, such as the observation that the second nodal point moves little on accommodation and therefore that angular resolution is expected to change little with accommodation. Further applications to retinal image formation are discussed in Chapters 6 and 9.

For accurate determinations of quantities such as large retinal image sizes and image quality due to aberrations, we need more realistic models than the paraxial schematic eyes. These are referred to as **finite** or **wide angle** schematic eyes. These include one or more of the following features: non-spherical refractive surfaces, a lack of surface alignment along a common axis, and a lens gradient refractive index.

Historically, paraxial schematic eyes have had uniform refractive indices, and it might be considered that schematic eyes with gradient indices must be finite eyes because the gradient index influences aberrations. However, replacing a uniform refractive index by a gradient index affects the paths of paraxial rays and hence paraxial properties, and thus gradient indices may be included in paraxial model eyes.

This chapter considers paraxial schematic eyes only. A discussion of finite model eyes is given in Chapter 16, following a review of the monochromatic aberrations of real eyes in Chapter 15.

Development of paraxial schematic eyes

The historical development of the understanding of the optical system of the human eye has been described in detail by Polyak (1957). The lens was believed to be the receptive element of the eye for 13 centuries following the work of Galen in 200 AD. Leonardo DaVinci (*c.* 1500 AD) proposed that the lens is only one element of the refractive system which forms a real image on the retina. In 1604, Kepler realized that the image is inverted; this was verified by Scheiner 15 years later. The first clear, accurate description of the eye's optical system was given by Descartes in 1637 in his *La Dioptrique*, which also included the first publication of what has become known as Snell's law of refraction.

The first physical model of the eye was probably that of Christian Huygens (1629–95). Smith (1738) described Huygens's eye as consisting of two hemispheres representing the cornea and retina respectively, with the retinal hemisphere having a radius of curvature three times that of the corneal hemisphere. The two hemispheres were filled with water and a diaphragm was placed between them.

Young (1801) discussed the optics of the eye and presented data, some of which are close to present day values. He gave the anterior corneal radius as 7.9 mm, and the anterior and posterior lenticular radii of curvature as 7.6 mm and 5.6 mm respectively. The anterior chamber depth was given as 3.0 mm. His refractive index for the aqueous and vitreous media was 1.333 (water), and that for the lens was 1.44.

According to Le Grand and El Hage (1980), Moser, in 1844, was the first to construct a schematic eye, but this was hypermetropic because it had a very low value for the refractive index of the lens. The first 'accurate' schematic eye has been attributed to Listing. In 1851, he described a three refracting surfaces schematic eye with a single surface cornea and a homogeneous lens, with an aperture stop 0.5 mm in front of the lens. Helmholtz (1909, p. 152) modified Listing's schematic eye by changing the positions of the lenticular surfaces. He also gave this model in a form accommodated to a distance of 130.1 mm in front of the corneal vertex. Helmholtz (1909, pp. 95–96) also described a much simpler schematic eye designed by Listing. This contains only one refracting surface (the cornea), and is called a **reduced** eye.

Tscherning (1900) published a four refracting surfaces schematic eye containing a posterior corneal surface, which he claimed to be the first to measure.

Gullstrand (1909) used a comprehensive analysis of ocular data to construct a six refracting surface schematic eye that used a four surface lens with the lenticular complexity aimed at accounting for refractive index variation within the lens. This schematic eye is referred to as Gullstrand's number 1 (exact) eye. Gullstrand presented this eye at two levels of accommodation. Gullstrand also presented a simplified version referred to as Gullstrand's number 2 (simplified) eye, also at two levels of accommodation. This simplified eye contains three refracting surfaces, with only one corneal surface and a zero lens thickness.

Emsley (1952) presented a modified version of Gullstrand's simplified eye. Emsley gave the lens the thickness that it has in Gullstrand's exact eye, and changed the aqueous, vitreous and lens refractive indices. This modified eye is sometimes called the Gullstrand–Emsley eye. Emsley also presented a reduced schematic eye.

As well as the Gullstrand exact eye, the Gullstrand–Emsley eye and Emsley's reduced eye, another popular schematic eye is Le Grand's 1945 four refracting surfaces eye, which is referred to as Le Grand's full theoretical eye (Le Grand and El Hage, 1980). It is a modification of Tscherning's schematic eye. Le Grand also presented a simplified three refracting surfaces model with a single corneal surface and a lens of zero thickness. The lack of lens thickness limits the usefulness of this particular model.

More recently, Bennett and Rabbetts (1988, 1989) presented a modification of the Gullstrand–Emsley eye, which they justified on the grounds that the data used to construct the earlier eye was from a restricted number of eyes and that the mean power is closer to 60 D than previously thought. They used the data from the study of Sorsby *et al.* (1957), which was based upon 341 eyes (mostly pairs of left and right eyes) with mean equivalent power of 60.12 ± 2.22 D.

Other schematic eyes have been proposed from time to time. For example, Swaine (1921) gave details of several eyes referred to as Matthiessen B, D and G eyes, and Laurance I and II eyes.

Blaker (1980) described an adaptive schematic eye. It is a modified Gullstrand number 1 paraxial schematic eye, in which the lens has been reduced to two surfaces but is given a gradient refractive index. The lens gradient index, lens surface curvatures, lens thickness and the anterior chamber depth vary as linear functions of accommodation. Blaker (1991) revised his model to include aging effects, with the lens curvatures, lens thickness and anterior chamber depth altering in the unaccommodated state as a function of age.

Some of the above mentioned eyes are discussed in greater detail later in this chapter, and constructional details of some eyes are given in Appendix 3.

Gaussian properties and cardinal points

One of the main applications of paraxial schematic eyes is predicting the Gaussian properties of real eyes. Of these, probably the most important are the equivalent power F, positions of the six cardinal points ($\mathbf{F}$, $\mathbf{F'}$, $\mathbf{P}$, $\mathbf{P'}$, $\mathbf{N}$ and $\mathbf{N'}$) and the positions and magnifications of the pupils. We can use the paraxial optics theory described in Appendix 1 to determine these properties. The Gaussian properties are given for specific schematic eyes in Appendix 3, and Table 5.1 shows a limited amount of data.

Equivalent power and cardinal points

The cardinal points are defined in Chapter 1 (*Cardinal points*). Figure 1.1 shows nominal positions of these in the emmetropic relaxed eye.

There are a number of useful equations connecting the cardinal points, including:

$$F = -n/\mathbf{PF} = n'/\mathbf{P'F'} \tag{5.1}$$

$$\mathbf{PN} = \mathbf{P'N'} = (n' - n)/F \tag{5.2}$$

$$\mathbf{FN} = \mathbf{P'F'} \tag{5.3a}$$

$$\mathbf{N'F'} = \mathbf{FP} \tag{5.3b}$$

where n and n' are the refractive indices of object space (air) and image space (the vitreous) respectively.

Table 5.1. Summary of Gaussian data. Distances are in millimetres and powers are in dioptres.

General

	length
Gullstrand number 1	24.385
Le Grand (full theoretical)	24.197
Le Grand (simplified)	24.192
Gullstrand–Emsley	23.896
Bennett and Rabbetts (simplified)	24.086
Emsley (reduced)	22.222

Relaxed eyes

	F	VE	VN	E'F' = E'R'	N'F' = N'R'	$\overline{m}$
Gullstrand number 1	58.636	3.047	7.078	20.720	17.054	0.823085
Le Grand (full theoretical)	59.940	3.038	7.200	20.515	16.683	0.813243
Gullstrand–Emsley	60.483	3.052	7.062	20.209	16.534	0.818128
Bennett and Rabbetts (simplified)	60.000	3.048	7.111	20.387	16.667	0.817532
Emsley (reduced)	60.000	0.0	50/9	22.222	16.667	0.750000

Accommodated eyes

	F	Accom.	VE	VN	E'R'	N'R'	F'R'	$\overline{m}$
Gullstrand number 1	70.576	10.870	2.668	6.533	21.173	17.539	3.371	0.795850
Le Grand (full theoretical)	67.677	7.053	2.660	7.156	20.942	17.041	2.265	0.791122
Gullstrand–Emsley	69.721	8.599	2.674	6.562	20.647	16.987	2.644	0.796683
Bennett and Rabbetts (10 D)	71.120	10.192	2.680	6.598	21.140	17.135	3.074	0.791439

Approximate mean values

Since the mean equivalent power of the eye is close to 60 D and the values of n and n' are 1.0 and 1.336 respectively, we can calculate expected approximate mean values of the above quantities. These are:

F = 60 D
FP = $N'F'$ = 16.67 mm
$P'F'$ = FN = 22.27 mm
PN = $P'N'$ = 5.6 mm.

The aperture stop and entrance and exit pupils

After the equivalent power and positions of the cardinal points, probably the next most important Gaussian properties of an eye are the aperture stop and pupil formation. The aperture stop of an eye is its iris. Reduced eyes do not have an iris, but we can place an aperture stop in the plane of the cornea or at some other suitable position. The image of the aperture stop formed in object space, that is, the image of the iris as seen through the cornea, is called the entrance pupil. The image of the aperture formed in image space is called the exit pupil. These concepts are discussed fully in Chapter 3.

Position and magnification of entrance pupil

For schematic eyes with a single surface cornea, the calculations are simple. In this case, we can use the lens equation given in Appendix 1,

$$n'/l' - n/l = F \qquad (5.4)$$

Figure 5.1 shows the path of a paraxial ray that can be used to locate the image of the iris. l is the anterior chamber depth, l' is the apparent anterior chamber depth, n is the refractive index of the aqueous, and n' is the refractive index of air (= 1.0). Solving for l' gives

$$l' = n'l/(n + lF) \qquad (5.5)$$

and the pupil magnification $\overline{M}_{EA}$, defined as the ratio of the entrance pupil diameter to that

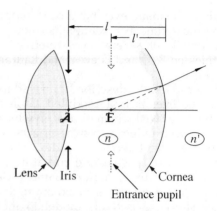

Figure 5.1. The formation of the entrance pupil of the eye and its relationship to the iris in a schematic eye with a single surface cornea.

of the stop, is given by

$$\overline{M}_{EA} = nl'/(n'l) \qquad (5.6)$$

The standard sign convention was used in the development of these equations, with distances to the left of the refracting surface being negative and distances to the right being positive. Distances l and l' are negative, although usually we express the final answers in a positive form.

Example 5.1: Calculate the position and magnification of the entrance pupil of the Gullstrand–Emsley simplified relaxed eye.

Solution: From the Gullstrand–Emsley schematic eye data given in Appendix 3, we have

n = 4/3
n' = 1
l = −3.6 mm and
F = 42.735 D.

Substituting these data into equations (5.5) and (5.6) gives

$$l' = \frac{1 \times (-3.6)}{[(4/3) + (-3.6) \times 42.735/1000]} = (-)3.052\text{mm}$$

and

$$\overline{M}_{EA} = \frac{(4/3) \times (-3.052)}{1 \times (-3.6)} = 1.1304$$

Thus the entrance pupil is 3.05 mm inside the eye, compared with a distance of 3.6 mm for the actual pupil. The entrance pupil is also 13 per cent larger than the actual pupil. The pupil position is shown in Table 5.1, along with the values for other schematic eyes.

Paraxial marginal ray and paraxial pupil ray

These are two special paraxial rays introduced and defined in Chapter 3 (*Entrance and exit pupils*). As can be seen from Figure 3.3, the paths of these rays depend upon the position of the object/image conjugates, field size and the position of the aperture stop and its diameter. Here, as a rule, we denote the marginal ray angles and heights by the respective symbols u and h and the paraxial pupil ray angles and heights by the respective symbols $\bar{u}$ and $\bar{h}$. The details of these rays (angles and heights) are given by Smith and Atchison (1997) for some schematic eyes with an entrance pupil diameter of 8 mm and a field-of-view of angular radius 5°.

Paraxial pupil ray angle ratio $\overline{m}$

A quantity that is useful in the calculation of retinal image sizes is the ratio $\overline{m}$ of the paraxial pupil ray angles

$$\overline{m} = \bar{u}'/\bar{u} \qquad (5.7)$$

The angles $\bar{u}$ and $\bar{u}'$ are the angles of the paraxial pupil ray in object and image space respectively, as shown in Figure 5.2. They are related by the paraxial refraction equation (Appendix 1)

$$n'\bar{u}' - n\bar{u} = -\bar{h}F \qquad (5.8)$$

where F is the equivalent power of the eye and $\bar{h}$ is the ray height at the principal planes. Equation (5.8) can be transposed to give

$$\overline{m} = [n - (\bar{h}/\bar{u})F]/n' \qquad (5.9)$$

where n has a value of 1 for air.

From Figure 5.2, within the paraxial approximation we have

$$\bar{h}/\bar{u} = -\textbf{PE} = -\bar{l} \qquad (5.10)$$

Therefore we have

$$\overline{m} = [n + \bar{l}\,F]/n' \qquad (5.11)$$

which shows that the value of $\overline{m}$ depends upon the refractive index of the vitreous which is fixed, the distance of the entrance pupil $\bar{l}$ from the front principal point and the equivalent power F. The values of both $\bar{l}$ and F depend upon accommodation level. For a typical schematic eye, $\bar{l} \approx 1.5$ mm, $F \approx 60$ D and $n' = 1.336$, giving $\overline{m} \approx 0.82$. Precise values for particular schematic eyes and at different levels of accommodation are given in Table 5.1. Equation (5.11) can be manipulated into the following form

$$\overline{m} = \frac{n}{n'\overline{M}_{\text{E'E}}} \qquad (5.11a)$$

where $\overline{M}_{\text{E'E}}$ is the pupil magnification = exit pupil diameter/entrance pupil diameter.

Effect of accommodation

The cardinal point positions of the relaxed (zero accommodation) and accommodated versions of schematic eyes can be compared in Figures 5.3, 5.4 and 5.5. Upon accommodation, the principal points move away from the cornea, the nodal points move towards the cornea, and the focal points move towards the cornea.

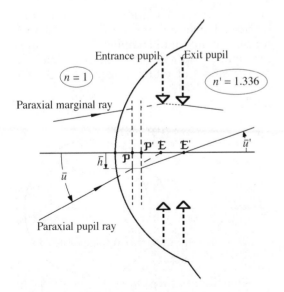

Figure 5.2. The paraxial pupil ray and its use in calculation of $\overline{m}$.

'Exact' schematic eyes

In the 'exact' schematic eyes, an attempt is made to model the optical structure of real eyes as closely as possible while using spherical surfaces. The minimum requirement of an 'exact' eye is that it must have at least four refracting surfaces, two for the cornea and two for the lens.

Gullstrand number 1 (exact) eye

This schematic eye takes into account the variation of refractive index within the lens (Figure 5.3). It is presented in both relaxed and accommodated versions. It consists of six refracting surfaces; two for the cornea and four for the lens. The lens contains a central nucleus (core) of high refractive index surrounded by a cortex of lower refractive index. The lens can be regarded as a combination of three lenses. The anterior and posterior lenses are thinner in the centre than at the edge, and may be erroneously considered to have negative power. However, they have positive power because the refractive index of the core lens is higher than that of the cortex.

Gullstrand placed the retina 0.39 mm short of the back focal point **F′** because he thought that the positive spherical aberration would lead to the best image plane being slightly in front of the paraxial image. However, this is arbitrary, because the level of spherical aberration depends upon pupil diameter, with primary wave spherical aberration depending upon the fourth power of this

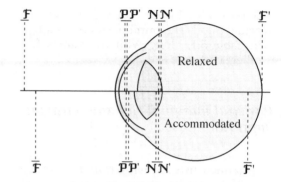

Figure 5.4. The Le Grand full theoretical schematic eye.

diameter. Furthermore, the role of spherical aberration may have been greatly exaggerated since real eyes have much less spherical aberration than schematic eyes. We adopt the usual practice of increasing the length of the eye so that the retina coincides with **F′**.

Le Grand full theoretical eye

The lens of this eye has a constant refractive index, and thus has only two refracting surfaces (Figure 5.4). The eye is presented in both relaxed and accommodated forms.

Simplified schematic eyes

For paraxial calculations, the Gullstrand number 1 eye and the Le Grand full theoretical eye are more complex than is required for many optical calculations, such as measurement of retinal image sizes. Simpler

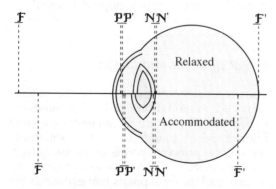

Figure 5.3. The Gullstrand number 1 schematic eye.

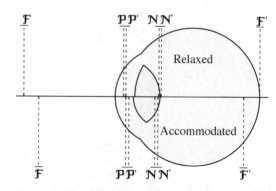

Figure 5.5. The Gullstrand–Emsley schematic eye.

eyes are now considered to be adequate. This is because errors that arise in using these simpler models are usually less than the expected variations between real eyes.

In simplified schematic eyes, the cornea is reduced to a single refracting surface and the lens has two surfaces with a uniform refractive index.

Gullstrand number 2 (simplified) eye as modified by Emsley – the Gullstrand–Emsley eye

Emsley (1952) modified Gullstrand's number 2 eye in order to simplify computation (Figure 5.5). The modifications included altering the aqueous and vitreous refractive indices to 4/3, altering the lens refractive index to 1.416 for both relaxed and accommodated eyes, thickening the lens and changing the accommodated lens surface radii of curvature to ±5.00 mm.

Le Grand simplified eye

Most of the parameters of this eye are different from those of Le Grand's full schematic eye. The lens is given a zero thickness. The eye has both relaxed and accommodated forms.

Bennett and Rabbetts simplified eye

Bennett and Rabbetts (1988, 1989) modified the relaxed version of the Gullstrand–Emsley eye (see Appendix 3). Rabbetts (1998) introduced forms for accommodation levels of 2.5, 5.0, 7.5 and 10 D. He introduced an 'elderly' version of the eye, which has a lower lens refractive index than do the other forms, and has a refractive error of 1 D hypermetropia (see Chapter 7).

Reduced schematic eyes

Further simplifications are possible which may give models accurate enough for some calculations, in particular, estimates of retinal image size.

Reduced eyes contain only one refracting surface, which is the cornea. In the exact and simplified eyes already presented, the two principal points and the two nodal points are each separated by values in the range 0.12–0.37 mm. In reduced eyes, the use of a single refracting surface means that its vertex must be at the principal points **P(P')** and its centre of curvature must be at the nodal points **N(N')**. To keep a power similar to that of the more sophisticated eyes, reduced eyes must have shorter axial lengths. As the cornea has absorbed the power of the lens, the radii of curvature are much smaller than real values. Since reduced eyes do not have a lens, they cannot be used to examine the optical consequences of accommodation.

Emsley's reduced eye (1952)

This eye has a corneal radius of curvature of 50/9 mm, a refractive index of 4/3 and a power of 60 D (Figure 5.6).

Bennett and Rabbetts (1988, 1989)

This eye has a corneal radius of curvature of 5.6 mm, a refractive index of 1.336 and a power of 60 D.

Variable accommodating eyes

While most of the above models have fixed accommodated forms, none has a variable level of accommodation. As mentioned previously, Blaker (1980) presented a variable accommodating paraxial eye which was later modified to consider aging effects (Blaker,

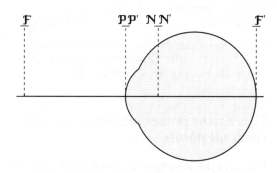

Figure 5.6. The Emsley reduced schematic eye.

1991). Navarro *et al.* (1985) presented a finite accommodating schematic eye which is suitable for easy paraxial calculations because the refractive index of the lens remains uniform, but we leave discussion of this eye until Chapter 16.

We present here a variable version of Gullstrand's number 1 schematic eye. The eye was specified at two levels of accommodation (zero and 10.87 D), but we can modify this eye to have a variable accommodation by assuming that the following individual parameters of this eye vary with accommodation:

anterior chamber depth
lens thicknesses
lens cortex anterior curvature
lens core anterior curvature
lens core posterior curvature
lens cortex posterior curvature.

To simplify the model, we relate the accommodation level A, measured at the corneal vertex, to a parameter x, where

$$x = 1.052A - 0.00531A^2 + 0.000048564A^3 \quad (5.12)$$

and the variable parameters of the eye are related to x by the equations

anterior chamber depth = $3.1 - (3.1 - 2.7)x/A_0$
lens

cortical anterior thickness	= $0.546 - (0.546 - 0.6725)x/A_0$
core thickness	= $2.419 - (2.419 - 2.655)x/A_0$
cortical posterior thickness	= $0.635 - (0.635 - 0.6725)x/A_0$
lens anterior curvature	= $1/10 - (1/10 - 1/5.333)x/A_0$
lens core anterior curvature	= $1/7.911 - (1/7.911 - 1/2.655)x/A_0$
lens core posterior curvature	= $-1/5.760 - [-1/5.760 - 1/(-2.655)]x/A_0$
lens posterior curvature	= $-1/6 - [-1/6 -1/(-5.333)]x/A_0$

where the distance unit is millimetres and A_0 is the level of the Gullstrand accommodated eye in dioptres, that is, 10.87013 D.

Equivalent power and positions of cardinal points

We can now assemble a schematic eye at any level of accommodation and, by paraxial ray-

tracing, calculate various quantities. For example:

$$F_a(A) = 58.636 + 11.940A/A_0 \text{ D}$$

$$\mathbf{N'R'}(A) = 17.054 - 0.485A/A_0 \text{ mm}$$

$$= 1/F_R - 0.485A/A_0 \text{ mm}$$

where F_R is the equivalent power of the relaxed eye. The values of $\overline{m}$ and the distances of the entrance pupil and the front nodal point from the anterior corneal vertex (**VE** and **VN**) are plotted as a function of accommodation in Figure 5.7.

Summary of main symbols

A	accommodation level at corneal vertex in dioptres
d	surface separations
F	equivalent power of the eye
$\overline{m}$	ratio $\overline{u}'/\overline{u}$ of paraxial pupil ray angles – this value is a constant for any particular eye at any particular level of accommodation
$\overline{M}_{EA}$	pupil magnification, the ratio of entrance pupil diameter to stop diameter
$\overline{M}_{E'E}$	pupil magnification, the ratio of exit pupil diameter to entrance pupil diameter

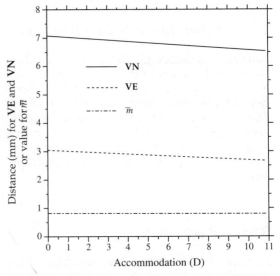

Figure 5.7. The effect of accommodation on $\overline{m}$, **VE** and **VN** of a variable accommodating version of the Gullstrand number 1 schematic eye.

n, n' refractive indices (usually of object and image space, respectively)

r radius of curvature

$\bar{u}$ paraxial pupil ray angle in object space (air)

$\bar{u}'$ paraxial pupil ray angle in image space (in the vitreous)

E, E' positions of entrance and exit pupils

F, F' front and back focal points

N, N' front and back nodal points

O, O' general object and corresponding image point

P, P' position of front and back principal points

R', R axial retinal point and corresponding conjugate in object space

References

Bennett, A. G. and Rabbetts, R. B. (1988). Schematic eyes – time for a change? *Optician*, **196 (5169),** 14–15.

Bennett, A. G. and Rabbetts, R. B. (1989). *Clinical Visual Optics*, 2nd edn. Butterworths.

Blaker, J. W. (1980). Toward an adaptive model of the human eye. *J. Opt. Soc. Am.*, **70**, 220–23.

Blaker, J. W. (1991). A comprehensive model of the aging, accommodative adult eye. In *Technical Digest on Ophthalmic and Visual Optics*, vol. 2, pp. 28–31. Optical Society of America.

Emsley, H. H. (1952). *Visual Optics*, vol. 1, 5th edn. Butterworths.

Gullstrand, A. (1909). Appendix II: Procedure of the rays in the eye. Imagery – laws of the first order. In *Helmholtz's Handbuch der Physiologischen Optik*, vol. 1, 3rd edn. (English translation edited by J. P. Southall, Optical Society of America, 1924).

Helmholtz, H. von (1909). *Handbuch der Physiologischen Optik*, vol. 1, 3rd edn. (English translation edited by J. P. Southall, Optical Society of America, 1924).

Le Grand, Y. and El Hage, S. G. (1980). *Physiological Optics* (translation and update of Le Grand Y. (1968). La dioptrique de l'oeil et sa correction. In *Optique Physiologique*, vol. 1), Springer-Verlag.

Navarro, R., Santamaría, J. and Bescós, J. (1985). Accommodation-dependent model of the human eye with aspherics. *J. Opt. Soc. Am. A*, **2**, 1273–81.

Polyak, S. L. (1957). *The Vertebrate Visual System*, Ch. 1. University of Chicago Press.

Rabbetts, R. B. (1998). *Bennett and Rabbetts' Clinical Visual Optics*, 3rd edn., pp. 209–13. Butterworth-Heinemann.

Smith, R. (1738). *A Compleat System of Opticks*, p. 25. Cornelius Crownfield.

Smith, G. and Atchison, D. A. (1997). *The Eye and Visual Optical Instruments*, Appendix 3. Cambridge University Press.

Sorsby, A., Benjamin, B., Davey, J. B. *et al.* (1957). *Emmetropia and its Aberrations*. Medical Research Council Special Report Series number 293. HMSO.

Swaine, W. (1921). Geometrical and ophthalmic optics – VII: paraxial schematic and reduced eyes. *The Optician and Scientific Instrument Maker*, **62**, 133–6.

Tscherning, M. (1900). *Physiologic Optics* (translated from the original French by C. Weiland). The Keystone.

Young, T. (1801). On the mechanism of the eye. *Phil. Trans. of the R. Soc. of Lond.*, **92**, 23–88 (and plates).

Section 2:

Image formation and refraction

6

Image formation: the focused paraxial image

Introduction

In this chapter, we consider in-focus image formation assuming the image forming rays behave as paraxial rays. The treatment is applicable to small angles only, as it ignores aberrations and the curvature of the retina.

The ability to predict retinal image size, given an object of known size, has many applications. For example, if the two eyes of a person with different levels of refractive error are corrected with ophthalmic lenses, the retinal image sizes of the two eyes may be different and this difference can lead to binocular vision problems (see *Binocular vision*, this chapter). A second example is the calculation of risks from radiation damage where, in the case of thermal damage (due to wavelengths longer than approximately 500 nm), the retinal image size affects the level of risk.

The general case

Figure 6.1 shows an axial point at **O** and an off-axis point at **Q** on the perpendicular plane through **O**. Beams of rays from each of these points pass into the eye through the cornea, iris and lens, and are imaged at **O′** and **Q′** respectively on the retina at **R′**. All the rays in each beam are concurrent (i.e. focus) at the appropriate points **O′** or **Q′**. According to the rules of paraxial optics, the point **Q′** lies on the plane passing through **O′** and perpendicular to the optical axis.

The points **O** and **Q** are at the edges of an object, and **O′** and **Q′** are at the edges of the

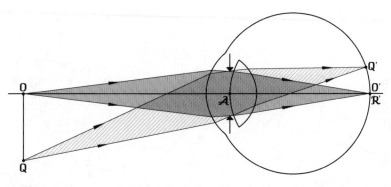

Figure 6.1. The general case of formation of the retinal image and image forming beams.

Point source
of light

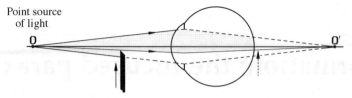

Figure 6.2. Demonstration that the retinal image is inverted (see text for explanation).

corresponding image. By noting the relative orientation of the object and image, we can deduce that the image is inverted. Extending this to two dimensions, we would note that the image is inverted in both horizontal and vertical directions (equivalent to a 180° rotation). The inversion is opposite to our perception, because a further inversion process occurs in the brain.

This retinal inversion can be demonstrated simply, without the use of optical ray-tracing. Figure 6.2 shows a slightly out-of-focus point source, with its image formed behind the retina. This can be achieved by bringing the point source within the nearest point of clear vision. This point source should appear as a circular patch of light. If a sharp edge is moved upwards as shown, it blocks the lower part of the beam. We observe the top edge being blocked, indicating that the brain inverts the retinal image. Since we observe the image erect, but the brain is inverting the image, it follows that the retinal image is inverted.

We cannot readily consider the image formation in a particular eye unless we know its construction details; in particular, surface radii of curvature, surface separations and

refractive indices. These data are not easy to determine. In many situations, all we need are reasonable estimates from a schematic eye. We can determine the image formation in the schematic eye either by tracing suitable paraxial rays or by using known positions of the cardinal points and pupils. Since these are readily available for the standard schematic eyes, we take this approach in the following discussion. The reader should be familiar with the properties of cardinal points and pupils as discussed in earlier chapters.

Figure 6.3 shows a beam of rays from an off-axis point **Q** being imaged to a point **Q'** on the retina of an eye with some level of accommodation. We have drawn two special paraxial rays, the **nodal ray** and the **paraxial pupil ray** (also **paraxial chief ray**). The nodal ray was introduced in Chapter 1. It is the ray from an off-axis object which is inclined at the same angle to the optical axis in both object and image spaces. In object space it is directed towards the first nodal point **N**, and in image space it is directed from the second nodal point **N'**. The paraxial pupil ray was introduced in Chapter 3. It is the ray which, in object space, is directed towards the centre of the entrance pupil **E**, and in image space is

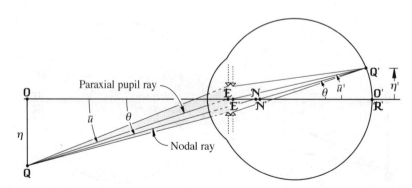

Figure 6.3. The formation of an off-axis image point, the paraxial pupil ray, and the nodal ray for an arbitrary level of accommodation.

directed from the centre of the exit pupil **E'**. Both of these rays can help us to determine the size of the retinal image.

We can use the nodal ray to find the size of the retinal image, using Figure 6.3. Within the limits of paraxial optics, the retinal image size η' is given by the equation

$$\eta' = \theta N'R' \tag{6.1}$$

where

$$\theta = -\eta/ON \tag{6.2}$$

The minus sign is present because, in the figure, η is negative and θ and the distance **ON** are positive. Combining these two equations gives

$$\eta' = -\eta N'R'/ON \tag{6.3}$$

To find the image size in a particular case, we need the object size η and distances **ON** and **N'R'**. The positions of the nodal points depend upon the level of accommodation of the eye, and estimates are available only for a limited range of accommodation for schematic eyes. If the positions are known, the use of the nodal rays to find the size or magnification of the image is straightforward.

An alternative method uses the paraxial pupil ray. One advantage of this ray is that it always (by definition) lies in the centre of the image-forming beam. From Figure 6.3, it follows that

$$\eta' = \bar{u}'E'R' \tag{6.4}$$

We can express the image size η' in terms of the angle $\bar{u}$ the pupil ray is inclined to the axis in object space. The angles $\bar{u}'$ and $\bar{u}$ are connected by equation (5.7), i.e.

$$\bar{u}'/\bar{u} = \text{a constant} = \overline{m} \tag{6.5}$$

with the value of the constant $\overline{m}$ depending upon the schematic eye used and level of accommodation. Combining these equations gives

$$\eta' = \bar{u}\,\overline{m}\,E'R' \tag{6.6}$$

where

$$\bar{u} = -\eta/OE \tag{6.7}$$

Therefore we can finally express the image size η' by the equation

$$\eta' = -\eta\,\overline{m}\,E'R'/OE \tag{6.8}$$

Values for $\overline{m}$ and the positions of the cardinal points for different schematic eyes are given in Table 5.1.

Example 6.1: Calculate the retinal image size of a letter of height 1 mm, seen at the near point of the accommodated Gullstrand number 1 schematic eye.

Solution: From Table 5.1 we have the following data:

N'R' = 17.539 mm
ON = 1000/10.870 + **VN** = 91.996 + 6.533 = 98.529 mm
$\overline{m}$ = 0.795850
E'R' = 21.173 mm
OE = 91.996 + **VE** = 91.996 + 2.668 = 94.664 mm.

Choosing a value of $\eta = -1$ mm, which is negative because the object is below the optical axis, and using equation (6.3) we have

$$\eta' = 1 \times 17.539/98.529 \text{ mm} = 0.178 \text{ mm}$$

Alternatively, using equation (6.8) we have

$$\eta' = 1 \times 0.795850 \times 21.173/94.664 \text{ mm} = 0.178 \text{ mm}$$

We note that the two values should be and are the same.

Retinal image size and perceived angular size in object space

In analysing visual images, we can specify the image size in two ways; one is the image size on the retina, and the other is as a perceived angular size in object space. These two quantities are related. Let us consider the situation in Figure 6.3, where an eye is looking at an object at **O** and this is imaged at **O'** on the retina at **R'**. The nodal points **N** and **N'** and the nodal ray are shown. The angle of inclination of this ray with the axis is the same in both object and image spaces. If the object subtends an angle θ at the front nodal point **N**, then the retinal image subtends the same angle at the back nodal point **N'**. For typical working distances, the distance to the object is large in comparison with the dimensions of the eye. Therefore, in determining the angular size of the object, we can take the reference point as the corneal vertex, the entrance pupil position or the front nodal point. In summary, we can conclude that the angular size of the perceived image is that angle subtended by the retinal image at the back nodal point. This conclusion is useful in some discussions on image sizes.

Eye focused at infinity

If the eye is focused at infinity, we can simplify the above equations. For an object at infinity (or very distant), its size can only be expressed as an angular measure, say θ. For the eye focused at infinity, the retinal point $\mathbf{R'}$ coincides with the back focal point $\mathbf{F'}$ and thus

$$\mathbf{N'R'} = \mathbf{N'F'} \tag{6.9}$$

Combining equations (5.1) and (5.3b) with $n = 1$ gives

$$\mathbf{N'F'} = 1/F \tag{6.10}$$

where F is the equivalent power of the eye. Combining equations (6.1), (6.9) and (6.10) gives

$$\eta' = \theta/F \tag{6.11}$$

The values of F for different schematic eyes are given in Table 5.1.

Alternatively, we can use the pupil ray equation (6.8). Because the object is at infinity, its angular size is independent of the point from which this angle is measured. Therefore we can write

$$\theta = -\eta/\mathbf{OE} \tag{6.12}$$

Thus equation (6.8) reduces to

$$\eta' = \theta \overline{m}\, \mathbf{E'F'} \tag{6.13}$$

We now use equations (6.11) and (6.13) in a numerical example.

Example 6.2: Calculate the retinal image size of the moon (angular diameter of 0.5°) using the Gullstrand number 1 relaxed schematic eye.

Solution: For the Gullstrand number 1 relaxed schematic eye, the relevant data are given in Table 5.1; in particular

$F = 58.636$ D
$\mathbf{E'F'} = 20.720$ mm and $\overline{m} = 0.823085$.

Substituting the relevant values and $\theta = 0.5° = 0.00872665$ radians into equation

(6.11) gives

$\eta' = 0.00872665/58.636$ m $= 0.14883$ mm

Substituting the relevant values into equation (6.13) gives

$\eta' = 0.00872665 \times 0.823085 \times 20.720032$
$\quad = 0.14883$ mm

Note that these two solution should be and are the same.

If we take an approximate value of the mean power of the eye of 60 D, then we can write equation (6.11) in the form

$$\eta' \approx 0.00485\theta \text{ mm} \tag{6.14}$$

where θ is in minutes of arc. This equation is a useful rule of thumb for working out expected retinal image sizes and indicates that 1 min arc is approximately equivalent to 0.005 mm on the retina, and 1 mm on the retina is approximately equivalent to 200 min arc.

Binocular vision

Stereopsis

The use of two eyes provides the potential for seeing depth in a scene. This perception of depth is called **stereoscopic vision** or **stereopsis**. The retinal images of that world, while flat two-dimensional images, are slightly different. This is explained with the help of Figure 6.4. Figure 6.4a shows, from above, the two eyes of a person who is looking at two points **A** and **B** in a horizontal plane. From an observer's point of view, **A** is imaged to the left of **B** by both eyes, and no perception of depth occurs. Figure 6.4b shows the person looking at **A** and **B**, which are now in line but at different distances. From the observer's point of view, **A** is imaged to the right of **B** for the left eye, but **A** is imaged to the left of **B** for the right eye – i.e. the two retinal images of **A** are closer together than are the two retinal images of **B**. This difference in relative position of the retinal images of **A** and **B** leads to the perception of depth.

Aniseikonia

Aniseikonia is usually defined as a relative

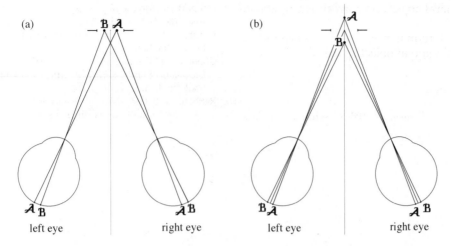

Figure 6.4. Binocular vision and the relative positions of the retinal images for two point objects.
a. Objects side by side.
b. One object behind the other.

difference in size and/or shape of the two retinal images (see, for example, Cline *et al.*, 1989). However, this is a simplification, as it is the brain which ultimately 'sees', rather than the eyes. A person can have different retinal image sizes and not have any problems, so we would like to replace the word 'retinal' by 'cortical' in the above definition. Most clinically significant cases of aniseikonia result from correcting anisometropia, which is where the two eyes have different refractive errors. Anisometropia is discussed at greater length in Chapter 10.

The symptoms of aniseikonia are usually indistinguishable from those caused by other binocular vision problems and by uncorrected refractive errors. The classical symptom is a distortion of spatial perception when both eyes are being used, but this occurs in relatively few patients (Bannon and Triller, 1944). Binocular vision must be well developed for aniseikonia to be a problem, and usually the clinician should consider other possible causes of symptoms before attempting to correct aniseikonia. Clinical treatments of aniseikonia, in order of increasing complexity, include the following:

1. Altering the prescription to reduce the amount of aniseikonia, for example, reducing high cylindrical corrections, omitting low cylindrical corrections, and reducing the difference in spherical powers.
2. Prescribing contact lenses rather than spectacles, because the former have much smaller effects on retinal image size.
3. Prescribing a pair of spectacle lenses called **isogonal lenses**, which have similar magnifications to each other.
4. Prescribing a pair of aniseikonic correcting lenses called **iseikonic (size) lenses**, according to results of the **eikonometer**, an instrument which measures aniseikonia.

Further information on aniseikonia is found in texts such as Borish (1970) and Rabbetts (1998).

Summary of main symbols

$\overline{m}$ ratio $\overline{u}'/\overline{u}$ of the angles of inclination of the paraxial pupil ray with the axis in image and object space, respectively. This ratio is a constant for any particular schematic eye at a particular level of accommodation

η, η' object and image sizes

θ angular size of object. This angle is assumed to be small so it can be regarded as a paraxial angle

E, E'   positions of entrance and exit pupils

N, N'   positions of front and back nodal points

O, O' general object and corresponding image point

R', R axial retinal point and corresponding conjugate in object space

References

Bannon, R. E. and Triller, T. (1944). Aniseikonia – a clinical report covering a 10-year period. *Am. J. Optom. Arch. Am. Acad. Optom.*, **21**, 171–82.

Borish, I. (1970). *Clinical Refraction*, 3rd edn., pp. 267–94. Professional Press.

Cline, D., Hofstetter, H. W. and Griffin, J. R. (1989). *Dictionary of Visual Science*, 4th edn., p. 36. Chilton Trade Book Publishing.

Rabbetts, R. B. (1998). *Bennett and Rabbetts' Clinical Visual Optics*, 3rd edn. Butterworth-Heinemann.

7

Refractive anomalies

Introduction

Ideally, when the eye fixates an object of interest, the image is sharply focused on the fovea. In paraxial optical terms, the object and fovea are conjugate. However, the object can only be focused sharply if it is within the accommodation range of the eye. If the accommodation range is inappropriate or too small, objects of interest cannot be focused sharply on the retina. In these cases, the retinal image is out-of-focus or blurred, and visual acuity is reduced. The effect of these focus errors on the retinal image is discussed in Chapter 9 and in Chapter 18.

An appropriate range of accommodation includes all reasonable object distances of interest. This includes distant objects, effectively at infinity, down to objects as close as a few centimetres.

An eye with a far point of distinct vision at infinity is called an **emmetropic** eye. The emmetropic eye is regarded as the 'normal' eye, provided that it has an appropriate range of accommodation. A refractive anomaly occurs if the far point is not at infinity. An eye whose far point is not at infinity is called an **ametropic** eye. The departure from emmetropia is often considered to be an error of refraction, and ametropias are also referred to as **refractive errors**. Emmetropia and ametropia may be regarded as opposites, but an alternative and more appropriate view is that emmetropia is part of the distribution of ametropias.

Another refractive anomaly occurs when the range of accommodation is reduced so that near objects of interest cannot be seen clearly. This is called **presbyopia** and is usually age-related.

Defocused retinal images may occur because the far point is closer to the eye than infinity or is beyond infinity. By beyond infinity, we mean that it is located behind a person's head. Defocused retinal images occur also when the refractive power of the eye varies with meridian. This is commonly due to one or more refractive surfaces in the eye being toroidal, transversely displaced or tilted. There are now two far points, one corresponding to each of two principal meridians. These errors are referred to as **astigmatic** or **cylindrical** refractive errors, in contrast to **spherical** refractive errors, which are present when the refractive error is the same in all meridians.

Refractive errors may occur as a result of surgery. The most obvious example of this is **aphakia**. In the aphakic eye, the lens has been removed, usually because of cataracts (semi-transparent and translucent formations in the lens) which absorb, reflect and scatter the image-forming light.

Whatever the cause of the refractive error, it can be corrected with appropriate **ophthalmic** lenses, which include spectacle, contact and intra-ocular lenses. When an ametropic eye is corrected by an ophthalmic lens, the equivalent power of the eye/ophthalmic lens system is different from the value of the uncorrected ametropic eye and hence there are shifts in the cardinal points. This causes changes in retinal image sizes, and hence produces magnification effects, which are discussed in Chapter 10.

Most ophthalmic practitioners do not make a distinction between the terms refractive error and **refractive correction**, a practice that we shall follow in this book, although from a purist perspective they should be opposites. Hence, we may refer to a myope having a –2 D refractive error whereas, strictly speaking, we should say either that the myope is corrected by a –2 D lens or requires a –2 D correction.

For a more intensive review of refractive error classification, see Rosenfield (1998).

Spherical refractive anomalies

Spherical refractive anomalies are categorized according to the position of the far point (the spherical refractive errors) or of the near point (presbyopia).

Spherical refractive errors

Emmetropia (normal sight)

We wrote in the previous section that the far point of the emmetropic eye is at infinity. This is not a practical definition in terms of deciding who is an emmetrope. An emmetropic range may be considered to include refractive errors smaller than the smallest measurement interval, which is usually 0.25 D – i.e. the far point is greater than 4 m away. For research purposes, a wider range may be used; for example, –0.25 D to +0.75 D.

Myopia (short sight)

If the far point is at a finite distance in front of the eye, as shown in Figure 7.1a, the eye is **myopic** or is said to suffer from **myopia**. This means also that the back focal point **F′** of the eye is in front of the retina as shown in the figure. An object at infinity is focused in the back focal plane at **F′** and is out of focus on the retina. This situation can be regarded as due to a mismatch between the length of the eye and its power – the eye can be regarded as being too powerful for its length, or as being too long for its power. The eye is not able to reduce its power in order to focus distant objects on the retina.

This eye can focus clearly on distant objects by viewing through a negative powered ophthalmic lens of appropriate power, as shown in Figure 7.2a. This lens forms a distant and virtual image at its back focal plane, which coincides with the far point of the eye.

Myopia can be classified in many different ways (Rosenfield, 1998). These include classification by rate of progression, magnitude (e.g. low, moderate, high), age of onset (e.g. juvenile), and the refractive component considered to be responsible.

Uncorrected myopes tend to complain of blurred distance vision, which is more notice-

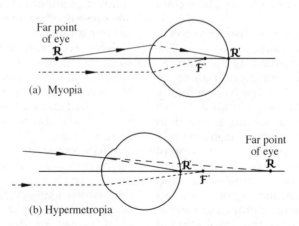

Figure 7.1. The (a) myopic and (b) hypermetropic eyes and their far points.

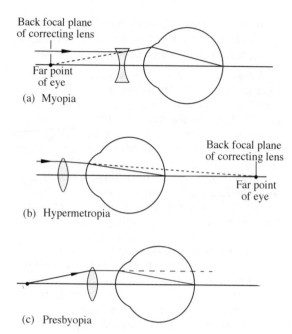

(a) Myopia

(b) Hypermetropia

(c) Presbyopia

Figure 7.2. The spectacle correction of (a) myopia, (b) hypermetropia, and (c) presbyopia.

able at night. Depending on the degree of myopia, they may notice that close objects appear blurred as well.

Hypermetropia (hyperopia)

In a hypermetropic eye, the far point lies behind the eye and the back focal point **F′** is behind the retina, as shown in Figure 7.1b. An object at infinity is focused in this back focal plane but, once again, the retinal image is defocused. This eye can bring the image into sharp focus if there is sufficient amplitude of accommodation. Once again, this situation can be regarded as due to a mismatch between the length of the eye and its power – the eye can be regarded as being too weak for its length, or as being too short for its power.

This eye can focus clearly on distant objects by viewing through a positive powered lens of appropriate power, as shown in Figure 7.2b. This lens forms a distant and real image on its back focal plane, which coincides with the far point of the eye.

Many young hypermetropes have difficulty relaxing their accommodation completely. A residual tonus in the ciliary muscle produces a degree of latent hypermetropia, which cannot be determined by subjective refraction without the use of cycloplegic drugs. **Total hypermetropia** can then be regarded as consisting of **manifest** and **latent** components. The part of the manifest hypermetropia that can be overcome by accommodative effort is referred to as **facultative** hypermetropia. Any deficit remaining is referred to as **absolute** hypermetropia. With increase in age and loss in amplitude of accommodation, the manifest component of total hypermetropia increases at the expense of the latent component. Similarly, the absolute component of manifest hypermetropia increases at the expense of the facultative component.

Uncorrected hypermetropes tend to complain of sore eyes and headaches associated with close visual tasks. This is because they must make more accommodative effort than emmetropes and myopes to view close objects. In addition, the degree of convergence they use is inappropriate for the level of accommodation demanded. They may also complain of blurred near and distance vision, depending on the level of hypermetropia and the amplitude of accommodation. The blurring is greater at near than at distance, because of the greater accommodative demand at near.

As hypermetropes may not be able to see distance objects clearly, the term **long sight** to describe hypermetropia should be discouraged.

Presbyopia

Presbyopia is the difficulty people have in performing close tasks because of the age-related decrease in amplitude of accommodation. The near point recedes from the eye so that it is close to or beyond the position at which a near task is performed. The onset of presbyopia is related to the degree of refractive errors, with uncorrected hypermetropes likely to have problems earlier in life than uncorrected myopes. Depending on the degree of myopia and the near task, the latter may not suffer from presbyopia. To compensate for presbyopia, ophthalmic lenses are required that are more positively powered or less negatively powered than the distance correction (Figure 7.2c). We discuss presbyopia further in Chapter 20.

Not surprisingly, uncorrected presbyopes usually complain of difficulty performing close tasks.

Astigmatic refractive errors

In many eyes, the refractive error is dependent upon meridian. This type of refractive error is known as an **astigmatic** refractive error (Figure 7.3). This is usually due to one or more refracting surfaces, most commonly the anterior cornea, having a toroidal shape. However, it may also be due to one or more surfaces being transversely displaced or tilted.

There are different types of astigmatism which may be related to the associated spherical refractive errors as follows:

1. **Myopic astigmatism** – the eye is too powerful for its length in one principal meridian for **simple myopic astigmatism**, and in both principal meridians for **compound myopic** astigmatism (as shown in Figure 7.3).
2. **Hypermetropic astigmatism** – the eye is too weak for its length in one principal meridian for **simple hypermetropic astigmatism**, and in both principal meridians for **compound hypermetropic astigmatism**.
3. **Mixed astigmatism** – the eye is too powerful for its length in one principal

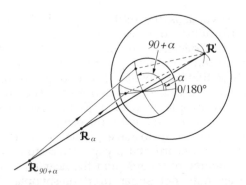

Figure 7.3. An astigmatic eye. The far points R_α and $R_{90 + \alpha}$ are imaged at the retinal point **R'**.

meridian (**myopic astigmatism**), and too weak for its length in the other principal meridian (**hypermetropic astigmatism**).

Astigmatism may also be classified by the axis direction. **With-the-rule** astigmatism is usually associated with a cornea that is steeper (i.e. has the greater surface curvature) along the vertical than along the horizontal meridian. It requires a correcting lens whose negative cylinder axis is within ±30° degrees of the horizontal meridian. Conversely, **against-the-rule** astigmatism is usually associated with a cornea that is steeper along the horizontal than along the vertical meridian, and requires a correcting lens whose negative cylinder axis is within ±30° degrees of the horizontal meridian. Astigmatism with axes more than 30° from the horizontal and vertical meridians is referred to as **oblique astigmatism**.

One further classification of astigmatism is related to its **regularity**. Astigmatism is usually **regular**, which means that the principal (maximum and minimum power) meridians are perpendicular to each other, and the astigmatism is correctable with conventional sphero-cylindrical lenses (see *The power of the correcting lens*, this chapter). **Irregular astigmatism** occurs when the principal meridians are not perpendicular to each other or there are other rotational asymmetries that are not correctable with the conventional lenses. It may occur in corneal conditions such as keratoconus.

Astigmatism is corrected with an astigmatic ophthalmic lens. Usually this has one spherical surface and one toroidal surface, the latter generally being the back surface. Astigmatic lenses are often referred to as **sphero-cylindrical** lenses for the historical reason that at one stage most astigmatic lenses had one spherical surface and one cylindrical surface.

To make analysis of large scale population data relatively easy, when astigmatism is present an **equivalent sphere** (also called the **mean sphere**) is used, which is the average refractive error of the two principal meridians.

People with astigmatism have blurred vision at all distances, although this may be worse at distance or near, depending on the type of astigmatism. They may complain of sore eyes and headaches associated with demanding visual tasks.

Anisometropia

This is the condition in which the refractive errors of the two eyes of a person are different. Sub-classifications include **anisomyopia**, in which both eyes are myopic, **anisohyper-metropia**, in which both eyes are hyper-metropic, and **antimetropia**, in which one eye is myopic and one eye is hypermetropic.

Spectacle lens correction of anisometropia may result in different retinal image sizes and different prismatic effects when looking through lens peripheries. These effects may compromise comfortable binocular vision. Some discussion of these side effects is provided in Chapter 10.

Distribution of refractive errors and ocular components

Distribution

The distribution of refractive errors is strongly age-dependent, particular in childhood (Hirsch and Weymouth, 1991). Neonates have a normal distribution of refractive errors (Hirsch and Weymouth, 1991; Goss, 1998; Zadnik and Mutti, 1998). From birth to maturity (about 11–13 years) the ocular components are growing, and the relationships among them must be co-ordinated so that emmetropia can be achieved and maintained (see review by Troilo, 1992). The term **emmetropization** is given to this fine-tuning of refraction, and it is thought that the process is visually regulated. A number of studies have been carried out on the distribution of ametropia in the adult population. Results of Strömberg's (1936), Stenstrom's (1948) and Sorsby *et al.*'s (1960) studies are shown in Figure 7.4. The mean refractive error is slightly hypermetropic, and the distributions are steeper than normal distributions (**leptokurtosis**). They have more pronounced tails in the myopic direction than in the hypermetropic direction (negative skewness). The distribution of refractive

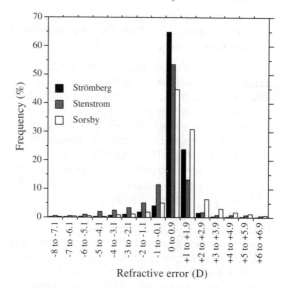

Figure 7.4. Population distribution of refractive errors. Data of Strömberg (1936), Stenstrom (1948) and Sorsby *et al.* (1960). Strömberg's data were obtained from Stenstrom (1948).

errors is fairly stable between the ages of 20 and 40 years, after which the distribution becomes less leptokurtic (Grosvenor, 1991).

The distributions of the main ocular parameters, such as axial length and corneal radius of curvature, are almost normal. Stenstrom (1948) found that the corneal power and radii were normally distributed, as were the depth of the anterior chamber, lens power and total power. He found that axial length was not normally distributed, but Sorsby *et al.* (1957) claimed that all components including axial length were normally distributed.

Sorsby *et al.* (1962) carried out an extensive study of the relationship between the various ocular parameters, and came to the following conclusions:

1. In emmetropic eyes, wide ranges of corneal power (39–48 D), lens power (16–24 D) and axial length (22–26 mm) occur.
2. In ametropic eyes with refractive errors in the range −4 D to +6 D, the same range of parameters occurred as for emmetropic eyes, but these were combined inadequately. Such eyes were referred to as **correlation ametropic** eyes.
3. For refractive errors outside the range of −4 D to +6 D, the axial length seemed to be the cause of the ametropia. It was too long in

myopia and too short in hypermetropia. These eyes were referred to as **component ametropic** eyes.

Component ametropia can be divided into **axial** and **refractive** categories by comparing dimensions of an eye with the range of values in the emmetropic population or with those of a schematic eye such as Gullstrand's number 1 eye. The refractive error is regarded as refractive in nature if the axial length is within an 'emmetropic' range, but the power of the eye or one of its components is outside the emmetropic range. The refractive error is regarded as axial in nature if the axial length is outside the emmetropic range, but the power of the eye and its components are within emmetropic ranges. Aphakia, in which the lens has been removed, is an obvious case of refractive ametropia. Most astigmatisms, including those caused by corneal conditions such as keratoconus, can be regarded as cases of refractive ametropia.

The ocular component most highly correlated with refractive error is axial length. Longitudinal studies indicate that axial elongation is the mechanism for juvenile and late onset myopia, and for the progression of myopia (Goss and Wickham, 1995). This suggests that most of the myopes that Sorsby and co-workers (1962) classified as correlation ametropes were actually axial component myopes.

If an eye is deprived of suitable visual stimuli early in its development, it grows to be unusually long, leading to myopia. This growth is controlled by local factors within the retina (Hodos *et al.*, 1991; Smith, 1991; Wallman, 1991). This indicates that a change in axial length is the main cause of emmetropization, with the eye increasing its length until emmetropia is achieved.

For reviews of hypotheses concerning emmetropization and of the possible roles of genetics and environmental factors in the development of refractive errors, see Troilo (1992) and Goss and Wickham (1995).

Astigmatism

As with spherical refractive errors (or spherical equivalents), the distribution of astigmatism changes with age. Considerable astigmatism, usually against-the-rule, exists in the first year of life and decreases quickly during early infancy. Most clinically measurable astigmatism is thereafter with-the-rule up to the age of 40 years, after which the prevalence of against-the-rule astigmatism increases (Goss, 1998).

The power of the correcting lens

This section explores the power of lenses required to correct a refractive error, starting with the thin lens case. While this approximation leads to some errors, it is satisfactory for simply examining trends. A thick lens treatment and its implications are supplied in a number of ophthalmic texts (e.g. Jalie, 1984; Fannin and Grosvenor, 1996).

In ophthalmic practice, the power of the correcting lens is determined by subjective techniques (using trial case lenses or refractor heads), or by objective techniques such as retinoscopy (described briefly in Chapter 8) or autorefraction. In none of these cases is the far point found directly, but mathematical analysis of the required lens power is made easier by reference to the far point distance. Consider a hypermetropic eye, as shown in Figure 7.5, in which the far point is a distance d behind the corneal vertex. The value of d must be given a sign. In our sign convention, d is positive if the far point is to the right of the corneal vertex and negative if it is to the left of the corneal vertex. Therefore, in the myopic eye d is negative, and in the hypermetropic eye d is positive. If a lens is now placed a distance h in front of the corneal vertex, the power $F_s(h)$ of the correcting lens, also called the spectacle refraction, is a function of vertex

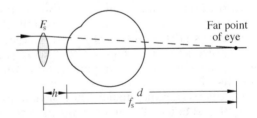

Figure 7.5. The power of the correcting lens (example of hypermetropia).

distance h, and is given by the equation

$$F_s(h) = 1/f_s = 1/(h + d)\qquad(7.1)$$

where the distance h is always regarded as positive. We can express equation (7.1) in the form

$$F_s(h) = R_e/(1 + hR_e)\qquad(7.2)$$

where

$$R_e = 1/d\qquad(7.3)$$

is the refractive error (or refractive correction) of the eye at the corneal plane. This is also referred to as the **ocular refraction**.

Example 7.1: Calculate the spectacle lens power, if the far point is 45 cm in front of the eye (i.e. a myopic error) and the spectacle lens vertex distance is to be 15 mm.

Solution: Here we have $h = 15$ mm and $d = -45$ cm. Substituting these values in equation (7.1) gives

$$F_s(15\ \text{mm}) = -2.30\ \text{D}$$

The sensitivity of the power to changes in distance h can be investigated by differentiating equation (7.1) with respect to h. If we do this, we have

$$\frac{dF_s(h)}{dh} = -\frac{R_e^2}{(1 + hR_e)^2} = -F_s^2(h)\qquad(7.4)$$

It follows that a small change δh in h leads to a change δF_s in F_s, given by the approximate equation

$$\delta F_s \approx -F_s^2(h)\delta h\qquad(7.5)$$

The above change in power δF_s is equivalent to a change in refractive error δR_e. Thus we have

$$\delta R_e \approx -F_s^2(h)\delta h\qquad(7.5a)$$

Example 7.2: Consider an eye requiring a $+12$ D spectacle lens placed at a vertex distance of $h = 12$ mm. If the lens is placed at 13 mm, estimate the induced refractive error.

Solution: In this problem, the change δh in h is $\delta h = +1$ mm, and substituting $F_s = +12$ D and $h = 12$ mm into equation (7.5a) gives the approximate induced refractive error

$$\delta R_e = -0.144\ \text{D}$$

In clinical practice it is common to determine the refractive error at one distance (say h_1) and prescribe for another (say h_2). A typical example is changing from spectacle lenses to contact lenses. Knowing $F(h_1)$, it can be shown using equation (7.1) that $F(h_2)$ is given by the equation

$$F(h_2) = \frac{F(h_1)}{(h_2 - h_1)F(h_1) + 1}\qquad(7.6)$$

Example 7.3: Consider the $+12$ D lens in Example 7.2. If the eye is to be corrected with a contact lens, calculate the power of that lens.

Solution: In this problem, h_1 is 12 mm, h_2 is 0 mm and $F_s = +12$ D. Substituting these values into equation (7.6) gives

$$F(0\ \text{mm}) = +14.0\ \text{D}$$

Astigmatic corrective powers

In the simplest mathematical model describing a cylindrical or astigmatic error in the eye, the power F of the eye can be thought of as varying with azimuth angle θ in the pupil according to the equation

$$F(\theta) = F_{sp} + F_{cy}\sin^2(\theta - \alpha)\qquad(7.7)$$

According to this equation, the correction is composed of a spherical component of power F_{sp} and a cylindrical component of power F_{cy} with the cylindrical axis along the direction α. The clinical representation of astigmatic corrections is

$$F_{sp}/F_{cy} \times \alpha$$

The axis notation most commonly used specifies the axis by the anticlockwise angle that it makes with the horizontal meridian. This is taken from the viewpoint of an observer looking at both lenses as worn in front of the two eyes. The axis varies between $0°$ and $180°$. A horizontal axis can be considered to be either $0°$ or $180°$, but is usually taken as the latter.

Thick lenses and the effect of thickness

Correcting lenses have some thickness, and therefore the above theory requires some modification in the case of real lenses. In ophthalmic optics, it is conventional to measure the distance of the lens from the eye by the back vertex distance, which is the distance from the back vertex of the lens (the vertex closest to the eye) to the corneal vertex. When this is done, the focal length f_s in Figure 7.5 and in the preceding equations becomes the back vertex focal length f'_v, and thus the power F_s in these equations becomes the back vertex power F'_v. Therefore, the equations (7.1) to (7.6) still apply, providing the distance h is the back vertex distance and the power F_s is replaced by the back vertex power F'_v.

However, when specifying the retinal image sizes in eyes corrected with ophthalmic lenses, it is the equivalent power rather than the back vertex power that sets the image size. When we go from thin to thick lenses we cannot take all the equations and simply replace the equivalent power by back vertex power. For image size calculations the situation becomes more complex, and we look at this problem in Chapter 10.

Effect of parameter changes on refractive errors

Refractive error and axial length

As already mentioned, spherical refractive errors are due to a mismatch between the refractive power of the eye and its axial length. In some cases, it is important to know how a change in axial length can affect the level of ametropia. This can be investigated using a schematic eye.

The lens equation for the eye can be written as

$$n'/l' - L = F \qquad (7.8)$$

where n' is the refractive index of the vitreous, F is the equivalent power of the eye and L (= $1/l$) is the vergence of the object, conjugate to the retina of the eye, relative to the first principal plane.

Suppose that the axial length changes by an amount $\delta l'$, as shown in Figure 7.6. This change $\delta l'$ leads to a change δL in the object vergence, given by differentiating equation (7.8) and using small changes to get

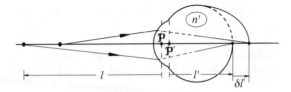

Figure 7.6. The change of axial length and corresponding change in refractive error.

$$-\frac{n'\delta l'}{l'^2} - \delta L = 0$$

Therefore

$$\delta l' = -\delta L l'^2/n' \qquad (7.9)$$

If the eye is initially emmetropic and relaxed, then $l = \infty$ and so

$$l' = n'/F$$

Therefore, equation (7.9) can be written as

$$\delta l' = -n'\delta L/F^2$$

or

$$\delta L = -\delta l' F^2/n' \qquad (7.9a)$$

This change in object vergence can be equated to the refractive error R_e. Thus

$$R_e = -\delta l' F^2/n' \qquad (7.10)$$

which shows that the relationship between changes or error in axial length and refractive error depends upon the equivalent power of the eye.

If we take an equivalent power for the eye of 60 D and a vitreous humour refractive index of 1.336, we have

$$R_e = -2.69 \, \delta l' \text{ D} \qquad (7.11a)$$

or

$$\delta l' = -0.371 R_e \text{ mm} \qquad (7.11b)$$

These two equations are useful as a guide in relating changes in axial length to changes in refractive error. They assume a value of 60 D for the equivalent power of the eye. If a more accurate value is available in a particular case, it can be substituted into equation (7.10).

Change in corneal curvature

The power F_c of the anterior surface of the cornea is given by the equation

$$F_c = (n-1)/r \tag{7.12}$$

where r is the radius of curvature of the surface and n is the refractive index of the cornea. A small change δr in radius of curvature r leads to a change δF_c in corneal power F_c given by the equation

$$\delta F_c \approx -(n-1)\delta r/r^2 \tag{7.13}$$

where r is the original corneal radius of curvature. This equation can also be expressed in the form

$$\delta F_c \approx -F_c{}^2 \delta r/(n-1) \tag{7.14}$$

If we measure the refractive error from the principal planes, the change in equivalent power is the refractive error. We need to relate the change in anterior corneal power to the equivalent power.

The equivalent power of the eye is due to the power of the cornea and lens. The above power of the cornea is only the anterior surface power, and does not include the posterior surface power. To relate this change in anterior corneal power to a change in equivalent power of the eye is not simple, and initially we will take a short cut and neglect the interaction of the posterior corneal power and the lens power. Later we will examine the error induced by this simplification.

With these approximations, the above change in corneal power is the same as the corresponding change in equivalent power, which in turn is the negative value of the induced refractive error δR_e. Therefore we have

$$\delta R_e \approx F_c{}^2 \delta r/(n-1) \tag{7.15}$$

Example 7.4: Using the Gullstrand number 1 eye, calculate the induced refractive error caused by an increase in corneal radius of 1 per cent.

Solution: For this eye, from data given in Appendix 3, $r = 7.7$ mm, $n = 1.376$ and the power of the corneal surface F_c is

$$F_c \approx (n-1)/r = 0.376/7.7 = 0.04883 \text{ mm}^{-1}$$

Also

$$\delta r = 0.01 \times 7.7 = 0.077 \text{ mm}$$

Substituting the values for F_c, δr and n into equation (7.16) gives

$$\delta R_e \approx 0.04883^2 \times 0.077/0.376$$
$$\approx 0.000488 \text{ mm}^{-1} \approx 0.488 \text{ D}$$

which, being positive, indicates that the induced refractive error is a hypermetropic error.

Other parameter changes

Using paraxial mathematical modelling and paraxial ray-tracing, we can investigate the effect of changes in any optical parameter on the refractive state of an eye. Table 7.1 shows the results of some calculations based upon the Gullstrand number 1 relaxed eye. The refractive error induced by a change of +1 per cent in anterior corneal radius is +0.483 D, which is only about 1 per cent different from the value given in Example 7.4. The major source of the difference is neglecting the effects of the lens and the posterior corneal surface in equation (7.15).

Table 7.1. Effects of small parameter changes on change in refractive error using the Gullstrand number 1 relaxed schematic eye with paraxial ray-tracing. Negative values indicate myopic refractive errors and positive values indicate hypermetropic refractive errors.

	$\delta R_e(D)$
Refractive index +1% increase	
cornea	+0.173
aqueous	−0.814
lens	−2.398
vitreous	+1.689
Radius of curvature +1% increase	
cornea anterior	+0.483
cornea posterior	−0.056
lens anterior	+0.039
lens posterior	+0.047
Distance +0.1 mm increase	
corneal thickness	−0.173
anterior chamber depth	−0.138
lens thickness (core)	−0.177
vitreous length	−0.256

Summary of main symbols

d distance of far point from the corneal vertex. This distance is negative for myopic eyes and positive for hypermetropic eyes

F equivalent power of the eye

F_c power of anterior surface of the cornea

F_s power of a correcting spherical lens. Also called the spectacle refraction

F_{cy} power of a cylindrical component of an astigmatic or sphero-cylinder lens

F_{sp} power of the spherical component of a sphero-cylinder lens

h vertex distance, i.e. the distance from the lens to corneal vertex (always positive)

l, l' object and image distances (from principal planes of refracting component)

L corresponding vergence ($= n/l$) of l

n, n' refractive indices (usually of object and image space)

r radius of curvature of cornea (anterior corneal surface)

R_e refractive error measured as the corneal plane. Also called the ocular refraction

α orientation of a cylindrical lens (usually the direction of the cylindrical axis)

θ azimuth angle for a sphero-cylinder lens

References

Fannin, T. E. and Grosvenor, T. E. (1996). *Clinical Optics*, 2nd edn. Butterworth-Heinemann.

Goss, D. A. (1998). Development of the ametropias. Chapter 3. In *Borish's Clinical Refraction*. (W.J. Benjamin, ed.), pp. 47–76. W. B. Saunders.

Goss, D. A. and Wickham, M. G. (1995). Retinal-image mediated ocular growth as a mechanism for juvenile onset myopia and for emmetropization. A literature review. *Doc. Ophthal.*, **90**, 341–75.

Grosvenor, T. (1991). Changes in spherical refraction during the adult years. In *Refractive Anomalies. Research and Clinical Applications* (T. Grosvenor and M. C. Flom, eds), pp. 131–45. Butterworth-Heinemann.

Hirsch, M. J. and Weymouth, F. W. (1991). Prevalence of refractive anomalies. In *Refractive Anomalies. Research and Clinical Applications* (T. Grosvenor and M. C. Flom, eds), pp. 15–38. Butterworth-Heinemann.

Hodos, W., Holden, A. L., Fitzke, F. W. et al. (1991). Normal and induced myopia in birds: models for human vision. In *Refractive Anomalies. Research and Clinical Applications* (T. Grosvenor and M. C. Flom, eds), pp. 235–44. Butterworth-Heinemann.

Jalie, M. (1984). *The Principles of Ophthalmic Lenses*, 4th edn. The Association of Dispensing Opticians.

Rosenfield, M. (1998). Refractive status of the eye. Chapter 1. In *Borish's Clinical Refraction*. (W.J. Benjamin, ed.), pp. 2–29. W. B. Saunders.

Smith, E. L. (1991). Experimentally induced refractive anomalies in mammals. In *Refractive Anomalies. Research and Clinical Applications* (T. Grosvenor and M. C. Flom, eds), pp. 246–67. Butterworth-Heinemann.

Sorsby, A., Benjamin, B., Davey, J. B. et al. (1957). *Emmetropia and its Aberrations. A Study in the Correlation of the Optical Components of the Eye*. Medical Research Council Special Report Series no 293. HMSO.

Sorsby, A., Leary, G. A. and Richards, M. J. (1962). Correlation ametropia and component ametropia. *Vision Res.*, **2**, 309–13.

Sorsby, A., Sheridan, M., Leary, G. A. and Benjamin, B. (1960). Vision, visual acuity, and ocular refraction of young men. *Br. Med. J.*, **9**, 1394–8.

Stenstrom, S. (1948). Investigation of the variation and correlation of the optical elements of human eyes. Part I and Part III (translated by D. Woolf). *Am. J. Optom. Arch. Am. Acad. Optom.*, **25**, 218–32 and 340–50.

Strömberg, E. (1936). Über Refraktion und Achsenlänge des menschlichen Auges. *Acta Ophthal.*, **14**, 281–93 (cited by S. Stenstrom, 1948).

Troilo, D. (1992). Neonatal eye growth and emmetropisation – a literature review. *Eye*, **6**, 154–60.

Wallman, J. (1991). Retinal factors in myopia and emmetropization: Clues from research on chicks. In *Refractive Anomalies. Research and Clinical Applications* (T. Grosvenor and M. C. Flom, eds), pp. 268–70. Butterworth-Heinemann.

Zadnick, K. and Mutti, D. O. (1998). Incidence and distribution of refractive errors. Chapter 2. In *Borish's Clinical Refraction*. (W. J. Benjamin, ed.), pp. 30–46. W. B. Saunders.

8

Measuring refractive errors

Introduction

This chapter is concerned with techniques for measuring refractive error. This is an area that has received wide coverage in ophthalmic texts, particularly regarding the subjective techniques. The emphasis here is on principles rather than on a detailed investigation of techniques or instruments. For descriptions of particular commercial instruments, readers can refer to texts such as Henson (1996), Rabbetts (1998) and Campbell *et al.* (1998).

The techniques for determining refractive error can be classified in three groups: those that are subjective, those that may be subjective or objective, and those that can be only objective. Some of the objective methods may be automated.

In subjective techniques, the patient makes a judgement of the correct focus. In the objective methods, the clinician or an instrument makes a judgement of the correct focus. The clinician makes the judgement in the case of manual or visual instruments, but with automatic optometers the clinician's role is limited to ensuring the correct alignment of the instrument. Automated instruments use an infrared source in the wavelength range 800–1000 nm, and the clinician is replaced by an electronic focus detector. These instruments have separate fixation targets, which are designed to encourage relaxation of accommodation.

Objective optometers rely upon the fact that some of the light incident upon the patient's fundus (including the retina, choroid and sclera) is reflected diffusely. Refractive error is determined either by measuring the vergence of light leaving the eye after fundus reflection, or by adjusting the vergence of light entering the eye so that a focused image of a target is formed on the fundus. With respect to objective refraction, we refer to the fundus image rather than the retinal image.

The measurement of refractive error has a number of inherent problems and potential sources of error. These are discussed later in this chapter (*Factors affecting refraction*).

Subjective-only refraction techniques

Simple perception of blur

The majority of refraction techniques are based on asking the patient to observe a suitable target, such as part of a letter chart, and make judgements about the best focus.

Conventional subjective refraction techniques

Conventional subjective refraction usually involves the patient reporting which of two views, seen through two slightly different combinations of lenses, gives a 'better' view of the target. The lens combinations may be placed as trial lenses into a trial frame, or as lenses in a refractor head (phoropter). These techniques include 'fogging' (also 'fan and block'), the cross-cylinder technique, and binocular balancing. As these techniques are covered in considerable detail by texts such as those by Michaels (1985), Grosvenor (1996), Rabbetts (1998) and Benjamin (1998), they are not discussed further here.

Optometers

An optometer contains a target moving in front of a suitable optical system, which is placed close to the eye. A simple optometer consists of a target T and a single positive lens. The vergence of the image in the lens depends upon the target position. Under the clinician's instruction, the patient moves the target towards the optometer lens from a position at which it is blurred to a position at which it first appears sharp. This point is taken as the measure of refraction. If the patient is emmetropic with relaxed accommodation, this point is at the front focal point F of the lens (Figure 8.1). For a hypermetrope, the point is farther away from the lens than is F. For a myope, it is closer. In the case of astigmatism, the refraction can be found by using a rotatable line target or a target consisting of a 'fan' of lines. The patient must identify the two positions at which one of the lines is in focus.

For the optometer shown in Figure 8.1a, l is the required end-point distance, F is the power of the optometer lens, and d is the distance between the lens and the eye. The vergence of the image in the lens, measured at the eye, is also the refractive error R_e. This is given by

$$R_e = \frac{1 + lF}{l(1 - dF) - d} \tag{8.1}$$

Such a design has several weaknesses. The ideal optometer should have the following properties:

1. The refractive error should be linearly related to the target displacement l from the lens, which allows easy and accurate calibration. Equation (8.1) shows that R_e is not linearly related to l for the arrangement shown in Figure 8.1.
2. The apparent size of the target should be independent of its position so that there is no size variation to stimulate accommodation.
3. The refractive error measuring range should be adequate.
4. The eye clearance (the distance from the back surface of the optometer to the eye) should be as large as possible so that the optometer's proximity to the eye does not stimulate accommodation.

The first two of these requirements are satisfied by the Badal optometer (Badal, 1876) which is shown in Figure 8.2. It is essentially the same as the optometer shown in Figure 8.1, but with the restriction that the eye must be placed at the back focal point F' of the lens. We can then substitute $1/F$ for d into equation (8.1) to obtain

$$R_e = -(1 + lF)F \tag{8.1a}$$

An alternative version of this equation is

$$R_e = -xF^2 \tag{8.1b}$$

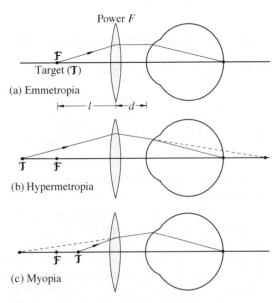

(a) Emmetropia

(b) Hypermetropia

(c) Myopia

Figure 8.1. Use of simple optometer in emmetropia, myopia and hypermetropia.

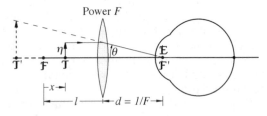

Figure 8.2. The simple Badal optometer.

where x is the target displacement from the front focal point **F**.

The apparent angular size θ of a target of physical size η is given by the equation

$$\theta = \eta F \qquad (8.2)$$

which is independent of target position.

There are different opinions of the appropriate ocular reference position for a Badal optometer, with candidates including the front focal point of the eye, its front nodal point, and the entrance pupil. The authors favour the entrance pupil, because the consistency of angular size occurs not only when the target is in focus but also when it is blurred.

A single lens Badal optometer may not satisfy requirements of range and eye clearance. While there is no theoretical upper limit to the hypermetropic range of the single lens Badal optometer, the maximum level of myopia occurs when the target is at the optometer lens. Putting $l = 0$ into equation (8.1a) or $x = -1/F$ into (8.1b) shows that the maximum myopic error measurable is $-F$, the negative of the power of the Badal lens. If we increase this power to improve the range of the instrument, there is a corresponding

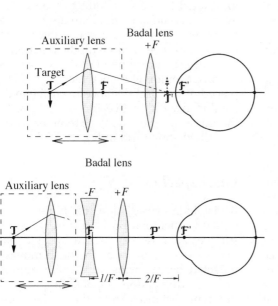

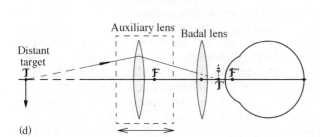

Figure 8.3. Variations of the Badal optometer:
a. Badal optometer with an auxiliary system to increase the negative power range.
b. Badal optometer with a second lens of equal and opposite power to the Badal lens to increase the distance between the Badal lens and the eye. The auxiliary system is needed to provide a negative vergence range.
c. Badal lens system with external principal points to increase the range of the optometer.
d. Badal optometer with a distant target and a movable auxiliary lens to overcome the problem of poor resolution with computer generated displays. The auxiliary lens power and sign can be selected according to the refractive error range required.

decrease in eye clearance $(1/F)$, which is clearly undesirable.

The negative range of the Badal optometer can be extended by various modifications. One simple example is by the addition of a moveable auxiliary system consisting of the target and a positive lens, which may provide a virtual target for the Badal lens (Atchison *et al.*, 1995) (Figure 8.3a). Another alternative is to use a multi-lens Badal system. One such solution is the inverse telephoto design suggested by Gallagher and Citek (1995). The Badal optometer is combined with a lens of equal and opposite power, with the second lens placed in front of the Badal lens – the lenses being separated by the focal length of the Badal lens (Figure 8.3b). As the equivalent power of a system of two lenses of power F_1 and F_2, separated by distance t in air, is given by

$$F_1 + F_2 - tF_1F_2 \qquad (8.3)$$

the equivalent power for this arrangement with the Badal lens of power F is

$$-F + F - (1/F)(-F)F = F$$

– that is, the same as the power of the Badal lens. The back principal plane of the system through **P'** is at a distance $1/F$ from the Badal lens. To place the Badal lens at the back focal point of the eye, this point must be a distance $2/F$ from the Badal lens. The advantage of such a system is that it increases the distance between the eye and the Badal lens (Gallagher and Citek, 1995). The two lenses do not give a negative vergence range because the front focal point **F** coincides with the negative lens, but this can be overcome in turn by using a moveable auxiliary system as shown in Figure 8.3b. One other solution to increasing the negative power range that avoids the use of the auxiliary system is to use a symmetric system, in which the principal points are outside the system, as shown in Figure 8.3c.

In the Badal system and its modifications described above, the target would usually be placed close to the system. This requires the target to be small. The development of computer-generated displays, with the limited resolution that this entails, requires a modification that allows a much larger target. This can be achieved by using a fixed, distant target and a moveable auxiliary lens (Figure 8.3d). The scale in dioptres is linear with movement of the lens (Atchison *et al.*, 1995).

Another variation of the use of the perception of blur to estimate refractive error is in some telescopic arrangements. Von Graefe used a Galilean telescope, varying the separation between the objective and eyepiece to alter the vergence of the emergent light (Rabbetts, 1998). Moving the eyepiece away from the eye produces a more convergent beam, while moving the eyepiece towards the objective produces a more divergent beam. The former movement can be used to measure hypermetropia, and the latter movement to measure myopia. The telescopic tube can be graduated to show the effective power as the eyepiece is moved. Unfortunately the scale is not linear, and the angular subtense of the image at the eye varies with the position of the eyepiece. Dudragne (1951) described a telescope optometer in which a +20 D lens, placed at its focal distance from the eye, was combined with a moveable –20 D lens. This is the same as the Badal optometer variation described above and in Figure 8.3d.

Laser speckle

If visible laser radiation (i.e. highly coherent light) is incident on a diffusely reflecting surface, an observer sees a speckle pattern that appears to move as the head moves. The reflected beam forms an infinite number of Fresnel diffraction (speckle) patterns at different distances from the surface, one of which is conjugate to the retina. If the pattern conjugate to the retina is not at the reflecting surface, any head movement produces a parallax effect. The rate of movement of the speckle pattern depends upon the position of the surface relative to the position at which the eye is focused. The rate of movement increases as the discrepancy of focus increases, and its direction depends upon the direction of discrepancy – a myope sees the speckle pattern moving in the opposite direction to head movement, while a hypermetrope sees the speckle pattern moving in the same direction as the head movement. When the surface and the plane of focus coincide, the pattern does not appear to move in any specific direction.

This phenomenon has been used in laser

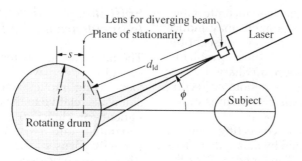

Figure 8.4. The laser optometer.

optometers (Figure 8.4). Instead of moving the head, the 'target' is moved by using the slowly rotating surface of a drum. Some correction needs to be made for the fact that the 'plane of stationarity' is inside rather than on the drum surface. Charman (1979) showed that s, the distance of the plane of stationarity from the drum rotation axis, is given in terms of d_{ld} (which is the inverse of the laser beam divergence at the drum), the radius of curvature of the drum r and the angle ϕ subtended by the laser and the eye at the drum, by the equation

$$s = \frac{r[d_{ld}\cos(\phi) + r\cos^2(\phi)]}{d_{ld}[1 + \cos(\phi)] + r\cos(\phi)} \tag{8.4}$$

Laser optometers have had wide research application. They allow the refractive error to be measured in dim conditions, and thus enable the resting point of accommodation to be determined easily.

Longitudinal chromatic aberration of the eye

The eye has approximately 2 D of longitudinal chromatic aberration between the wavelengths of 400 nm and 700 nm (see Chapter 17). If a small white light is viewed through a piece of cobalt glass, only red and blue light are transmitted, with the blue light focused in front of the red light inside the eye (Figure 8.5). If the light is a long distance away, an emmetrope sees a purple disc, because the red and blue images are approximately equal in size. A myope of moderate degree (say 2 D) sees a red central spot surrounded by a blue annulus. Conversely, a hypermetrope sees a blue central spot sur-

rounded by a red annulus. The strongest positive or weakest negative lens placed close to the eye that reduces the coloured fringes to a single purple disc gives the refractive correction. With appropriate modification in technique, astigmatic refractive errors can be corrected.

The cobalt filter is rarely used, but the eye's chromatic aberration is often used in the **duochrome test**, in which the patient compares the sharpness of letters presented on red and green backgrounds. This technique is used often near the end of a refraction. Refraction is adjusted until the letters on the two coloured backgrounds appear equally clear, or until the letters on one of the backgrounds are slightly clearer.

Subjective/objective refraction techniques

Remote refraction and relay systems

Positioning equipment close to the face means that the clinician is not able to see the patient's

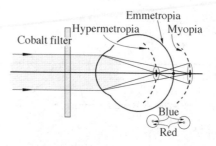

Figure 8.5. Chromatic optometer, showing the appearance of a distance spot viewed by emmetropes, myopes and hypermetropes.

face. The patient may also feel uncomfortable. The proximity of the equipment may induce 'instrument' myopia in some susceptible individuals. To overcome these problems, some instruments use an auxiliary lens or mirror system to image a remote correcting lens at the eye. The auxiliary system is thus a relay system.

Figure 8.6a shows a correcting lens of power F, which is imaged by an auxiliary lens of power F_a to the eye. The target at **T** for the correcting lens may be the real object, or it may be the image of the real target, in which case it may be referred to as the 'intermediate' target. A concave mirror may replace the auxiliary lens (Humphrey, 1976; Bennett, 1977; Alvarez, 1978).

Another system that might be considered to be remote refraction uses a −1× telescope consisting of two lenses of equal power separated by twice their focal lengths. The correcting lens is placed at the first focal point of the first telescope element, and the eye is placed at the second focal plane of the second telescope element (Figure 8.6b).

A full description of the imaging properties of these relay systems is beyond the scope of this book.

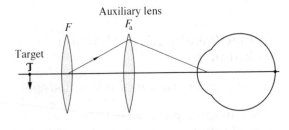

(a)

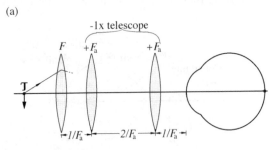

(b)

Figure 8.6. Remote refraction systems:
a. Remote refraction with an auxiliary lens.
b. Remote refraction with a −1× telescope system.

Split image and vernier acuity (coincidence method)

The target using this method has at least one straight edge, which is split into two. Defocusing moves one part of this edge sideways relative to the other part, so that the patient (or clinician) sees the straight edge separated into two. When the system is correctly focused, the two parts are aligned (that is, in coincidence). The principle works well because the patient (for subjective instruments) or the clinician (viewing light reflected from the fundus for objective instruments) is very sensitive to vernier misalignment.

A subjective instrument using the coincidence principle is the polarizing optometer (Simonelli, 1980). A pair of crossed polarized filters is placed over the target, and another pair is placed over the pupil of the eye. The second pair is cut at right angles to the first pair – for example, if the first pair join along the horizontal meridian, then the second pair join along the vertical meridian (Figure 8.7). The beam from half of the target enters only half the pupil, and the beam from the other half of the target enters the other half of the pupil. The target is moved until its two halves appeared aligned.

Scheiner principle

When an unaccommodating, emmetropic patient views a target through a disc with two holes in it, the target appears doubled if it is beyond the focal point of the lens (Figure 8.8a). If the pinholes are aligned vertically, the upper hole corresponds to the spot appearing higher up (lower retinal projection). When the target is placed closer than the focal point of the lens, the target again appears doubled, with the upper hole corresponding to the spot appearing lower down (Figure 8.8b). When the target is placed at the focal point of the lens, the target appears single (Figure 8.8c).

A simple optometer incorporating this doubling or Scheiner principle consists of a moveable target, which is usually a small light spot, and a Scheiner disc, which is an opaque disc with two pinhole apertures about 2 mm apart. The patient moves the target towards

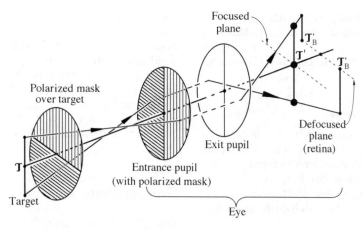

Figure 8.7. Coincidence method of focusing using polarized filters.

the optometer lens from a position at which the target appears double to a position at which it appears single. This position is the measure of the refraction. For astigmatism, the axis of the two image points coincides with that of the pinholes only when the pinhole axis coincides with one of the principal meridians.

The Scheiner principle has been incorporated into some automated optometers. In one configuration, two infrared sources replace the two pinholes and are imaged in the plane of the patient's pupil. The target is a moveable diaphragm. Two blurred images of the diaphragm are produced at the fundus at different positions, one from each of the two infrared sources, except when the diaphragm is conjugate with the fundus. Radiation from the fundus passes out of the eye to a detector unit, which senses this difference in position and controls the movement of the target so that only one fundus image is formed.

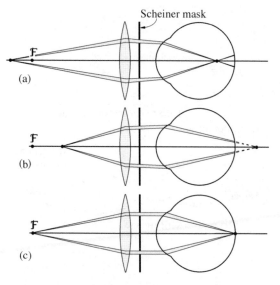

Figure 8.8. Imagery of a point source for an unaccommodating emmetrope using a Scheiner disc optometer:
a. Target beyond far point of lens
b. Target closer than focal point of lens
c. Target at focal point of lens.

Objective-only refraction techniques

Retinoscopy

Retinoscopy is probably the most common method of measuring refractive error. In this technique, the fundus of the eye acts as a screen over which a spot or streak of light is moved by tilting an instrument called a retinoscope back and forth. The clinician watches the shape and movement of the patch of reflected light within the patient's pupil. The patch is known as the 'reflex'. By placing trial lenses in front of the patient's eye, the speed of movement of the reflex is modified until it moves infinitely fast (or as close to this as can be judged). This condition is known as 'reversal'. At this position, the fundus of the patient's eye is conjugate with the sight hole of the retinoscope, so that there is an almost instantaneous cut-off of the return beam entering the examiner's eye as the light patch moves over the patient's fundus. As this is a well-known clinical technique, we refer readers to texts such as Grosvenor (1996) and Rabbetts (1998).

Automated optometers

Retinoscopy has been modified for use in some automated optometers, with a detector system with two photodetectors replacing the sight hole and the clinician. Refractive error is determined by the phase shift between the signals reaching the two detectors from the fundus.

Parallax movement between object and image

The instrument used for this technique is a modification of the single lens indirect ophthalmoscope (Figure 8.9). The image S_2' of the intermediate (off-axis) source S_1' is formed near the edge of the patient's pupil. A test object **T** on the common optical axis of the patient's eye and the optometer occludes the illuminating beam along the ray path $TS_2'T_1'S_1'$.

Viewing at an angle to the axis of illumination, the clinician sees the original test object **T** and its aerial image T_2' laterally displaced. Moving **T** along the axis of the instrument alters S_2' and the angle of incidence of the ray through **T**, causing T_1' to move across the fundus. At the same time, image T_2' moves laterally. When **T** is focused on the fundus, T_1' is on the axis of the system, and T_2' coincides with **T**. Thus T_2' appears to move in parallax as **T** is moved back and forth.

Grating focus

The grating focus principle is similar to the perception of blur, but here an automated optometer analyses the intensity of a signal to determine refractive error. The object is a square wave infrared intensity pattern (grating) (Figure 8.10). This is imaged into the eye. Radiation reflected by the fundus is imaged on a photodetector through a square wave grating mask. Either the mask or the

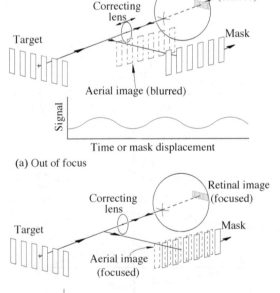

(a) Out of focus

(b) In focus

Figure 8.10. The grating focus principle. See text for details.

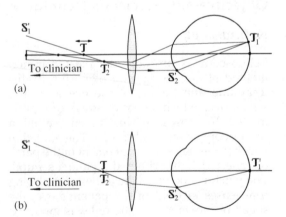

(a)

(b)

Figure 8.9. The parallax optometer (based on Bennett and Rabbetts, 1989, Figure 18.3).
a. Target **T** is not conjugate with its fundus image at T_1'. The clinician sees T_2' displaced laterally relative to **T**.
b. Target **T** has been moved so that it is now conjugate with fundus image T_1'. The clinician sees T_2' aligned with **T**.

target moves transversely, with the former situation being shown in Figure 8.10. The spatial frequency of the mask and the aerial image are matched. The signal from the photodetector modulates with the mask (or target) movement. The maximum modulation occurs when the aerial image is focused at the mask – this corresponds to the object being focused at the fundus (Figure 8.10b). The signal modulation is monitored as an optometer lens moves along the optical axis. An estimate of the refraction is given by the optometer lens position corresponding to the maximum modulation. To obtain the full refractive state of the eye, measures are made in a number of meridians.

Photography

The use of photography for determining the refraction of the eye is termed **photorefraction** (Howland and Howland, 1974). Its main application is screening of infants and young children. A flash photograph is taken of the eyes, with the flash source near the plane of the camera. The size and location of the pupil reflex recorded by the camera indicate the degree and direction of refractive error. Variations of the technique include **orthogonal**, **isotropic** and **eccentric** photorefraction (Campbell *et al.*, 1998).

In its simplest form, known as isotropic photorefraction (Howland *et al.*, 1979), a small flash source of light is mounted in front of a camera with a lens system such that one or both eyes are imaged with the pupil large enough to allow analysis. The source is imaged on the fundus of each eye. If the eye is focused at the source, the light leaving the eye returns to the source and is occluded from the camera lens. Thus the pupil appears dark. When the eye is not focused at the source, a blur circle (in spherical errors) or an ellipse (in astigmatism) is formed at the fundus. In turn, this produces an illuminated zone around the source, so that light enters the camera. The pupil appears illuminated, with the size of the film image depending upon the refractive error relative to the plane of the source. The sign of the refractive error cannot be determined by this basic technique, so Howland and co-workers took photographs with the camera focused both in front of and behind the patient's pupil plane. Using simple geometrical optics, the refractive error can be determined from the film image sizes, the pupil size and other dimensions of the camera setup.

The refractive error range that can be measured by the isotropic method is limited. Larger errors can be measured with eccentric photorefraction, which is similar to retinoscopy. In this method, an eccentric point source of light is used. Some of the light reflected from the fundus is vignetted by the camera, and this produces an image shaped like the profile of a biconvex lens. In hypermetropia relative to the light source, the image is on the side of the pupil opposite to the flash; myopia relative to the light source produces an image on the same side of the pupil as the source. From the placement of the camera, flash and patient, the refractive error can be determined. For measurement of astigmatism errors, different meridians must be investigated. Bobier and Braddick (1985), Howland (1985) and Crewther *et al.* (1987) evaluated this technique. More recently, the technique has been used with videotape or digital cameras replacing film (Campbell *et al.*, 1998). This has the advantage that the images can be viewed immediately, and retaken if necessary.

Visual evoked response

The visual evoked response (VER) is the response of the visual cortex to visual stimulation, primarily reflecting activity at the central retinal area. An active electrode is placed on the occipital scalp region, and an inactive electrode is placed in another part of the scalp. Pre-amplifiers, recorders, and a computer averaging technique are used to obtain electrical responses. With appropriate targets, the amplitude of the VER depends upon the refractive status of the eye. It is a useful, but not precise, method for patients who cannot be assessed by more conventional methods.

Factors affecting refraction

The reliability of subjective refraction is about ±0.3 D in young patients with good visual acuity (Jennings and Charman, 1973; Rosenfield and Chiu, 1995). Rounding prescriptions off to the nearest 0.5 D step had no effect on their acceptability to Appleton's patients (Appleton, 1971). Refraction and its reliability are influenced by various target, optical and neural factors.

Target factors

Different refraction methods may give systematically different results because of the different conditions under which the refractions are determined – for example, different luminances, spatial frequency distributions and spectral distributions. These interact with ocular factors such as aberrations and pupil size.

Optical factors

Subjective depth-of-field decreases, or subjective reliability increases, with increase in pupil diameters up to approximately 5 mm, and then remains fairly constant. This is discussed further in Chapter 19.

Many automated optometers have a minimum pupil size requirement; the pupil needs to be a certain size to pass the radiation from the stimulus into and out of the eye, and the electronic signals provided by the detectors need to have sufficient strength to be distinguished from background noise.

Monochromatic aberrations, particularly spherical aberration, may affect refraction through their interaction with pupil size and target factors. With large pupils, spherical aberration may cause the refraction to be dependent upon target spatial distribution, with positive spherical aberration causing the refraction to move in the myopic direction for targets having considerable low spatial frequency components. This is discussed further in Chapter 15. Large monochromatic aberrations can decrease the reliability of refraction techniques through their influence on depth-of-field.

Refraction is influenced by the spectral distribution of the target, through its influence on accommodation. For objective refraction, refraction is also influenced by the spectral distribution of the radiation reflected by the fundus of the eye. This is a consequence of longitudinal chromatic aberration, which is discussed in Chapter 17.

Eccentric viewing

Retinoscopy is usually performed at a small angle to the visual axis. Provided this angle is within 10°, the peripheral power errors introduced should be less than 0.25 D (see Chapter 15). When there is eccentric fixation or heterotropia, the clinician may need to direct the patient's gaze to the most appropriate axis.

Site of fundus reflectance in objective refraction

This is affected by the spectral distribution and by any polarization of the radiation source. The longer the wavelength, the deeper into the retina and choroid are the main reflecting layers.

Accommodation

It is important for the eye's accommodation to be relaxed during refraction. This may be attempted by the following methods:

1. Placing positive lenses in front of the non-tested eye so that accommodation blurs the image.
2. Ensuring that the axes of both right and left eye channels are parallel in instruments so that convergence cannot stimulate accommodation.
3. Using a blue fixation target, which provides a reduced stimulus to accommodation because the eye has greater power for blue light than for other visible wavelengths.
4. Using cycloplegic drugs.

Maximum potential visual acuity

Attenuation of high spatial frequency contrast by defocus is generally greater than that of low spatial frequencies. Thus, high visual acuities may give a greater reliability of subjective refraction than lower visual acuities.

Discrepancies between subjective and objective refraction

Discrepancies occur between objective and subjective measures of refraction if the main reflecting layers for the radiation used in objective refraction do not coincide with the subjectively preferred focal plane, which we may expect to be at or near the photoreceptors. The dominant reflecting layers depend on the wavelength of radiation used, whether the radiation is polarized, and the age of patients.

A major problem with manual optometers is that there is not sufficient control over the patient's accommodation. The targets are visible to the patient, and the stimulus to accommodation is altered as vergence from the target is altered.

The disadvantage of the near-infrared sources used in automated optometers is that there is considerable choroidal scattering of the radiation because the retinal pigment epithelium is fairly transparent at these wavelengths. This gives the reflection site increased depth and size. Because of the longitudinal chromatic aberration of the eye, the eye is more hypermetropic for the near-infrared wavelengths than for visible wavelengths. This is counteracted to some extent because the infrared wavelengths penetrate further than visible wavelengths into the retinal and choroidal layers. To reduce these sources of error, manufacturers of automated optometers calibrate their instruments using subjective refractions.

Summary of main symbols

R_e	refractive error
l	distance from lens to object
d	distance from lens to eye
F	power of lens
F_a	power of auxiliary lens
x	distance from front focal point of lens to object
θ	angular subtense of image of target at eye
t	distance between lenses
η	object size
r	radius of curvature of drum (laser speckle optometer)
d_{ld}	distance between laser and drum
s	distance of plane of stationarity from drum axis
ϕ	direction of laser beam from line of sight
F, F'	front and back focal points of lens or optical system
P, P'	front and back principal points of lens or optical system
$S, S_1' S_2'$	positions of source and its conjugates
$T, T_1' T_2'$	positions of target and its images

References

Appleton, B. (1971). Ophthalmic prescription in half-diopter intervals. Patient acceptance. *Arch. Ophthal.*, **86**, 263–7.

Atchison, D. A., Bradley, A., Thibos, L. N. and Smith, G. (1995). Useful variations of the Badal Optometer. *Optom. Vis. Sci.*, **72**, 279–84.

Alvarez, L. W. (1978). Development of variable-focus lenses and a new refractor. *J. Am. Optom. Assoc.*, **49**, 24–9.

Badal, J. (1876). Optomètre métrique international du Dr Badal. Pour la mesure simulanée de la réfraction et de l'acuité visuelle même chez les illetrés. *Ann. Ocul.*, **5**, 101–17.

Benjamin, W. J. (1998). Monocular and binocular subjective refraction. Chapter 19. In *Borish's Clinical Refraction* (I. Borish and W. J. Benjamin, eds), pp. 629–723. W. B. Saunders.

Bennett, A. G. (1977). Some novel optical features of the Humphrey Vision Analyser. *Optician*, **173**(4481), 7–16.

Bennett, A. G. and Rabbetts, R. B. (1989). *Clinical Visual Optics*, 2nd edn., p. 423. Butterworth-Heinemann.

Bobier, W. R. and Braddick, O. J. (1985). Eccentric photorefraction: optical analysis and empirical measures. *Am. J. Optom. Physiol. Opt.*, **62**, 614–20.

Campbell, C. E., Benjamin, W. J. and Howland, H. C. (1998). Objective refraction: retinoscopy, autorefraction, and photorefraction. Chapter 18. In *Borish's Clinical Refraction* (W. J. Benjamin, ed.), pp. 559–628. W. B. Saunders.

Charman, W. N. (1979). Speckle movement in laser refraction. I. Theory. *Am. J. Optom. Physiol. Opt.*, **56**, 219–27.

Crewther, D. P., McCarthy, A., Roper, J. and Costello, K. (1987). An analysis of eccentric photorefraction. *Clin. Exp. Optom.*, **70**, 2–7.

Dudragne, R. A. (1951). Optomètre à variation continue

de puissance. *International Optical Congress 1951,* pp. 286–98. British Optical Association.

Gallagher, J. T. and Citek, K. (1995). A Badal optical stimulator for the Canon Autoref R-1 optometer. *Optom. Vis. Sci.,* **72**, 276–8.

Grosvenor, T. P. (1996). *Primary Care Optometry: Anomalies of Refraction and Binocular Vision,* 3rd edn., pp. 285–307. Butterworth-Heinemann.

Henson, D. B. (1996). *Optometric Instrumentation,* 2nd edn. Butterworth-Heinemann.

Howland, H. (1985). Optics of photoretinoscopy: results from ray tracing. *Am. J. Optom. Physiol. Opt.,* **62**, 621–5.

Howland, H. C. and Howland, B. (1974). Photorefraction: A technique for study of refractive state at a distance. *J. Opt. Soc. Am.,* **64**, 240–49.

Howland, H. C., Atkinson, J. and Braddick, O. (1979). A new method of photographic refraction of the eye. *J. Opt. Soc. Am.,* **69**, 1486.

Humphrey, W. E. (1976). A remote subjective refractor employing continuously variable sphere-cylinder corrections. *Opt. Engr.,* **15**, 286–91.

Jennings, J. A. M. and Charman, W. N. (1973). A comparison of errors in some methods of subjective refraction. *Ophthal. Opt.,* **13**, 8–11, 18.

Michaels, D. D. (1985). *Visual Optics and Refraction: A Clinical Approach,* 3rd edn. Mosby.

Rabbetts, R. B. (1998). *Bennett and Rabbetts' Clinical Visual Optics,* 3rd edn. Butterworth-Heinemann.

Rosenfield, M. and Chiu, N. N. (1995). Repeatability of subjective and objective refraction. *Optom. Vis. Sci.,* **8**, 577–9.

Simonelli, N. M. (1980). Polarized vernier optometer. *Behav. Res. Meth. Inst.,* **12**, 293–6.

9

Image formation: the defocused paraxial image

Introduction

In Chapter 6 we examined image formation for the focused eye. However, often the eye is not focused on the object of interest. This may be because of an uncorrected refractive error. Also, when there is a poor stimulus – such as a bright empty field or in low luminances – the accommodation system tends to settle towards an intermediate resting state or tonic accommodation level (Rosenfield *et al.*, 1993). This corresponds to about 1.5 D of accommodation for habitually corrected young people.

The effect of such focus errors on vision is important. A focus error affects the quality of the retinal image, and hence visual performance (see, for example, Westheimer and McKee, 1980; Simpson *et al.*, 1986; Pardhan and Gilchrist, 1990). Of particular clinical importance is the effect of defocus on visual acuity (Prince and Fry, 1956; Atchison *et al.*, 1979; Simpson *et al.*, 1986; Smith, 1991 and 1996). Its effect on image size is of considerable interest (see, for example, Pascal, 1952; Marsh and Temme, 1990; Smith *et al.*, 1992). To fully understand the effect of defocus in these situations, the optics of defocused vision must be understood, and this is developed in this chapter.

Let us consider the situation shown in Figure 9.1, which shows the eye focused to the plane at **R**, but observing an object point **Q** in the perpendicular plane at **O**. Following a beam of rays from **Q** through the pupils, this beam focuses at the point **Q′** on the perpendicular plane at **O′** in front of the retina, but continues to the retina. Thus, the retinal image **Q′** of this object is out of focus. If we

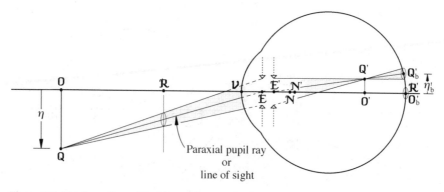

Figure 9.1. The formation of the blurred image of a distant point by an eye focused at some finite distance.

ignore the effects of aberrations and diffraction, the light distribution of Q' on the retina is uniform and the area illuminated is the projection of the exit pupil at E', through Q' onto the retina at Q_b'. Therefore, the beam cross-section on the retina has the same shape as the pupils. It is assumed that the normal pupil of the eye is circular, and therefore the light distribution at Q_b' is called the **defocus blur disc** for the object point Q. Similarly, the circle centred on R' is the defocus blur disc for the object point O.

The centre of the defocus blur disc is at Q_b', and this is the intersection of the paraxial pupil ray (the **line of sight**) with the retina. We can see from Figure 9.1 that the retinal image of the object OQ is blurred or defocused, and it is a different size from the focused image $O'Q'$ formed in front of the retina. In this chapter, we explore the effect of such a defocus on the apparent size of the blurred retinal image and the size of the defocus blur disc. We start with the retinal image size of the object OQ.

Retinal image size

Consider the points O and Q shown in Figure 9.1 as the ends of a line object. Each point on this line is imaged as a defocus blur disc (assuming a circular pupil), but only the blur discs for the points O and Q are shown. We could define the size of the blurred image of OQ as being measured from the bottom of the blur disc centred on O_b' to the top of the blur disc centred on Q_b'. However, with this definition the defocused image size depends

upon pupil size, and it is preferable to have a definition that is independent of pupil size. A definition that satisfies this criterion is the image size measured from the centres of the defocused blur discs at O_b' and Q_b', that is, the distance η_b' where the pupil rays from O and Q meet the retina.

In this case of a defocused retinal image we should not use the nodal ray to determine the image size, as we did in Chapter 6 for focused images. The nodal ray is not the central ray of the beam, and may not be part of the image-forming beam. It can be seen in Figure 9.1 that, if the pupil diameter is small enough, the rays through the nodal points are blocked and do not reach the retina. The likelihood of this happening increases as Q moves further away from the axis. When we investigate the size of a defocused image, we should use pupil rays only. We can find equations for this image size and its magnification relative to the focused image.

The size of the defocused image

Figure 9.2 shows the eye focused on the point O_2, but observing the scene at the plane at O_1. From this figure, the size η_b' of the defocused image is

$$\eta_b' = \bar{u}_2' E_2' R' \tag{9.1}$$

Now the angles $\bar{u}_2'$ and $\bar{u}_2$ shown in Figure 9.2 are connected by equation (5.7). Therefore

$$\bar{u}_2' = \overline{m}_2 \bar{u}_2 \tag{9.2}$$

with the value of the constant $\overline{m}_2$ depending upon the actual schematic eye used, in

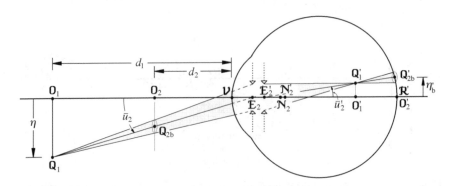

Figure 9.2. The retinal image and perceived angular sizes of defocused images.

particular the equivalent power and positions of the pupils and principal planes. Combining the above two equations gives

$$\eta_b' = \overline{m}_2 \overline{u}_2 E_2' R' \tag{9.3}$$

where

$$\overline{u}_2 = -\eta/O_1 E_2 \tag{9.4}$$

is the angular size of the object, measured at the entrance pupil. Equation (9.3) shows that the retinal image size (whether focused or not) is proportional to the angular size of the object measured at the entrance pupil at E_2.

More meaningful than the defocused image size η_b' is its size relative to the size η' of the image if it were in focus. This ratio is the magnification M

$$M = \eta_b'/\eta' \tag{9.5}$$

The size of focused images was discussed in Chapter 6, and equation (6.6) is relevant. Here we have

$$\eta' = \overline{m}_1 \overline{u}_1 E_1' R' \tag{9.6}$$

where the subscript '1' refers to the quantities measured for the eye focused on the point O_1 instead of O_2. Equation (9.5) can now be written as

$$M = \frac{\overline{m}_2 \overline{u}_2 E_2' R'}{\overline{m}_1 \overline{u}_1 E_1' R'} \tag{9.7a}$$

Using equation (9.4), we can express this equation in terms of the distance d_1 and d_2 of the focused planes from the corneal vertex as

$$M = \frac{\overline{m}_2 (d_1 + VE_1) E_2' R'}{\overline{m}_1 (d_2 + VE_2) E_1' R'} \tag{9.7b}$$

As the eye changes its refractive state, there is a change in entrance and exit pupil positions. This in turn leads to changes in most of the above quantities.

An eye focused at a finite distance, looking at an object at infinity

Before deriving an equation for the expected change in the image size, we will examine the optics of this process. As the eye accommodates, the equivalent power increases and, according to equation (6.11), the in-focus image size must decrease. However, because the object is at infinity, this focused image is formed in front of the retina as shown in Figure 9.3. Therefore, we may expect that the perceived image also decreases in size. However, in Figure 9.3, the height of the retinal image is set by the position where the pupil ray intersects the retina, and this position is higher than the image point Q'.

To determine whether the observed image actually decreases or increases with accommodation, it is possible to derive a suitable equation directly from first principles using Figure 9.3. Equation (9.3) still applies, and for the focused image we can use equation (6.11), with the angle θ replaced by the angle $\overline{u}_1$ and the power here written as F_e. Thus

$$\eta' = \overline{u}_1/F_e \tag{9.8}$$

Since the object is at infinity, $\overline{u}_1 = \overline{u}_2$, and if we now substitute for η_b' from equation (9.3) and

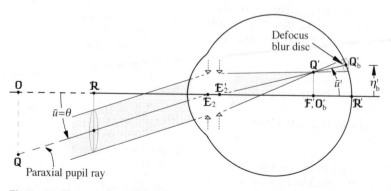

Figure 9.3. The retinal image and perceived angular sizes of defocused images (as in Figure 9.2), but with the object at infinity.

for η' from the equation (9.8), equation (9.5) becomes

$$M = \overline{m}_2 E_2' R' F_e \tag{9.9}$$

Example 9.1: Compare the retinal image sizes of the moon for the two extreme states of accommodation of the Gullstrand number 1 eye.

Solution: Equation (9.9) is used, with the following data from Table 5.1,

For the relaxed eye: $F_e = 58.636100$ D
For the
accommodated eye: $\overline{m}_2 = 0.795850$
        and $E_2' R' =$
        21.173464 mm

Substituting these values into equation (9.9) gives

$$M = 0.795850 \times 0.058636100 \times 21.173464$$
$$= 0.98807$$

The value of 0.98807 correspond to a 1.2 % decrease in image size.

Thus, if the eye accommodated by 10 D while looking at the moon, the moon's image would decrease by only 1.2%, showing that the retinal image size is remarkably stable with focus error.

The use of artificial pupils

The results of this section show that the effect of a focus error on retinal image size depends upon the position of the entrance pupil of the eye. In some experimental situations, the eye's natural pupil is dilated and artificial pupils are placed close to the spectacle plane about 12–15 mm in front of the eye. The artificial pupil becomes the effective aperture stop and the entrance pupil of the eye, and its position and size affect the size of defocused images.

Size of the defocus blur disc

The geometrical aberration-free defocus blur disc

Calculations of the diameter of the defocus blur disc, whether by physical or geometric optics, have traditionally used schematic eye models (e.g. van Meeteren, 1974; Charman

and Jennings, 1976; Obstfeld, 1982). These calculations use a schematic eye with a given refractive power (often that of Gullstrand's number 1 model eye) and a specific pupil diameter. Appropriate rays are traced to the retina to determine the diameter of the defocus blur circle on the retina. The expected or perceived angular diameter of this blur disc is then found by calculating the angular diameter of the retinal image subtended at the back nodal point. This method has the disadvantage that schematic eyes are only specified in the relaxed or in a greatly accommodated state, usually about 10 D, and thus defocus calculations at other levels of accommodation are not readily found.

If the retinal image diameter is not required, the expected perceived angular diameter can be found by a very simple equation which, although approximate, may be accurate enough for many circumstances. Smith (1982) showed two derivations of this equation, the second and simpler of which is presented here.

In Figure 9.4, an eye with its front principal plane at **P** is focused on a plane at **R** a distance l_R from **P**. If the eye views a point **O** at distance l while still focused on **R**, the point **O** appears as a blur circle or disc superimposed on the plane at **R**. The longitudinal focus error δl is

$$\delta l = l - l_R \tag{9.10}$$

and the physical linear diameter ϕ_b of the blur circle using similar triangles can be shown to be

$$\phi_b = D_P \delta l / l = D_P (l - l_R)/l \tag{9.11}$$

where D_P is the diameter of the beam at the principal planes. The expected perceived or visual angular diameter Φ of this disc must be measured at the front nodal point **N**, as shown in the figure. Thus,

$$\Phi = \phi_b / (l_N - l_R)$$

that is

$$\Phi = \frac{D_P(l_R - l)}{l(l_N - l_R)} \tag{9.12}$$

In terms of vergences, this equation can be written

$$\Phi = \frac{D_P(L - L_R)}{(1 - L_R l_N)} \tag{9.13}$$

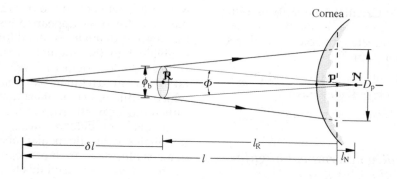

Figure 9.4. The formation of the perceived diameter of the defocus blur disc.

The sign is not important since the angle Φ corresponds to a diameter.

The beam diameter D_P is not in general the diameter D of the entrance pupil. The relation between these two quantities can be found by referring to Figure 9.5. From this figure, the two quantities are related by the equation

$$D = D_P(l - T)/l$$

that is,

$$D_P = D/(1 - LT) \qquad (9.14)$$

where T is the distance between the front principal plane and the entrance pupil. This distance depends upon the level of accommodation, and is 1.7 mm in the relaxed Gullstrand number 1 eye and 0.9 mm in the accommodated version. If D_P in equation (9.13) is replaced by D using equation (9.14), then

$$\Phi = \frac{D(L_R - L)}{(1 - LT)(1 - L_R l_N)} \qquad (9.15)$$

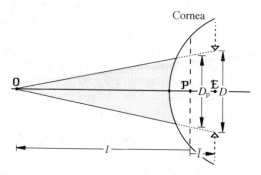

Figure 9.5. The difference between beam diameter at the front principal plane and the entrance pupil.

For low to medium levels of refractive error, we can make some useful approximations as follows:

1. If T is neglected the fractional error is T/l, and its value depends upon the level of accommodation and the distance l of the out-of-focus object. However, if this distance is infinite, the error is zero.
2. The quantity l_N can be neglected if the quantity $L_R l_N \ll 1$. While l_N depends upon the equivalent power of the eye and hence accommodation level, its value is about 5 mm. For a value of L_R of 10 D, the error induced in neglecting this term is about 5%, but for $L_R = 0$, the error is zero.

If we accept these two approximations, equation (9.15) reduces to

$$\Phi = (L_R - L)D \qquad (9.16)$$

If $(L_R - L)$ is replaced by the focus error ΔL, the above equation can be re-expressed as

$$\Phi = \Delta L \, D \text{ radian} \qquad (9.17)$$

which expresses the visual angular subtense Φ of the defocus blur disc in terms of the dioptric level of defocus ΔL and the pupil diameter D. Thus, within the limits of the approximations made in deriving this equation, the angular diameter of the defocus blur disc is independent of the constructional parameters of the schematic eye and the acccommodation level.

If we express the pupil diameter in milli-metres and defocus in dioptres and Φ in minutes of arc, we have

$$\Phi = 3.483 \, \Delta L \, D_{mm} \text{ min. arc} \qquad (9.17a)$$

Example 9.2: Calculate the defocus blur disc size for an object at infinity viewed by a 1 D uncorrected myopic eye with a 4 mm diameter pupil.

Solution: We substitute $\Delta L = 1$ and $D_{mm} = 4$ into equation (9.17a), to give

$$\Phi = 3.483 \times 1 \times 4 = 13.8 \text{ min. arc}$$

Experimentally determined angular diameter of the blur discs

The accuracy of equation (9.17) relative to the more accurate equation (9.15) is shown in Figure 9.6, where we have plotted the values for a 4.2 mm diameter pupil and an eye focused at different distances but viewing a scene at infinity – i.e. $L = 0$. The values of T and l_N are taken from the Gullstrand relaxed number 1 eye data in Appendix 3. The approximate equation gives values that are too high, but by only a few per cent.

Smith (1982) suggested that the perceived angular diameters of the blur discs can be measured using two small light sources, such as illuminated optical fibres, whose separation is adjustable. When these sources are defocused, they are seen as blur discs. The separation between the sources is varied until the two blur discs appear to just touch, and the angular diameter of one blur disc is then equivalent to the angular separation of the sources. At low defocus levels the blur disc takes on an irregular star-shaped pattern, which is due to ocular aberrations, making it difficult to locate the edge of the blur discs. At high levels of defocus, where the defocus dominates over the ocular aberrations, the defocus blur discs are more regular.

Chan *et al.* (1985) used this technique to test the accuracy of equation (9.17). Six observers were used, and since the differences between observers were small, the mean data are shown in Figure 9.6. The spectacle plane lens power was converted to an equivalent power at the front principal plane of the eye. There is good agreement between theory and measurements at intermediate levels of refractive error (3–9 D). However, at lower refractive errors the theoretical values are too low, while at higher refractive errors the theoretical values are too high. At the lower levels of refractive error, the discrepancy is because of the effects of ocular aberrations and diffraction, which give a wider spread of light than expected by aberration-free geometrical optics. At the higher levels of refractive error, the deviations can be explained by equation (9.17) being only approximate. The more accurate equation (9.15) agrees well with the measured values at these levels.

Defocus ratio

The level of defocus can be quantified by the diameter ϕ_b' of the defocus blur disc in the image, the diameter ϕ_b of the defocus blur disc in object space, or its corresponding angular size Φ. Alternatively, if we want to study the effect of a defocus on the visibility of an object of a certain size Φ, a more appropriate quantity is the defocus ratio, which we define by the equation

$$\text{Defocus ratio} = \phi_b'/\eta' = \phi_b/\eta \qquad (9.18)$$

In angular terms in object or visual space we have

$$\text{Defocus ratio} = \Phi/\theta \qquad (9.19)$$

where θ is the angular size of the object.

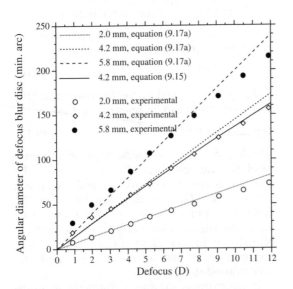

Figure 9.6. The diameter Φ of defocused blur discs measured by Chan *et al.* (1985), corresponding values predicted by the approximate equation (9.17a), and values for a 4.2 mm diameter pupil using the exact equation (9.15), with $L = 0$.

Example 9.3: Calculate the defocus blur ratio for the situation given in Example 9.2, if the eye is observing a 6/6 letter, i.e. one that subtends 5 min arc.

Solution: Substitute $\Phi = 13.8$ min arc and $\theta = 5$ min arc into equation (9.19) to give

Defocus ratio $= 13.8/5 = 2.76$

Other effects of defocus

Alignment of two targets at different distances

In some visual experiments, the eye is aligned by asking the subject to subjectively align two targets at different distances. Figure 9.7 shows points Q_1 and Q_2 aligned along the visual axis. If these points are so aligned, do they appear superimposed in the visual field? In other words, are their retinal images superimposed? By analysing the situation shown in Figure 9.7, we can deduce that the targets do not appear to be aligned. This shows the point Q_2 imaged, in focus, at Q_2' on the retina. The other point Q_1 is imaged in front of the retina at Q_1' and is therefore defocused at the retina. The retinal image of Q_1 is the defocus blur disc centred on the point Q_{1b}', which is laterally displaced with respect to the in-focus image Q_2'. Therefore, while the two points are aligned along the visual axis, their retinal images are transversely displaced.

If the points are to appear superimposed, the two targets must lie along the paraxial pupil ray (i.e. the line of sight) rather than the visual axis.

Effect on visual acuity

Defocus reduces the quality of the retinal image and hence various aspects of visual performance. Uncorrected visual acuity correlates with refractive error. However, the correlation is not perfect, even after pupil size is taken into account (Atchison *et al.*, 1979). The relationship has been quantified from time to time by various investigators fitting regression equations to clinical data. Perhaps the most common equation used is of the form

$$\log(A) = a + b \log(\Delta L) \tag{9.20}$$

where A is the (uncorrected) visual acuity in minimum angle of resolution in min arc, ΔL is the refractive error (say in dioptres), and a and b are constants. This equation is not based upon any theoretical optics justification. In contrast, an argument based upon the defocus blur circle model described in the preceding section suggests that the minimum angle of resolution should be linearly related to refractive error, except for low levels of refractive errors. Smith (1991) used the defocused blur disc concept and the optical transfer function to show that, for typical pupil diameters and for refractive errors greater than about 1 D, the expected relationship is a simple one of the form

$$A = kD\Delta L \tag{9.21}$$

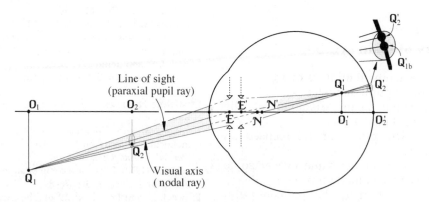

Figure 9.7. The alignment of two targets along the visual axis. Their retinal images are not superimposed, and hence they do not appear to be aligned.

where D is the pupil diameter and k is a constant whose value depends on the structure of the acuity target and the recognition rate (e.g. 50 per cent, 75 per cent, etc). For letters of the alphabet and a 50 per cent recognition rate, the value of k is approximately 650 for A in minutes of arc, D in metres and ΔL in dioptres (Smith, 1996).

For low levels of defocus, aberrations and diffraction dominate the quality of the retinal image, but these factors are beyond the scope of the paraxial optics discussion of this chapter. The influence of these factors is considered in Chapter 18.

The value of k and the corresponding defocus ratio

From the above value of k, we can estimate the defocus ratio of alphabetical characters at the 50 per cent threshold of visibility.

The letter size is regarded as five times the minimum angle or detail in the letter. Using this value, transforming equation (9.21) to the threshold letter size H in radians gives

$$H = 5A = 5 \times 650 \times D\Delta L \times \pi/(180 \times 60)$$
$$= 0.945 \, D\Delta L \text{ radians}$$

and since

$$\Phi = D\Delta L,$$

from equation (9.17), it follows that

$$\text{Defocus ratio} = \Phi/H = 1.06 \qquad (9.22)$$

which indicates that a letter may be recognized at a 50 per cent success level when the defocus blur disc is about the same diameter as the letter height.

Summary of main symbols

A	visual acuity in minutes of arc
D	entrance pupil diameter
D_P	equivalent beam diameter at the principal planes
F_e	equivalent power of eye focused on infinity
F_a	the power of the same eye at some level of accommodation
$\overline{m}$	ratio $\overline{u}'/\overline{u}$ of angles that paraxial pupil ray subtends at axis in image and object space, respectively

l, l'	object and image distances from front and back principal planes, respectively
L	corresponding vergence of the distance l
ΔL	refractive error
l_N	distance of nodal point from principal plane
l_R	distance of object, conjugate with the retina, from principal plane
L_R	vergence corresponding to l_R
$\overline{l}$	distance of entrance pupil from front principal plane
η_b'	defocused image size at retina
η, η'	object and image sizes
θ	angular size of object
$\phi_\mathrm{b}', \phi_\mathrm{b}$	diameter of defocus blur disc on retina and its conjugate in object space
Φ	corresponding perceived angular diameter of defocus blur disc, measured at the nodal points (always positive)
E, E'	position of entrance and exit pupils
N, N'	position of front and back nodal points
O, O'	general object point and corresponding image point
P, P'	positions of front and back principal points
R, R'	axial retinal point and corresponding conjugate in object space

References

Atchison, D. A., Smith, G. and Efron, N. (1979). The effect of pupil size on visual acuity in uncorrected and corrected myopia. *Am. J. Optom. Physiol. Opt.*, **56**, 315–23.

Chan, C., Smith, G. and Jacobs, R. J. (1985). Simulating refractive errors: source and observer methods. *Am. J. Optom. Physiol. Opt.*, **62**, 207–16.

Charman, W. N. and Jennings, J. A. M. (1976). The optical quality of the monochromatic retinal image as a function of focus. *Br. J. Physiol. Opt.*, **31**, 119–34.

Marsh, J. S. and Temme, L. A. (1990). Optical factors in judgements of size through an aperture. *Human Factors*, **32**, 109–18.

Obstfeld, H. (1982). *Optics in Vision*, 2nd edn. Butterworths.

Pardhan, S. and Gilchrist, J. (1990). The effect of monocular defocus on binocular contrast sensitivity. *Ophthal. Physiol. Opt.*, **10**, 33–6.

Pascal, J. I. (1952). Effect of accommodation on the retinal image. *Br. J. Ophthal.*, **36**, 676–8.

Prince, J. H. and Fry, G. A. (1956). The effect of errors of refraction on visual acuity. *Am. J. Optom. Arch. Am. Acad. Optom.*, **33**, 353–73.

Rosenfield, M., Ciuffreda, K. J., Hung, G. K. and Gilmartin, B. (1993). Tonic accommodation: a review. I. Basic aspects. *Ophthal. Physiol. Opt.*, **13**, 266–84.

Simpson, T. L., Barbeito, R. and Bedell, H. E. (1986). The effect of optical blur on visual acuity for targets of different luminances. *Ophthal. Physiol. Opt.*, **6**, 279–81.

Smith, G. (1982). Angular diameter of defocus blur discs. *Am. J. Optom. Physiol. Opt.*, **59**, 885–9.

Smith, G. (1991). Relation between spherical refractive error and visual acuity. *Optom. Vis. Sci.*, **68**, 591–8.

Smith, G. (1996). Visual acuity and refractive error. Is there a mathematical relationship? *Optometry Today*, **36** (17), 22–7.

Smith, G., Meehan, J. W. and Day, R. H. (1992). The effect of accommodation on retinal image size. *Human Factors*, **34**, 289–301.

van Meeteren, A. (1974). Calculations on the optical modulation transfer function of the human eye for white light. *Optica Acta*, **21**, 395–412.

Westheimer, G. and McKee, S. P. (1980). Stereoscopic acuity with defocused and spatially filtered retinal images. *J. Opt. Soc. Am.*, **70**, 772–8.

10

Some optical effects of ophthalmic lenses

Introduction

When an eye is corrected by an ophthalmic lens in the form of spectacles or contact lenses, aspects of the retinal image are changed as well as the image being focused. Most noticeably, the lens affects the size of the retinal image. This change in image size can be measured in two different ways. One of these is the **spectacle magnification**, which is the ratio of the image sizes after and before correction. The second, which is of limited use, is called **relative spectacle magnification**. This is the corrected or focused retinal image size compared with that of a 'standard' eye. These magnifications are associated with other effects. For example, a positive power lens produces a magnified image and a blank part of the visual field called a **scotoma**. Image magnification of spectacle lenses is associated with prismatic effects and changes in the required eye rotation to look at an object which is not on the lens optical axis. There are also effects on binocular vision. In anisometropia the two eyes are corrected by different lens powers, and differential effects between eyes, for example different amounts of eye rotations, may produce eyestrain.

In this chapter we investigate some of these effects, but consider only thin lenses. While this leads to some approximation and inaccu-

racies, the equations are simple and readily show trends. Aberrations associated with the lenses are not considered. We refer readers who want a full thick lens treatment, or to consider effects of aberrations, to texts such as Jalie (1984) and Fannin and Grosvenor (1996).

Most of the equations in this chapter apply to both spectacle and contact lenses. Exceptions are the equations dealing with rotational magnification and field-of-view in the section *Effects on far and near points and accommodation demand*. The equations assume a rotating eye behind a fixed lens, which is not applicable for contact lenses, which rotate with the eye. Most of the effects described have much smaller magnitudes for contact lenses than for spectacle lenses, because of the small distance between contact lenses and relevant ocular reference positions such as the entrance pupil.

Spectacle magnification

Spectacle magnification SM is defined as

$$SM = \frac{\text{retinal image size after correction}}{\text{retinal image size before correction}} \quad (10.1)$$

An equivalent definition is

$$SM = \frac{\text{angular subtense of image in correcting lens at eye}}{\text{angular subtense of object at eye before correction}} \quad (10.1a)$$

In both cases, the pupil ray is used as the reference ray because it determines the centre of the defocused image (neglecting aberrations).

The following equation is derived for spectacle magnification using Figure 10.1. An object of height η is at a distance q from the entrance pupil of the eye at **E** (Figure 10.1a). It subtends an angle ω at the entrance pupil of the eye, given by

$$\omega = \eta/q \qquad (10.2)$$

In Figure 10.1b, a correcting lens of power F_s has been placed in front of the eye. The object is a distance l from the lens, and the eye's entrance pupil is a distance h_e from the lens. The object subtends an angle ϕ at the lens, given by

$$\phi = \eta/l \qquad (10.3)$$

The image of the object in the lens has height η' and is a distance l' from the lens. From the figure, η' is given by

$$\eta' = \phi l' \qquad (10.4)$$

Substituting the right-hand side of equation (10.3) for ϕ into equation (10.4) gives

$$\eta' = \eta l'/l \qquad (10.5)$$

The angle ω' subtended by the image at the entrance pupil **E** is given by

$$\omega' = \eta'/(l' - h_e) \qquad (10.6)$$

Substituting the right-hand side of equation (10.5) for η' into equation (10.6) gives

$$\omega' = \eta l'/[l(l' - h_e)] \qquad (10.7)$$

From the definition of equation (10.1a), *SM* is

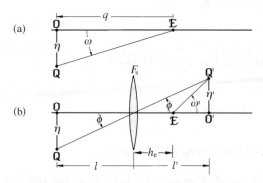

Figure 10.1. The optics of spectacle magnification and the angular size of the images:
a. The uncorrected eye looking at an object.
b. The eye looking at the object through a correcting spectacle lens.

given by

$$SM = \omega'/\omega \qquad (10.8)$$

Substituting the right-hand sides of equations (10.2) and (10.7) for ω and ω', respectively, into equation (10.8) gives

$$SM = l'q/[l(l' - h_e)] \qquad (10.8a)$$

If we replace l and l' by their corresponding vergences $L \ (= 1/l)$ and $L' \ (= 1/l')$, we obtain

$$SM = qL/(1 - h_e L') \qquad (10.8b)$$

Given that L is known, L' is found simply by the refraction equation $L' = L + F_s$. For the object at infinity, it can easily be shown that

$$SM = 1/(1 - h_e F_s) \qquad (10.8c)$$

Equations (10.8b) and (10.8c) can be extended to the thick lens case, with F now the equivalent power of the lens and L and L' determined relative to the front and back principal planes, respectively, of the lens.

Examination of equation (10.8c) shows:

1. For positive lens powers, spectacle magnification is greater than 1, i.e. the observed object is enlarged. For negative power lenses, spectacle magnification is less than 1.
2. The departure of spectacle magnification from a value of 1 is increased with increase in distance between the lens and the eye.

In ophthalmic optics, it is more convenient to measure the back vertex power rather than the equivalent power of a lens. For the object at infinity, it can be shown (see, for example, Jalie, 1984) that

$$SM = \frac{1}{1 - tF_1/n} \cdot \frac{1}{1 - h_{ve}F_v'} \qquad (10.9)$$

where t is lens thickness, n is lens refractive index, h_{ve} is the distance between the lens back vertex and the eye's entrance pupil, F_1 is the front surface power of the lens, and F_v' is the back vertex power of the lens. This equation shows how *SM* is dependent on the parameters of the lens. The expressions $(1 - tF_1/n)^{-1}$ and $(1 - h_{ve}F_v')^{-1}$ on the right-hand side of the equation are referred to as the shape factor and power factor, respectively.

Example 10.1: An object is 30 cm in front of the corneal vertex of the eye. A correcting thin lens of power -5 D is placed 12 mm in front of the eye. What is the spectacle magnification?

Solution: Refer the positions of the lens and the object to the entrance pupil of the eye. As this is approximately 3 mm inside the eye (3.05 mm for the Gullstrand number 1 relaxed eye),

$q = -(0.3 + 0.003) = -0.303$ m

and

$h_e = 0.012 + 0.003 = 0.015$ m

From Figure 10.1,

$l = q + h_e = -0.303 + 0.015 = -0.288$ m

L is given by

$L = 1/l = -1/0.288 = -3.472$ D

From the lens equation (A1.21)

$L' = -3.472 - 5 = -8.472$ D

Substituting the values obtained for q, h_e, L, and L' into equation (10.8b) gives

$SM = (-0.303 \times -3.472)/[1 - (0.015$
$\qquad \times -8.472)] = 0.933$

The object is perceived to be minified by 0.067 or 6.7 per cent by the spectacle lens. *Note*: q and l (or L) are always negative if the object is not at infinity, and h_e is always positive.

Example 10.2: If the object in the previous example is now at infinity, what is *SM*?

Solution: Using $h_e = 0.015$ and $F_s = -5$ D, in equation (10.8c)

$SM = 1/[1 - (0.015 \times -5)] = 0.930$

The object is seen to be minified by 0.003 or 0.3 per cent relative to the previous example.

Pupil position and magnification

Figure 10.2 shows the effect of the correcting ophthalmic lens on the position of the entrance pupil of the eye. The ray from the centre of the actual entrance pupil is refracted by the lens, and the image of this entrance pupil (the new effective entrance pupil of the lens/eye system) is displaced from the original pupil and is also different in size. Application of the lens equation allows us to

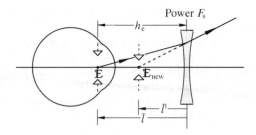

Figure 10.2. The effect of the correcting spectacle lens on pupil position and size.

determine the new pupil position and the magnification.

The lens equation applied to the ray shown in Figure 10.2 is

$1/T' - 1/T = F_s$ \hfill (10.10)

and solving for T' gives

$T' = T/(1 + TF_s)$ \hfill (10.11)

The magnification $\overline{M}$ of the pupil defined as

$$\overline{M} = \frac{\text{new pupil diameter}}{\text{old pupil diameter}} \hfill (10.12)$$

is given by the lens equation

$\overline{M} = T'/T$

and therefore

$\overline{M} = 1/(1 + TF_s)$ \hfill (10.13)

However,

$T = -h_e$

with the negative sign present because h_e is always positive and T is negative in the figure. It then follows that

$\overline{M} = 1/(1 - h_e F_s)$ \hfill (10.14)

The right-hand side expression is the same as that of the spectacle magnification given by equation (10.8c). Thus pupil magnification is the same as spectacle magnification of a distant object.

Retinal image illuminance

The above equations show that, for positive power lenses, the effective entrance pupil is enlarged, and this allows an increase in the amount of luminous flux entering a system. The amount of luminous flux entering is proportional to the area of the pupil, and is thus proportional to the square of the pupil diameter – or, in this case, the increase is proportional to the square of the pupil magnification. However, this does not lead to a change in image brightness, because the image has the same magnification as the pupil, and the area of the retinal image changes by the same amount. Thus the effects of spectacle magnification and pupil magnification on retinal illuminance cancel each other out. However, there is some light loss due to surface reflections of lenses without anti-reflection coatings (approximately 8 per cent for a lens with a refractive index of 1.5).

Relative spectacle magnification

In this section, for simplification, it is assumed that the object is at infinity.

Relative spectacle magnification, denoted here by the symbol *RSM*, is defined as

$$RSM = \frac{\text{retinal image size in the corrected ametropic eye}}{\text{retinal image size in a standard emmetropic eye}} \quad (10.15)$$

with both images in focus and when viewing the same object at the same distance.

The in-focus image size η' of a distant object of angular subtense ω is given by the equation (6.11), i.e.

$$\eta' = \omega/F \quad (10.16)$$

where F is the power of the eye. Therefore

$$RSM = F_e/F_t \quad (10.17)$$

where F_e is the equivalent power of the emmetropic eye, and F_t is the equivalent power of the combined system of the ophthalmic lens and ametropic eye. For the corrected ametrope,

$$F_t = F_a + F_s - h_p F_a F_s \quad (10.18)$$

where F_a is the equivalent power of the uncorrected eye, h_p is the distance between the (back principal point of the) ophthalmic lens and the front principal point of the ametropic eye, and F_s is the equivalent power of the correcting ophthalmic lens (Figure 10.3). Thus

$$RSM = \frac{F_e}{F_a + F_s - h_p F_a F_s} \quad (10.19)$$

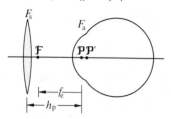

Figure 10.3. Parameters for calculation of relative spectacle magnification.

Axial ametropia

If the difference between an uncorrected ametropic eye and the standard eye is the axial length only, they have the same powers. Substituting F_e for F_a in equation (10.19) gives

$$RSM = \frac{F_e}{F_a + F_s - h_p F_a F_s} = \frac{1}{1 - (h_p + f_e)F_s} \quad (10.20)$$

where f_e is the anterior focal length $(-1/F_e)$ of the eye. Typical values of h_p are 15–20 mm, while $f_e = -16.67$ mm for an eye of power +60 D. If h_p is equal and opposite to f_e, the previous equation reduces to

$$RSM = 1 \quad (10.21)$$

This is **Knapp's law**, which states that a spectacle lens placed at the anterior focal point of an axially ametropic eye has the same retinal image size as that of a standard emmetropic eye.

Refractive ametropia

If the length of an uncorrected ametropic eye is the same as that of the standard eye, their powers must be different. The effective power of the ophthalmic lens at the eye, together with the power of the ametropic eye, is the same as that of the standard eye, that is

$$F_e = F_s/(1 - h_p F_s) + F_a = (F_a + F_s - h_p F_a F_s)/ \\ (1 - h_p F_s) \quad (10.22)$$

Substituting the right-hand side of this equation for F_e into equation (10.19), after some simplification gives

$$RSM = 1/(1 - h_p F_s) \qquad (10.23)$$

RSM is now similar to the spectacle magnification given by equation (10.8c), except that the distance between the lens and the entrance pupil of the eye has been replaced by the distance between the lens and the front principal plane of the eye. The difference in positions of the entrance pupil and the front principal plane is approximately 1.5 mm (1.70 mm for the Gullstrand number 1 relaxed eye).

Further comments

The concept of relative spectacle magnification has limited use for three reasons:

1. It is not always known whether the ametropia is axial or refractive. The distinction is useful for anisometropia known to be caused by differences in a single parameter, for example axial length.
2. The concept of a standard emmetropic eye power is of limited value. The power of emmetropic eyes can vary over a wide range (Sorsby *et al.*, 1962). This is unimportant in cases of anisometropia, where the ratio of the relative spectacle magnifications of the two eyes does not even require a definition of a standard eye.
3. The relative spectacle magnification difference in anisometropia is not necessarily a good indicator of the likelihood of magnification problems. A good example of this is axial anisometropia – spectacles may provide equal retinal image sizes according to Knapp's law, but this does not mean that the brain's cortical images are the same sizes. A stretching of the retina that may accompany elongation of the eye in myopia may move the retina's receptors further apart. Alternatively, there may be 'rewiring' occurring between the retina and the brain. Some evidence for these possibilities was provided by Winn *et al.* (1988), who measured **aniseikonia**, which is a measure of differences in cortical image sizes (Chapter 6), in myopic axial anisometropes. They found smaller aniseikonia with contact lenses, for which *RSM* > 1, than for spectacle lenses, which would be

expected to have *RSM* values close to 1 as in equations (10.20) and (10.21).

Atchison (1996) developed further equations that give relative retinal image sizes of a pair of corrected eyes. These are useful in calculations involving anisometropia and/or refractive surgery.

Effects on far and near points and accommodation demand

The farthest and closest positions of clear vision are called the far point and near point, respectively. These positions are different for the eye–ophthalmic lens system than for the uncorrected eye alone. The accommodation demand, that is, the amount of accommodation required to focus clearly to an object, is also affected by a correcting ophthalmic lens.

For correcting distance vision, the far point of the eye–ophthalmic lens system is placed at infinity. Consider what happens to the near point. Figure 10.4 shows a spectacle lens imaging a point **O** to **O′**. Take the point **O′** to be the near point of the uncorrected eye. The object and image distances can be related using the lens equation. For the situation shown in the Figure 10.4, the lens equation is

$$\frac{1}{d_{np} + h_v} - \frac{1}{(d_{np})_{new} + h_v} = F_s \qquad (10.24)$$

where d_{np} and $(d_{np})_{new}$ are the near point distances in uncorrected and corrected vision respectively, F_s is the lens power and is assumed to be a function of position, and h_v is the distance from the lens to the corneal vertex. Solving for $(d_{np})_{new}$,

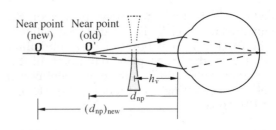

Figure 10.4. The effect of the correcting lens on the near point.

$$(d_{np})_{new} = \frac{d_{np} + h_v}{[1 - (d_{np} + h_v)F_s]} - h_v \qquad (10.25)$$

This equation (and Figure 10.4) shows that negative ophthalmic lenses push the effective near point of myopes away from the eye. For positive power lens and hypermetropes, the near point comes closer to the eye.

Accommodation through a correcting lens

The presence of an ophthalmic lens in front of the eye changes the apparent position of the object and therefore changes the demand on

accommodation. In equation (10.25), we replace d_{np} and $(d_{np})_{new}$ by general distances W and W' respectively. If we then replace these distances by their corresponding vergences W and W', we can obtain

$$W' = \frac{(1 + h_v W)F_s + W}{1 - h_v F_s - h_v^2 F_s W} \qquad (10.26)$$

Now the effective spectacle refraction at the corneal vertex F_{so} is given by

$$F_{so} = \frac{F_s}{1 - h_v F_s} \qquad (10.27)$$

The **ocular accommodation demand** $A(W)$, referenced to the corneal vertex, is simply given by

$$A(W) = F_{so} - W' \qquad (10.28a)$$

which can be shown to be

$$A(W) = \frac{-W}{(1 - h_v F_s)(1 - h_v F_s - h_v^2 F_s W)} \qquad (10.28b)$$

Sometimes the accommodation demand is referred to the spectacle lens plane. In this case, we can set h_v to zero and replace W in the above equation by L, which is the vergence of the object relative to the spectacle plane. We then have the spectacle accommodation demand $A(L)$, which is

$$A(L) = -L \qquad (10.28c)$$

Hence the **spectacle accommodation demand** is simply the absolute value of the inverse of the distance of the object from the lens.

Example 10.3: An eye looks at an object 30 cm away through a distance correction of –5 D placed 12 mm in front of the cornea. What are the ocular and spectacle accommodative demands?

Solution: We can make the following substitutions into equation (10.28b):

$W = -1/0.3 = -3.333$ D, $h_v = 0.012$ m and $F_s = -5$ D

to give the ocular accommodative demand as

$$A(W) = \frac{3.333}{[1 - 0.012 \times (-5)][1 - 0.012 \times (-5) - 0.012^2 \times (-5) \times (-3.333)]} = 2.97 \text{ D}$$

The object is a distance $-(0.3 - 0.012) = -0.288$ m away from the lens, which makes the object vergence relative to the lens

$$L = -1/0.288 = -3.47 \text{ D}$$

from which, using equation (10.28c), the spectacle accommodative demand is

$$A(L) = 3.47 \text{ D}$$

If we repeat the above exercise for a +5 D lens, we obtain an ocular accommodation demand of 3.76 D. This tells us that corrected hypermetropes have greater ocular accommodation demands than do corrected myopes. Thus, all other things being equal, corrected hypermetropes experience presbyopia earlier in life than do corrected myopes.

Rotational magnification, field-of-view and field-of-vision

Rotational magnification

The magnification effect of ophthalmic lenses influences the eye's rotation to look at off-axis objects of regard. We quantify this by the **rotational magnification**, which we define as

$$RM = \frac{\text{angle of rotation of eye looking through lens } (\theta')}{\text{angle of eye rotation without lens } (\theta)} \qquad (10.29a)$$

This is similar to determining spectacle magnification (*SM*) at the beginning of this chapter (*Spectacle magnification*), except that the ocular reference point is the centre-of-rotation rather than the entrance pupil. In line with equation (10.8b), *RM* is given by

$$RM = q_c L/(1 - h_c L') \qquad (10.29b)$$

where q_c is the distance from the object to the centre-of-rotation of the eye, and h_c is the distance from the spectacle lens to the centre-of-rotation. Because h_c is approximately twice the value of h_e in equation (10.8b), values of *RM* are much further from 1 than are values of *SM*. For the object at infinity, it can easily be shown that

$$RM = 1/(1 - h_c F_c) \qquad (10.29c)$$

Field-of-view

Apparent and **real fields-of-view** are shown for positive and negative power lenses in Figure 10.5. The apparent field-of-view is the maximum ocular rotation θ'_{max} of the eye, about its centre-of-rotation **C**, for which the eye can look through a lens at an object of regard. The real field-of-view is given by the angle θ_{max}. From Figure 10.5, the apparent field-of-view is

$$\theta'_{max} = D_s/(2h_c) \qquad (10.30)$$

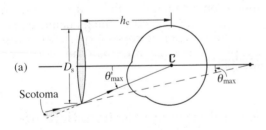

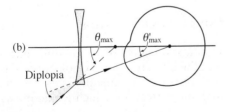

Figure 10.5. Real and apparent fields-of-view:
a. Corrected hypermetropia.
b. Corrected myopia.

Combining equations (10.29a) and (10.29b), but using θ_{max} and θ'_{max} instead of θ' and θ, gives the equation

$$\theta_{max} = \theta'_{max}(1 - h_c L')/(q_c L) \qquad (10.31a)$$

Substituting the right-hand side of equation (10.30) for θ'_{max} into equation (10.31a) gives

$$\theta_{max} = D_s(1 - h_c L')/(2h_c q_c L) \qquad (10.31b)$$

For a distant object, this equation reduces to

$$\theta_{max} = D_s(1 - h_c F_s)/(2h_c) \qquad (10.31c)$$

Comparing the last equation with equation (10.30) shows clearly that the real field-of-view is less than the apparent field-of-view for positive lens powers (corrected hypermetropia). This gives a scotoma (blind area) of magnitude $(\theta'_{max} - \theta_{max})$ in the field of vision (Figure 10.5a). This can be a considerable problem for moderate and high power hypermetropes.

The real field-of-view is greater than the apparent field-of-view for negative lens powers (corrected myopia). This gives a region of diplopia (double vision) of magnitude $(\theta_{max} - \theta'_{max})$ in the field-of-vision (Figure 10.5b), but this does not seem to inconvenience corrected myopes.

As these are first order equations, which ignore the influence of the aberration distortion on the real field-of-view, we caution their use with large angles.

Field-of-vision

This is similar to field-of-view, except that the eye is stationary and looking through the centre of the lens. Limits correspond to the field seen by the periphery of the eye through the lens. A similar set of equations to equations (10.30)–(10.31c) apply, except that we revert to using the distances q and h_e, that were used for the spectacle magnification calculations in the *Spectacle magnification* section, instead of q_c and h_c.

Summary of main symbols

h_e distance from ophthalmic lens to the entrance pupil of eye (always positive)

h_c distance from ophthalmic lens to the

centre-of-rotation of eye (always positive)

h_p distance from ophthalmic lens to the front principal point of eye (always positive)

h_v distance from ophthalmic lens to the corneal vertex (always positive)

D_s diameter of spectacle lens

l distance from ophthalmic lens to object (always negative)

l' distance from ophthalmic lens to image

L, L' vergences corresponding to l and l'

q distance between entrance pupil of eye and the object (always negative)

q_c distance between centre-of-rotation of eye and the object (always negative)

d_{np} distance from corneal vertex to near point of uncorrected eye

$(d_{np})_{new}$ distance from corneal vertex to near point of corrected eye

F_s equivalent power of ophthalmic lens

F_a equivalent power of the ametropic eye

F_e equivalent power of the emmetropic eye

F_t equivalent power of ophthalmic lens and ametropic eye together

$A(W)$ ocular accommodation demand

ω angular diameter of the object

θ_{max} real field-of-view through a spectacle lens

θ'_{max} apparent field-of-view through a spectacle lens

SM spectacle magnification

$\overline{M}$ pupil magnification

RSM relative spectacle magnification

RM rotational magnification

References

Atchison, D. A. (1996). Calculating relative retinal image sizes of eyes. *Ophthal. Physiol. Opt.*, **16**, 532–8.

Fannin, T. E. and Grosvenor, T. (1996). *Clinical Optics*, 2nd edn. Butterworth-Heinemann.

Jalie, M. (1984). *Principles of Ophthalmic Lenses*, 4th edn. Association of Dispensing Opticians.

Sorsby, A., Leary, G. A. and Richards, M. J. (1962). Correlation ametropia and component ametropia. *Vision Res.*, **2**, 309–13.

Winn, B., Ackerley, R. G., Brown, C. A. *et al.* (1988). Reduced aniseikonia in axial anisometropia with contact lens correction. *Ophthal. Physiol. Opt.*, **8**, 341–4.

Section 3:

Light and the eye

11

Light and the eye: introduction

Introduction

Since the eye is the organ of light sense, how the eye interacts with light is of great importance in understanding the visual process and the limits to vision. As we see in the next few chapters, not all the light entering the eye forms the intended image on the retina. Some light is reflected, scattered and absorbed, with a small part of the absorbed light being re-emitted in the form of fluorescence.

Intense levels of light can cause damage to the eye. Furthermore, other nearby bands of the electromagnetic spectrum (ultraviolet and infrared radiation) interact with the eye and these can also cause damage.

Since the eye is essentially a detector of light, we need to understand the nature of light. In this chapter we discuss the nature of light, how it is quantified, and different aspects of it that affect vision.

Radiation and the electromagnetic spectrum

Light is a small part of the electromagnetic spectrum. The complete electromagnetic spectrum is shown schematically in Figure 11.1. The range of wavelengths that cover the ultraviolet, visible and infrared ranges is called **optical radiation**. The limits of the optical radiation bands are 100–380 nm (ultraviolet), 390–780 nm (visible) and 780–10^6 nm (infrared).

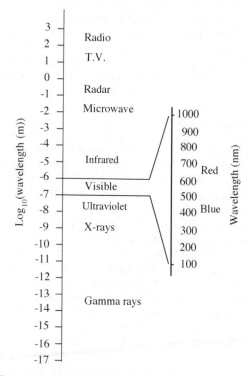

Figure 11.1. The electromagnetic spectrum.

If a beam of electromagnetic energy has a spectral radiant flux denoted by $F_R(\lambda)$, the amount of **radiant power** or **flux** F_R in the beam is given by the integral

$$F_R = \int_0^\infty F_R(\lambda)d\lambda \quad \text{watt} \tag{11.1}$$

where $F_R(\lambda)$ has the unit of watt/unit of wavelength.

Light

The *Penguin Dictionary of Physics* (1977) defines light as

> The agency that causes a visual sensation when it falls on the retina of the eye. Light forms a narrow section of the electromagnetic spectrum ...

While this is correct, agencies other than the narrow band of the electromagnetic spectrum that we normally call light can produce a visual sensation. Our sense of light arises usually from stimulation of the cones and rods in the retina and by signals being transmitted from them to the visual centres of the brain through a number of different types of nerve cells and pathways. If any of these cells or centres are stimulated by other means, a visual sensation still occurs. For example, these cells may be activated by chemicals, X-rays and pressure from a knock on the head.

Light can be defined simply as that band of the electromagnetic spectrum that produces a visual response, and this band is from about 380–780 nm. The eye is not equally responsive to all wavelengths in this band. The spectral visual response curve is approximately 'bell'-shaped, with its shape and position depending upon the light level. Two extreme forms of the spectral response curve are identified; one for moderate to high light levels, and one for low light levels. For moderate to high light levels, the cones dominate vision, we see colour and the spectral response is referred to as the **photopic** response. For low light levels, the rods dominate vision, we are unable to distinguish colour, and the spectral response is referred to as the **scotopic** response. The range of light levels intermediate between these two extremes, where both cones and rods operate, is called the **mesopic** range. Throughout this book, the photopic case is assumed unless stated otherwise.

Photopic vision

The amount of light F (luminous flux) in an electromagnetic beam of radiation is given by

the equation

$$F = K_m \int_0^\infty F_R(\lambda)V(\lambda)\,d\lambda \ \text{ lumen} \qquad (11.2)$$

where the constant K_m is known as the **maximum spectral luminous efficacy of radiation for photopic vision**. It has a value of 683.002 lm/W (CIE, 1983). $V(\lambda)$ is known as the **spectral luminous efficiency function for photopic vision**. It was determined from the average response of many subjects across a small number of studies and was defined by the Commission Internationale de l'Eclairage (CIE) in 1924. $V(\lambda)$ has a maximum value of 1 at 555 nm. Figure 11.2 shows the $V(\lambda)$ function.

The $V(\lambda)$ function is too low below about 450 nm because of shortcomings in the studies from which it was developed, but the advantages to be gained from correcting it are considered to be outweighed by the practical inconvenience. It should be appreciated that individuals' photopic relative sensitivities differ for a number of reasons, including the following:

1. Luminous efficiency is the combined effect of the three types of cones (containing short, medium and long wavelength sensitive photopigments), so that while the

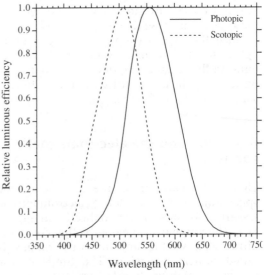

Figure 11.2. The relative luminous efficiency functions $V(\lambda)$ – photopic and $V'(\lambda)$ – scotopic. The peaks of these functions are at 555 nm and 507 nm, respectively.

spectral sensitivity of the cones may be the same for each individual, the relative number of cones may vary. In addition, colour defective people have a missing cone type (dichromasy) or a cone type whose photopigment has an altered spectral sensitivity (anomalous trichromats).

2. Variations in spectral transmittance by the ocular media and variations in the density of a yellow pigment (xanthophyll) in the macula of the retina. In particular, as we age our sensitivity to blue light decreases because our lenses absorb more blue light and there are neural changes associated with the short wavelength-sensitive cones (Werner *et al.*, 1990).

Mesopic vision

As the light level decreases from photopic towards scotopic levels, there is a change in relative spectral sensitivity accompanying the transition from cone to rod vision. This transition region is called the mesopic region and the shift in relative spectral sensitivity is called the **Purkinje shift**.

Scotopic vision

The CIE defined the spectral luminous efficiency function for scotopic vision $V'(\lambda)$ in 1951. This function has a maximum value of 1 at 507 nm. It is shown, along with $V(\lambda)$, in Figure 11.2. If we convert radiant energy into light using $V'(\lambda)$, we use equation (11.2) with $V'(\lambda)$ replacing $V(\lambda)$ and K'_m, the **maximum spectral luminous efficacy of radiation for scotopic vision**, replacing K_m. The value of K'_m is 1700.06 lm/W (CIE, 1983), which is derived from the definition that 1 photopic lumen = 1 scotopic lumen for a monochromatic source with a frequency of 540×10^{12} Hz. The ratio of the two K_m values is the ratio of the $V(\lambda)$ and $V'(\lambda)$ values at a wavelength of 555.016 nm in air with a refractive index of 1.00028.

Since there is only one class of cells (the rods) operating at scotopic light levels, we would expect less variability between individuals for scotopic relative sensitivity than for photopic relative sensitivity.

Photopic, mesopic and scotopic limits

There are no sharp divisions between the boundaries of these three ranges. The lower luminance limit of photopic vision is approximately 3 cd/m^2, with mesopic vision extending from this level to 0.03 cd/m^2, after which scotopic vision starts (see next section for unit of luminance).

Photometric quantities, units and example levels

There are four fundamental photometric quantities: luminous flux, luminous intensity, luminance and illuminance.

Luminous flux (F)

Luminous flux is the measure of the total amount of light in a beam, and has the unit of lumen (lm).

If we think of a light source as emitting so many watts of electromagnetic radiation, it emits a certain amount of lumens of light. The ratio of lumens to watts of a particular light source is known as its luminous efficacy. For example, there are about 10 lumens for each watt of a tungsten filament light source (giving about 600 lumens for a 60 W light bulb), about 40 lumens per watt for a fluorescent tube, and about 95 lumens per watt for sunlight.

Luminous intensity (I)

Luminous intensity is a measure of the brightness of a point source of light, and has the unit of candela (cd). It is a measure of luminous flux density. The luminous intensity in a given direction is the quotient of the luminous flux (δF), contained in an infinitesimally narrow cone in the given direction, by the solid angle ($\delta \Omega$) of the cone (Figure 11.3). That is

$I = \delta F / \delta \Omega$ lumen/steradian or candela (cd)

(11.3)

In the above example of the 60 W light bulb, the 600 lumens is not emitted nor distributed

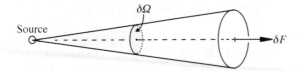

Figure 11.3. Luminous intensity $I = \delta F / \delta \Omega$.

evenly in all directions in space. For many light sources, it is more important to know the luminous intensity emitted in a given direction rather than the total luminous flux emitted. In practice, luminous intensity is used only for sources of small angular subtense.

The luminous intensity of a common wax candle is about 1 cd, and this is the origin of the word 'candela'. Traffic signal lights have axial luminous intensities of about 200–600 cd, or even higher. The axial luminous intensity of a car headlight on full beam can be about 20,000 cd. Marine lighthouses have intensities of millions of candelas.

Luminance (L)

Luminance is the objective measure of the 'brightness' of an extended source, and has the unit of candela per square metre (cd/m^2).

For a small element of an extended source, luminance can be related to the luminous intensity of the element and a direction. Referring to Figure 11.4, if the source is a small plane element of area δA with luminance $L(\theta)$ in a direction θ, the luminous intensity $I(\theta)$ in that direction is given by the equation

$$I(\theta) = L(\theta)\, \delta A \cos(\theta)$$

That is

$$L(\theta) = \frac{I(\theta)}{\delta A \cos(\theta)} \text{ cd/m}^2 \qquad (11.4)$$

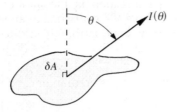

Figure 11.4. Relationship between luminance (*L*) and luminous intensity (*I*).

Some sources have the same 'brightness' or luminance in all directions, i.e. luminance is independent of θ. These sources are refered to as **Lambertian**.

Many sources of light, such as the sky, are effective sources because they scatter incident light. A perfectly diffusing surface scatters incident light equally in all directions, which means that the surface luminance is the same for all directions, and it acts as a Lambertian source. Magnesium oxide, soot, barium sulphate and roughened chalk (calcium carbonate) come close to being perfect diffusers. For a Lambertian source or surface

$$L(\theta) = \text{constant} = L \qquad (11.5)$$

and the luminous intensity is given by

$$I(\theta) = L\, \delta A \cos(\theta) \qquad (11.6a)$$

For normal viewing, $\theta = 0°$ and

$$I = L\, \delta A \qquad (11.6b)$$

For a perfect **specular surface**, which is the opposite of a perfect diffusing surface, all the incident light is reflected according to Snell's law. All surfaces have both specular and diffusing properties, thus lying somewhere between the two extremes.

The luminance of the sun depends upon its elevation above the horizon and the scattering, reflection and absorption by water vapour, dust and other substances in the atmosphere. The scatter and absorption by atmospheric molecules is wavelength-dependent, thus producing the blue sky and the reddish sun at sunset. Under clear atmospheric conditions, the luminance of the sun at high elevations is about 1.5×10^9 cd/m^2 and the luminance of the moon is about 2000 cd/m^2.

Illuminance (E)

Illuminance is a measure of the luminous flux density incident on a surface, and has the unit of lumens per square metre (lm/m^2 or lux).

Since illuminance can vary over a surface, it is best defined in terms of small elements of area δA. Thus

$$E = \delta F / \delta A \text{ lux} \qquad (11.7)$$

On a clear day with the sun high in the sky,

the illuminance at the earth's surface can be as high as 50,000 lux. The illuminance at a desk in a well-lit office is about 200–1000 lux.

Some useful relationships

The four basic photometric units are connected within the preceding definitions, but there are other relationships that are useful in a number of different situations. We discuss two of these in this section.

Luminous intensity and illuminance: the inverse square law

The illuminance E on a surface at a distance d from a small source of light, described by its luminous intensity I, is given by the inverse square law equation

$$E = \frac{I}{d^2} \cos(\theta) \tag{11.8}$$

where θ is the angle of inclination of the surface normal to the direction of the source.

This equation assumes that the source is a point source. Since all sources have some size, this equation is only an approximation. If the angular subtense of the longest dimension of the source is less than 5° at the distance d, the error in this equation is less than 1 per cent.

Luminance and illuminance

Visual performance in any task is related to light level, and it is the stimulus luminance that is the important measure of light level. For many stimuli that reflect light, such as a visual acuity chart, the luminance depends upon the illuminance in the plane of the stimulus. The relationship between the two quantities depends on the scattering properties of the stimulus material. If the stimulus is perfectly diffusing and reflects a fraction r of the incident light, luminance L is related to illuminance E by the simple equation

$$L = rE/\pi \tag{11.9}$$

Which quantity to use

Since visual performance is dependent upon light level, we may need to specify light levels for particular tasks. We need to know which of the four photometric quantities of luminous flux, luminous intensity, illuminance and luminance is most relevant to each task.

Threshold detection

The threshold light level for detection of a light stimulus with a small angular subtense depends upon the total amount of light collected by the retina – that is, the luminous flux. This is because the light from this stimulus falls on a few photoreceptors, which pool their input. This is known as spatial summation. Since this pooled amount of light is the product of local illuminance and the area, the amount of light collected is the luminous flux. Under such circumstances, **Ricco's law** states that

luminance × area = constant

but more strictly speaking this should be

local illuminance × area = luminous flux
= constant

For a large source, whose retinal image is much larger than the region of spatial summation, detection thresholds depend upon the stimulus luminance (or retinal illuminance) and not on stimulus size. The detection threshold depends upon the luminance contrast of the stimulus relative to its background.

In between the extremes of size, thresholds vary approximately with the square root of the product of luminance and area (**Piper's law**).

Supra-threshold visibility of sources with a small angular subtense

For light levels well above threshold, the visibility of a small 'point' source is related to its luminous intensity. For example, the performances of signal and warning lamps such as traffic signal lamps are specified by their luminous intensities.

Supra-threshold visibility of sources with a large angular subtense

The visibility of a source with a large angular subtense is usually correlated with its luminance. For example, the performances of pedestrian road crossing signals are specified by their luminances.

Measurement of ambient light level

In general, visual performance improves with increase in light level. Most realistic scenes contain many objects of various sizes, luminances and luminous intensities. We need a consistent, repeatable method of measuring the ambient light level of such scenes. The obvious approach is to measure the amount of light entering an observer's eye, i.e. the luminous flux. However, this requires knowing the pupil size of the observer. This problem can be avoided by using the illuminance at the pupil plane of the observer.

Other comments

While thresholds and levels of visibility depend upon the light level reaching the retina, we can measure accurately only the photometric properties of the source itself and corresponding light levels (e.g. illuminance) at any distance from the source. However, the light level reaching the retina is dependent upon pupil size, and therefore threshold and supra-threshold levels depend upon pupil diameter. We discuss how pupil size affects retinal light level in Chapter 13.

Summary of main symbols

λ	wavelength
$F_R(\lambda)$	spectral radiant flux
F_R	radiant power or radiant flux (integrated over all wavelengths)
$V(\lambda)$, $V'(\lambda)$	spectral luminous efficiency functions for photopic and scotopic vision
K_m, K'_m	maximum spectral luminous efficacies of radiation for photopic and scotopic vision
F	luminous flux
I	luminous intensity
L	luminance
E	illuminance
Ω	solid angle
A	area
d	distance
θ	direction relative to the normal of a surface
r	reflectance fraction

References

CIE (1983). *The Basis of Physical Photometry*. Publication CIE No. 18.2 (TC-1.2). Commission Internationale de l'Éclairage.

Penguin Dictionary of Physics (1977). (V. H. Pitt, ed.), p. 219. Penguin Books Ltd.

Werner, J. S., Peterzell, D. H. and Scheetz, A. J. (1990). Light, vision, and aging. *Optom. Vis. Sci.*, **67**, 214–29.

12

Passage of light into the eye

Introduction

Not all the light entering the eye forms the retinal image. A significant amount is lost from the beam by the following processes:

1. Some light is specularly reflected at the four major refracting surfaces.
2. Some light is elastically scattered (no change in wavelength) by the ocular media. In some other chapters we refer to diffusely reflected light (e.g. Chapter 8), but in this chapter we refer to the light which is diffusely reflected as back-scattered light, to distinguish it from forward-scattered light.
3. Some light is absorbed and is then either
   a. re-emitted at other (longer) wavelengths, which is known as inelastic scattering or as fluorescence, or
   b. converted to other forms of energy

Both 2 and 3a above are causes of veiling glare (also straylight). Veiling glare from elastically scattered light is not usually uniform and has an angular distribution, which we discuss further in Chapter 13. By contrast, fluorescence produces a uniformly distributed veiling glare, and we discuss the source of this fluorescence later in this chapter.

Of the above three causes of light loss, specular reflection by the refracting surfaces makes up only a small proportion. Most of this occurs at the cornea, and this is useful in determining the radii of curvature of these refracting surfaces. However, this may be annoying because it produces veiling glare for the clinician during direct ophthalmoscopy. Light scattered by the ocular media plays a similar dual role. Light specularly reflected or back-scattered out of the eye helps clinicians to delineate the different components of the eye during internal eye examination with the slit-lamp, particularly in examination of the lens and the cornea. However, any forward-scattered light produces a veiling glare at the retina and reduces scene contrast. This is a problem particularly when bright lights are present in otherwise dark fields and in low contrast fields, and increases with age. While the loss of light due to absorption reduces the amount of light reaching the retina, it protects the retina from light of shorter wavelengths, which may be damaging to ocular structures.

Light is able to reach the retina after passage through the iris and sclera. Van den Berg et al. (1991) determined that, for eyes with light irises, the effective transmission is between 0.2 per cent (green) and 1 per cent (red), and that the eye wall around the iris transmits a significant amount of light. This light makes a small contribution to veiling glare at large angles.

Specular reflection

Some light is reflected at each interface in the eye. Since the surfaces are smooth, the specularly reflected light is image forming.

The fractions of reflected and transmitted light depend on the refractive indices on each side of the surface, and these fractions are given by the Fresnel equations. If the refractive indices are n and n' on the incident and refracted sides respectively, for normal incidence the reflectance (i.e. fraction of light reflected) R and the transmittance (i.e. the fraction of light transmitted) T are given by the equations

$$R = [(n' - n)/(n' + n)]^2 \text{ and } T = 4nn'/(n' + n)^2 \tag{12.1}$$

We may note that from these equations

$$R + T = 1 \tag{12.2}$$

implying that there is no absorption of light at the surface. However, there is some absorption by the bulk tissue. Since the eye contains four main reflecting surfaces, there are four main reflected images. These are called Purkinje–Sanson or Purkinje images, and are often denoted by the symbols P_I, P_{II}, P_{III} and P_{IV}.

The above equations apply strictly only to a simple smooth surface between two homogeneous media with well-defined refractive indices n and n'. In biological systems, this ideal situation does not exist. For example, in the case of the anterior corneal surface, the boundary consists of a number of layers (see Chapter 2) of different refractive indices. The outermost layer (the tear film) has an index of approximately 1.336, compared with a value of 1.376 for the bulk of the cornea. The lens surfaces are also complicated by the presence of the capsule, and are not as smooth as the cornea, and this makes their Purkinje images more diffuse than those of the cornea. A rigorous analysis of the reflectance of surfaces would have to take into account the fine structure of the capsular matrix.

The positions, sizes and brightnesses of the Purkinje images depend upon the position of the light source and the optical structure of the eye. Table 12.1 has these details for the Gullstrand number 1 relaxed schematic eye and an axial, distant light source. Figure 12.1 shows the positions and sizes of the images of this schematic eye.

These images can be used to determine the positions and curvatures of the intra-ocular surfaces and, in particular, those of the lens. Measuring Purkinje image sizes allows us to monitor lens changes due to accommodation and aging in the lens.

The Purkinje images are useful also in locating the different axes of the eye (see Chapter 4) and for monitoring eye movements. The brightness of Purkinje images has also been used to determine the spectral transmission of the lens (Said and Weale, 1959; Johnson *et al.*, 1993).

Images formed by multiple reflections

The Purkinje images discussed above are formed from single reflections. Some light suffers more than one reflection, but the amount of light in a multi-reflected beam is rapidly attenuated as the number of reflections increases. If there is an odd number of reflections, the beam exits the eye. On the other hand, if the beam suffers an even number of reflections, it finally reaches the retina and forms an image somewhere along its path. There are six possible combinations of double reflection images, and the brightest are the three involving the anterior corneal surface. However, to see any of these double reflections, the image has to be formed near the retina and has to arise from a bright source in a dim or dark field.

The degree of focus at the retina of these higher order Purkinje images depends upon the distance of the source, the structure of a particular eye, and the level of accommodation. If the source is about 25 cm in front of

Table 12.1. The Purkinje images of the relaxed Gullstrand number 1 eye for a distant light source.

Purkinje image	Relative size	Distance from corneal pole (mm)	Relative brightness
P_I (anterior cornea)	1.000	3.850	1.000
P_{II} (posterior cornea)	0.882	3.765	0.00826
P_{III} (anterior lens)	1.967	10.620	0.0128
P_{IV} (posterior lens)	−0.760	3.979	0.0128

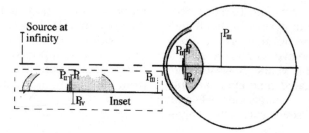

Figure 12.1. The positions and relative sizes of the Purkinje images for the Gullstrand number 1 relaxed eye, for the light source at infinity.

the cornea, the reflections from the posterior lens surface and the anterior corneal surface are in focus close to the retina and form an erect image.

Specular reflections may occur that are not Purkinje images. For example, the lenticular cortex shows a small steady increase in back-scatter with age, which may be because of the specular reflections from the ever increasing zones of discontinuity in the cortex (Weale, 1986).

Transmittance

There have been several studies measuring the transmittance of the eye, particularly of the lens. These include psychophysical and physical methods. Physical methods include comparing the relative intensities of the third and fourth Purkinje images, and *in vitro* measurements of individual parts of the eye or the whole of the eye.

Spectral transmittance of the whole eye

Figure 12.2 shows spectral transmittances of the whole eye (which includes the cornea, aqueous, lens and vitreous) from the work of Ludvigh and McCarthy (1938), Boettner and

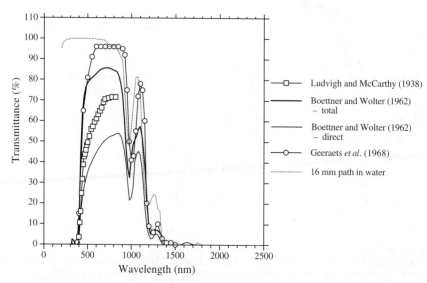

Figure 12.2. The spectral transmittance of the whole eye from Ludvigh and McCarthy (1938), Boettner and Wolter (1962), Geeraets and Berry (1968), and 16 mm of water. The data of Boettner are for a young child/young adult, except for wavelengths less than 380 nm, where they are those for a young child.

Wolter (1962) and Geeraets and Berry (1968). The mean age of the four eyes of Ludvigh and McCarthy was 62 years, but they adjusted the transmittances as if the eyes contained lenses of a mean age of 21.5 years. Boettner and Wolter (1962) investigated nine eyes ranging from 4 weeks to 75 years of age. Geeraets and Berry (1968) measured seven eyes, whose ages were not given.

Since the ocular components scatter light, the measured transmittance depends upon the amount of scattered light that is collected by the instrument. Boettner and Wolter (1962) measured the transmittance under two conditions; first, light collected only within a 1° cone centred on the transmitted beam, and second, light collected within a 170° cone. The first condition simulated directly transmitted light plus a small amount of scattered light, and the second condition included most of the forward-scattered light and measured total transmittance. Boettner and Wolter's results show a strong dependency on age. Ludvigh and McCarthy (1938) and Geeraets and Berry (1968) did not state their collecting angles.

The transmittance of the whole eye can be found by removing the sclera, choroid and retina in the region of the fovea. However, Boettner and Wolter calculated their whole eye values from the transmittances of individual components. Their individual component transmittances, as well as data from other sources, are discussed below.

Spectral transmittance of each ocular component

The cornea

Figure 12.3a shows the spectral transmittances of the cornea (Boettner and Wolter, 1962; Beems and van Best, 1990; van den Berg and Tan, 1994). Boettner and Wolter stated that the total transmittance (scattered plus direct light) was representative of six eyes with no age effect, and that the direct (scattered light excluded) transmittance for the 53-year-old eye was close to the mean of eight eyes. They found that the direct transmittance is age-dependent, but Beems and van Best (1990) and van den Berg and Tan (1994) did not find an age dependency.

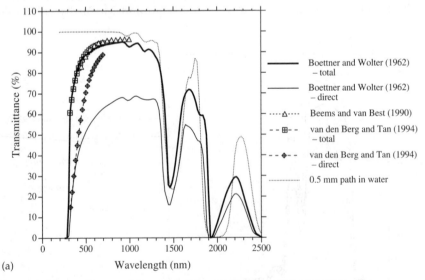

(a)

Figure 12.3. The spectral transmittances of the ocular components from various sources:
a. The cornea, from Boettner and Wolter (1962) for a 53-year-old subject, Beems and van Best (1990) mean data for 22–43 years and 67–87 years groups, and van den Berg and Tan (1994) from their equation (1).
b. The aqueous, from Boettner and Wolter (1962), both direct and total.
c. The lens, from Said and Weale (1959) mean of ages 21–45 years, Boettner and Wolter (1962) for a young child, and Mellerio (1971) estimated mean of 19–32 years and 46–66 years groups.
d. The vitreous, from Boettner and Wolter (1962).

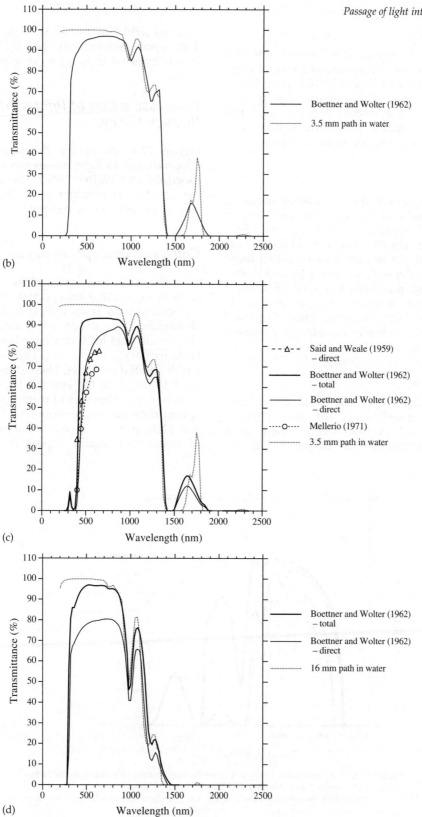

(b)

(c)

(d)

The aqueous

Figure 12.3b shows the mean spectral transmittance of the aqueous of several eyes, from Boettner and Wolter (1962). They found no differences in transmission due to age. They found no difference between total and direct transmittance, indicating that there is no significant scattering in the aqueous.

The lens

Figure 12.3c shows spectral transmittance of the lens (Said and Weale, 1959; Boettner and Wolter, 1962; Mellerio, 1971). The data for Said and Weale (1959) and for Mellerio are estimated means of their results, which show a strong age-dependence. Boettner and Wolter (1962) found that both the total and direct transmittances decrease with age, particularly at the short wavelengths. This decreased transmittance at shorter wavelength produces the yellowing of the lens with age.

The vitreous

Figure 12.3d shows the total and direct spectral transmittances of the vitreous (Boettner and Wolter, 1962). There is a measurable amount of scattering in the vitreous, which does not seem to be dependent upon wavelength. No differences in transmittance due to age were found.

Progressive loss of light as it passes through the eye

Figure 12.4 shows the decrease in direct transmittance as light passes through the eye (Boettner and Wolter, 1962). The data shows the spectral transmittance at the posterior surface of each ocular component.

Causes of absorption bands

Since the major component of the eye is water, we may expect that the spectral absorption of the ocular media is strongly influenced by the absorption properties of water. Spectral absorption data for water have been given by Hulburt (1945), Curcio and Petty (1951), and Smith and Baker (1981). These data have been used to calculate the spectral transmittances of different thicknesses of water samples, and appropriate curves are plotted on Figures 12.2 and 12.3a–d. Since the eye is not made totally of water, we would expect that, for any

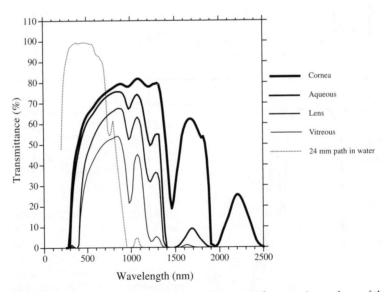

Figure 12.4. The cumulative spectral transmittances at the posterior surfaces of the ocular components, from Boettner and Wolter (1962). These data are for direct transmittance and for a young child/young adult, except for wavelengths less than 380 nm, where they are those for a young child.

component, the best match occurs for a length of water shorter than the eye component thickness. We would expect a good match for the aqueous, which has the highest concentration of water, and the worst match for the cornea and lens. For the eye as a whole, it appears that a 16 mm thickness of water matches the whole eye fairly well.

Examination of the transmittance curves for water in Figures 12.2 and 12.3a–d shows that the spectral absorption of the eye is dominated by water for wavelengths greater than about 600 nm. Absorption of energy by water at these wavelengths leads to heating of the water and surrounding tissue, and this may pose a risk of thermal damage.

For shorter wavelengths, the ocular tissue is far more absorbing than a similar path length of water, indicating that the absorption properties of proteins and other cellular components are dominating the absorption process. Since these materials dominate the absorption, there is a risk that they will be damaged by the radiation.

Figures 12.2–12.4 show that there is strong absorption for wavelengths less than about 400 nm. The cornea absorbs all radiation below 290 nm. Wavelengths less than 300 nm are potentially damaging to the cornea, and it is most sensitive to damage at a wavelength of about 270 nm, where the threshold for observable damage is about $50 \, \text{J/m}^2$ (Pitts, 1978). The lens absorbs radiation strongly between 300 nm and 400 nm, with the shortest wavelength reaching the retina being approximately 380 nm.

Luminous transmittance

The above data describe the spectral transmittance of the ocular media. Of equal importance is the transmittance for a given light source. This can be calculated, given the spectral transmittance and the spectral output of the particular light source, as

$$\text{Luminous transmittance} = \frac{\int S(\lambda)T(\lambda)V(\lambda)\mathrm{d}\lambda}{\int S(\lambda)V(\lambda)\mathrm{d}\lambda}$$

$$(12.3)$$

where $S(\lambda)$ is the spectral output of the light source, $T(\lambda)$ is the spectral transmittance of the eye, $V(\lambda)$ is the photopic relative luminous efficiency value, λ is wavelength and the region of integration is over the visible spectrum, typically 380–780 nm.

Scatter

Scatter is due to spatial variations in the refractive index within a medium, usually on a microscopic scale. Scatter is due to a combination of diffraction, refraction and reflection. For example, light incident on a transparent object embedded in a medium of a different refractive index is scattered. Some of this light reflects from the incident surface, some passes through the surface and is refracted in a forward direction, and some is reflected inside the object a number of times and is finally refracted, either backwards or forwards. Finally, light outside the object but near its edge is diffracted in a forward direction.

The angular distribution of this scatter depends upon a number of factors; in particular, the size and shape of the scattering particles, the refractive index mismatch, the scale of the inhomogeneities relative to the wavelength, and whether the inhomogeneities have any regularity. Thus, the angular distribution of scattered light may be complex. The complexity increases if the light is scattered more than once. In biological media, the angular distribution can be so complex that it is not usually possible to predict the amount of forward-scatter from measures of back-scatter. This is particularly important in visual optics, because it is easy to measure back-scattered light objectively but impossible to measure forward-scatter objectively in the living eye. Forward-scattered light is usually measured subjectively using psychophysical measures (see Chapter 13).

Since the cornea and lens consist of cells and connective tissue, which contain inhomogeneities on the scale of the order of the wavelength of light, it is surprising that they have a high transparency. By contrast, other cells (such as those in the skin) scatter light strongly. We need to understand why the normal cornea and lens have such a high transparency. The aqueous and vitreous humours are much more homogeneous, and are therefore less likely to scatter light.

Even in healthy eyes scatter within the eye is usually sufficient to cause a reduction in visual performance in the presence of bright light sources (veiling glare), but this is much worse if cataracts are present. Cataracts are due to an aggregation of lens proteins, which lead to an increase in inhomogeneity and anisotropy of the lens. The forward-scatter from cataracts produces a veiling glare, while back-scatter from them reduces the amount of light reaching the retina.

The effect of forward-scattered light may be partly mitigated by the directional sensitivity of the receptors – the Stiles–Crawford effect, which is described in Chapter 13. The Stiles–Crawford effect relates mainly to the cones, and is thus mainly a photopic phenomenon. It does not greatly reduce the effects of scattered light under low light level conditions.

Scattering theory

For particles whose dimensions are much smaller than the wavelengths under consideration, and for which the scattering particles are mutually incoherent and independent, Rayleigh theory may be used to describe the scattering process. This theory assumes that the scattering particles are polarizable. Incident radiation polarizes the electronic structure of each particle into the form of a dipole, in which the electrons are pushed towards one side of the particle, leaving a positive change on the opposite side. These dipoles oscillate in time with the incident radiation. According to classical physics, oscillating dipoles must radiate energy; thus they absorb energy from the incident field and re-radiate it. The re-radiated energy is maximally radiated in a direction perpendicular to the dipole axis, and zero energy is radiated along the axis of the dipole.

Rayleigh scattering predicts the following:

1. The radiation scattered at 90° to the directly transmitted beam is completely polarized.
2. The amount of scattered light is proportional to the inverse of the fourth power of the wavelength. Therefore, blue light of 400 nm is scattered 9.4 times more strongly than red light of 700 nm wavelength.
3. The amount of forward- and backward-scattering are the same.

Rayleigh theory does not apply when the sizes of scattering particles are comparable or greater than the wavelength under consideration, and in this case one has to use more complex scattering models. The significance of particle size is as follows:

1. If the oscillating dipole is much longer than the wavelength, the calculation of the amount of radiation emitted in any direction must take into account the radiation from each point of the dipole. Since these are now at different distances, and hence have different phases with respect to an observer or detector, interference from the different points on the dipole must be taken into account.
2. If a scattering particle is much longer than the wavelength along the direction of light travel, there are a number of oscillating dipoles in the particle which interfere in a constructive manner in the forward direction, but tend to interfere destructively in the backwards direction. These trends become more pronounced with increase in particle size. Therefore, as the particle size increases, forward-scatter increases at the expense of backward-scatter.

The prediction of the scattering properties of particles of arbitrary size and shape is very difficult, if not impossible, but solutions are available for simple shapes. Because the amount of scattered light is proportional to the amount of light incident on the particle, the greater the cross-sectional area of the particle, the greater the scatter. For example, Mie theory explains the scattering by spheres of any size. For very large spheres, the scattering is independent of wavelength, and the amount of scattered light is twice that incident on the cross-section of the particle. For example, in liquid water aerosols the scattering is proportional to the total cross-sectional area of the droplets. This means that, for a given volume of water in droplet form, the scattering is inversely proportional to the droplet radius or proportional to $N^{1/3}$, where N is the number of droplets.

A third scattering theory is the Rayleigh–Gans theory, or Rayleigh–Deybe theory according to Kerker (1969). This theory applies when the refractive index of the scattering particles is close to that of the medium in which they are imbedded. Applied to spherical scattering particles, this theory predicts that, for spheres, forward-scatter increases and back-scatter decreases with increase in size.

The above scattering theories can be readily applied when the scattering particles are independent of each other. This assumes that they are weakly scattering and/or randomly ordered. These assumptions do not apply to the cornea, which has an ordered structure.

Cornea

The bulk of the cornea is the corneal stroma (Chapter 2). The stroma contains 200–250 or more layers (lamellae) of long cylindrical collagen fibrils, with the thickness of each lamella being about 2.0 μm (Hogan *et al.*, 1971). Fibrils within each lamella have diameters of 32–36 nm, and are separated by 20–50 nm. The fibrils within a layer are parallel to each other, and uniform in size and spacing (Hogan *et al.*, 1971). The fibrils within a layer are inclined at large angles to fibrils in adjacent lamellae. The refractive index of fibres is about 1.47, and the surrounding ground substance has a refractive index of about 1.354 (Maurice, 1969).

Hart and Farrell (1969), using a theoretical model of scattering by arrays of cylindrical structures with the degree of regularity found in real corneas, argued that the transparency of the cornea is due to the regularity of the fibril separation. Their theoretical predictions for the rabbit cornea closely matched experimental measures of transparency. Their theory was based upon the diffraction/interference from regular arrays. According to their theory, for an infinite array of equally spaced point-scattering particles, with a separation that is negligible compared to wavelength, the scattered light destructively interferes in all directions for all wavelengths except in the direction of the incident beam. However, because the fibrils have finite diameters, their array is not perfectly regular and infinite, and because the spacing is not negligible compared with the wavelength, there is some residual scattering that is wavelength-dependent. It follows that, if this regularity is disrupted further, scattering increases.

McCally and Farrell (1988) investigated the wavelength dependency of scatter within the cornea and concluded that the range of the ordering of the fibrils (e.g. short distance versus long distance order) would affect scatter. They argued that if the order is short range, the dependency is proportional to the inverse of the cube of the wavelength (i.e. $1/\lambda^3$). This was supported experimentally for the rabbit cornea. This cubic dependency is in contrast with the Rayleigh fourth power (i.e. $1/\lambda^4$) dependency, which assumes no regularity of the scattering particles and that the particles have negligible dimensions compared with the wavelength.

Lens

Because the lens is much thicker than the cornea and is composed of cells, we expect it to scatter more light than the cornea. This happens, with scatter increasing with age, and the forward-scatter being greater than the back-scatter (Bettelheim and Ali, 1985). Hemenger (1988, 1992) argued that the scattering is caused by the lens fibre lattice.

Fluorescence

Fluorescence is the absorption of radiation by a medium at one wavelength, and the immediate re-emission of radiation at longer wavelengths. The re-emission is isotropic and therefore, in the eye, tends to produce a uniform veiling glare on the retina.

Fluorescence occurs mostly in the lens, and increases with age and in people with cataract (Lerman and Borkman, 1976; Bleeker *et al.*, 1986; Siik *et al.*, 1993). The lens contains at least three fluorescent compounds; one called tryptophan, with a maximum sensitivity at 290 nm, and at least two fluorogens, with maximum sensitivities at 370 nm and 430 nm. Figure 12.5 shows the spectral emission properties of these compounds. Tryptophan is present at birth, and does not change greatly with age, but the two fluorogens are not present at birth and accumulate throughout life.

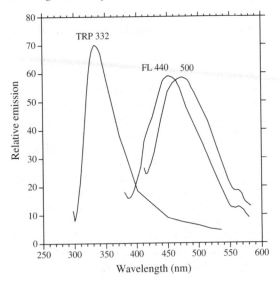

Figure 12.5. The fluorescent emission profiles of tryptophan and two fluorogens for a 78-year-old human lens (from Lerman and Borkman, 1978).

The veiling glare produced by fluorescence can lead to a small loss in visual acuity of low contrast targets, an effect that increases with age (Elliott *et al.*, 1993). The level of fluorescence depends upon the spectral sensitivity of the fluorescent compound and the spectral profile of the incident radiation–i.e. how much ultraviolet radiation and blue light is contained in the illuminating source. The contribution from tryptophan is minimized, because the cornea absorbs much of the activating wavelengths.

Birefringence

Optical materials such as water and glass are **isotropic**, which means that their physical properties are the same in all directions. This is because of the lack of atomic or molecular order. In contrast, many crystals have a well-defined atomic order. In some crystals, such as calcite, the physical properties (in particular the speed of light) depend upon direction of travel. This is referred to as **anisotropy**. Materials are called **birefringent** when the speed of light (or refractive index) depends not only on direction of travel, but also on the orientation of the electric field. This can occur in glass and plastics when they are placed under stress.

If unpolarized light enters a birefringent material, a phenomenon called double refraction occurs. The incident ray splits into two parts on entering the material, with the electric vectors of the rays at right angles to each other. These rays are now completely linearly polarized. One ray is refracted according to Snell's law and is called the ordinary ray. The other ray is called the extra-ordinary ray, and does not obey this law. Some materials have a particular direction or axis for which double refraction does not occur, and crystals with this property are called uniaxial crystals. They have two refractive indices, n_o for the ordinary ray and n_e for the extra-ordinary ray. The level of birefringence is quantified by the difference $(n_e - n_o)$ between these two refractive indices.

In biological materials there is usually little crystal-like atomic order, but there is sometimes order at the tissue structural level. This is called **form birefringence**, to allow differentiation from the **intrinsic birefringence** due to molecular arrangement. The eye exhibits some birefringence, mostly due to form birefringence. This can occur only where there is some regularity to the structure, and it occurs only in the cornea, lens and retina. In this section, we look at birefringence in the cornea and lens. Birefringence of the retina is covered in Chapter 14.

Cornea

As mentioned in the above *Scatter* section, the bulk of the cornea consists of the approximately 200 lamellae of the stroma, in which the fibrils are cylindrical in shape and are usually regularly spaced. The fibrils in adjacent layers lie at large and different angles. Thus, we would expect each layer of fibrils to exhibit form birefringence. According to Bour (1991), Wiener (1912) showed that an assembly of parallel rods immersed in a medium of lower index acts as a uniaxial crystal, with a positive birefringence with the optical axis in the direction of the rods. However, because of the large number of layers and their wide-ranging orientation, a light beam incident normally on the cornea would not encounter fibrils with any overall preferred orientation. Therefore, the cornea would not appear to be birefringent. On the other hand, a beam inclined to the corneal surface would undergo a slight birefringence. Bour and Lopez Cardozo (1981) estimated corneal birefringence to be +0.0020.

In contrast with the uniaxial model of the cornea, van Blokland and Verhelst (1987) argued that the cornea acts as a biaxial crystal, with the faster principal axis lying normal to the cornea and the slower axis lying nasally downwards.

Lens

The structure of the lens is different from that of the cornea. The lens consists of fibres (about 8 μm in diameter) that are laid down radially, rather than being parallel as in the cornea. Therefore, we would not expect the same level of birefringence. Weale (1979) gave values varying between -0.5×10^{-6} and -3.5×10^{-6}.

Summary of main symbols

n, n' refractive indices on the incident and refracted side of a surface
R Fresnel reflectance at a surface
T Fresnel transmittance at a surface

References

Beems, E. M. and van Best, J. A. (1990). Light transmission of the cornea in whole human eyes. *Exp. Eye Res.*, **50**, 393–5.

Bettelheim, F. A. and Ali, S. (1985). Light scattering of normal human lens III. Relationship between forward and backward scatter of whole excised lenses. *Exp. Eye Res.*, **41**, 1–9.

Bleeker, J. C., van Best, J. A., Vrij, L. *et al.* (1986). Autofluorescence of the lens in diabetic and healthy subjects by fluorophotometry. *Invest. Ophthal. Vis. Sci.*, **27**, 791–4.

Boettner, E. A. and Wolter, J. R. (1962). Transmission of the ocular media. *Invest. Ophthal.*, **1**, 776–83.

Bour, L. J. (1991). Polarized light and the eye. In *Vision and Visual Dysfunction*, vol. 1 of *Visual Optics and Instrumentation* (W. N. Charman, ed.), pp. 310–25. MacMillan.

Bour, L. J. and Lopez Cardozo, N. J. (1981). On the birefringence of the living human eye. *Vision Res.*, **21**, 1413–21.

Curcio, J. A. and Petty, C. C. (1951). The near infrared absorption spectrum of liquid water. *J. Opt. Soc. Am.*, **41**, 302–4.

Elliott, D. B., Yang, K. C. H., Dumbleton, K. and Cullen, A. P. (1993). Ultraviolet-induced lenticular fluorescence: intraocular straylight affecting visual function. *Vision Res.*, **33**, 1827–33.

Geeraets, W. J. and Berry, E. R. (1968). Ocular spectral characteristics as related to hazards from lasers and other light sources. *Am. J. Ophthal.*, **66**, 15–20.

Hart, R. W. and Farrell, R. A. (1969). Light scattering in the cornea. *J. Opt. Soc. Am.*, **59**, 766–74.

Hemenger, R. P. (1988). Small-angle intraocular light scatter: a hypothesis concerning its source. *J. Opt. Soc. Am. A.*, **5**, 577–82.

Hemenger, R. P. (1992). Sources of intraocular light scatter from inversion of an empirical glare function. *Applied Optics*, **31**, 3687–93.

Hogan M. J., Alvarado J. A. and Weddell J. E. (1971). *Histology of the Human Eye. An Atlas and Textbook*, p. 89. W. B. Saunders.

Hulburt, E. O. (1945). Optics of distilled and natural water. *J. Opt. Soc. Am.*, **35**, 698–705.

Johnson, C. A., Howard, D. L., Marshall, D. and Shu, H. (1993). A non-invasive video-based method of measuring lens transmission properties of the human eye. *Optom. Vis. Sci.*, **70**, 944–55.

Kerker, M. (1969). *The Scattering of Light*, p. 414. Academic Press.

Lerman, S. and Borkman, R. F. (1976). Spectroscopic evaluation and classification of the normal, aging and cataractous lens. *Ophthal. Res.*, **8**, 335–53.

Lerman, S. and Borkman, R. F. (1978). Ultraviolet radiation in the aging and cataractous lens. A survey. *Acta Ophthal.*, **56**, 139–49.

Ludvigh, E. and McCarthy, E. F. (1938). Absorption of visible light by the refractive media of the human eye. *Arch. Ophthal.*, **20**, 37–51.

McCally, R. L. and Farrell, R. A. (1988). Interaction of light and the cornea: light scattering versus transparency. In *The Cornea: Transactions of the World Congress on the Cornea III.* (H. D. Cavanagh, ed.), pp. 165–71. Raven Press.

Maurice, D. M. (1969). The cornea and sclera. In *The Eye*, vol. 1, 2nd edn. (H. Davson, ed.), pp. 486–600. Academic Press.

Mellerio, J. (1971). Light absorption and scatter in the human lens. *Vision Res.*, **11**, 129–41.

Pitts, D. G. (1978). The ocular effects of ultraviolet radiation. *Am. J. Optom. Physiol. Opt.*, **55**, 19–35.

Said, F. S. and Weale, R. J. (1959). The variation with age of the spectral transmissivity of the living human crystalline lens. *Gerontologia*, **3**, 213–31.

Siik, S., Airaksinen, P. J., Tuulonen, A. and Nieminen, H. (1993). Autofluorescence in cataractous human lens and its relationship to light scatter. *Acta Ophthal.*, **71**, 388–92.

Smith, R. C. and Baker, K. S. (1981). Optical properties of the clearest natural waters (200–800 nm). *Applied Opt.*, **20**, 177–84.

van Blokland, G. J. and Verhelst, S. C. (1987). Corneal

polarization in the living human eye explained with a biaxial model. *J. Opt. Soc. Am. A*, **4**, 82–90.

van den Berg, T. J. T. P., IJspeert, J. K. and de Waard, P. W. T. (1991). Dependence of intraocular straylight on pigmentation and light transmission through the ocular wall. *Vision Res.*, **31**, 1361–7.

van den Berg, T. J. T. P. and Tan, K. E. W. P. (1994). Light transmittance of the human cornea from 320 to 700 nm for different ages. *Vision Res.*, **34**, 1453–6.

Weale, R. A. (1979). Sex, age and the birefringence of the human crystalline lens. *Exp. Eye. Res.*, **29**, 449–61.

Weale, R. A. (1986). Real light scatter in the human crystalline lens. *Graefe's Arch. Clin. Exp. Ophthal.*, **224**, 463–6.

Wiener, O. (1912). Allgemaine Sätze über die Dielektrizitätskonstanten der Mischkörper. *Abh. Sächs. Ges. Akad. wiss. Math.-Phys. Kl.*, **32**, 574 (cited by Bour, L. J. (1991) and Weale, R. A. (1979)).

13

Light level at the retina

Introduction

In the previous chapter, we considered the transmittance of the ocular media. Given the spectral transmittance data of the media, we can determine the amount of radiation and light reaching the retina from a source of known spectral output. The results shown in Figure 12.2 indicate that 50–90 per cent of the light entering the eye reaches the retina as image-forming light (although it is important to be aware that results from different studies vary considerably, and there is considerable age-dependence).

Ideally, the spectral and spatial light distribution in the retinal image should be proportional to that in the object. In reality this is not so, because of the effects of aberrations, absorption, diffraction and scatter. Absorption and diffraction are wavelength-dependent, and aberrations, diffraction and scatter affect the spatial distribution. In this chapter, we assess the spatial light distribution in the image.

Retinal illuminance: directly transmitted light

In this section, we present equations that can be used to calculate the retinal light level or illuminance, given the brightness of the object (luminance of large area sources or luminous intensity for effectively point sources). We assume that the eye is correctly focused on that object, and therefore the equations are not strictly valid if the object is out of focus. If the level of defocus is small compared with the size of the object, the defocus has little effect on retinal illuminance except near the edge of the object. On the other hand, if the defocus is large compared to the size of the object, the equations give very misleading results. This is particularly so for point sources. Campbell (1994) presented a scheme for extended sources that can be used whether the eye is focused or not. Campbell's scheme is for calculating retinal irradiance, not retinal illuminance, but the equations apply equally to illuminance.

In this section, we consider only directly transmitted light, i.e. image forming light. To determine the retinal illuminance of images formed from this directly transmitted light, it is most convenient to divide this section into two parts; one dealing with on-axis imagery, and the other dealing with off-axis imagery.

On axis

Large area sources

For large area sources, small angle scatter, aberrations and diffraction can be neglected, and then the light distribution in the image has the same form as the object. When the eye is observing an object of large angular subtense which has a luminance L (cd/m^2), the corresponding retinal illuminance E' is given by the equation (Smith and Atchison, 1997)

$$E' = \tau \pi L n'^2 \sin^2(\alpha') \text{ lux} \qquad (13.1)$$

where τ is the transmittance of the ocular media (≈ 0.6 to 0.9) taking into account light losses due to reflection, absorption and scatter, n' is the refractive index of the vitreous humour (usually taken as 1.336), and α' is the half angular subtense of the exit pupil measured at the retina. We can re-express this equation in terms of the (entrance) pupil diameter D rather than the angle α' as

$$E' = \tau \pi L D^2 F^2 / 4 \text{ lux} \qquad (13.2a)$$

where F is the equivalent power of the eye and has a value of about 60 D.

We can also express the retinal illuminance in terms of area A of the (entrance) pupil, instead of its diameter D, as

$$E' = \tau L A F^2 \text{ lux} \qquad (13.2b)$$

Since the power of the average eye is close to 60 D, and if we take D and A in millimetre units, the above two equations can be approximated by the equations

$$E' \approx 0.002830 \tau L D^2_{mm} \text{ or} \approx 0.003600 \tau L A_{mm} \text{ lux} \qquad (13.2c)$$

The troland

The retinal illuminance is sometimes expressed in terms of trolands, which are the product of the object luminance L measured in cd/m^2 and the area A of the pupil measured in square millimetres. Thus the retinal illuminance E'_T in trolands for a source of luminance L and viewed through a pupil of area A_{mm} in square millimetres is give by the equation

$$E'_T = L A_{mm} \text{ trolands} \qquad (13.3a)$$

and since

$$A_{mm} = \pi D^2_{mm}/4$$

then

$$E'_T = \pi L D^2_{mm}/4 \text{ trolands} \qquad (13.3b)$$

Relationship between troland and lux

We can relate retinal illuminance E' in lux with retinal illuminance E'_T in troland by equation (13.2a) and equation (13.3b). In relating these two equations, we must use the same units for pupil diameter, and if we replace the pupil diameter D in equation (13.2a) (which is in metres) with the diameter D_{mm} in millimetres, we have

$$E' = \tau F^2 E'_T / 10^6 \text{ lux} \qquad (13.4a)$$

or

$$E'_T = 10^6 E' / (\tau F^2) \text{ troland} \qquad (13.4b)$$

If we now use the approximation that the power F is 60 D, we can write these equations as

$$E' = 0.0036 \tau E'_T \text{ lux} \qquad (13.5a)$$

or

$$E'_T = (278 / \tau) E' \text{ troland} \qquad (13.5b)$$

The point source – diffraction limited

The preceding equations do not apply for very small sources imaged without any aberration. In this case, the geometrical optical image is smaller than the diffraction limited point spread function, which has an angular radius

$$\theta = 1.22 \lambda / D \qquad (13.6)$$

In general, while the point spread function is affected by aberrations and diffraction, only the diffraction effect is easily predicted for any optical system.

The total luminous flux in the image of a point source, whether aberrated or not, is given by the equation (Smith and Atchison, 1997)

$$Flux = \frac{\tau \pi I D^2}{4 d^2} \qquad (13.7)$$

where d is the distance of the source and I is the luminous intensity of the source.

For the diffraction limited (i.e. aberration-free) image, the peak value of the illuminance is given by the equation (Smith and Atchison, 1997)

$$E' = \tau I \left[\frac{\pi F}{4 n' d \lambda} \right]^2 D^4 \qquad (13.8)$$

These equations demonstrate two useful results:

1. The total luminous flux in a point spread function is proportional to the square of the pupil diameter (i.e. proportional to pupil area).

2. The peak illuminance is proportional to the fourth power of the pupil diameter or the square of the area.

The point source – aberrated

The light distributions in real eyes and the effect of aberrations and diffraction are discussed in detail in Chapter 18.

Off-axis or peripheral sources

The retinal illuminance of off-axis sources is a little more complicated than for on-axis sources. In conventional optical systems such as a camera, the image plane illuminance decreases as the fourth power of the cosine of the peripheral angle, a result often known as the $\cos^4$ law. This is due to a combination of the following:

1. The reduction in apparent size of the peripheral pupil (proportional to cos (angle)).
2. The increase in distance from the exit pupil to the image on the image plane (the inverse square law, proportional to $\cos^2$ (angle)).
3. The inclination of the image plane to the direction of the incident beam (tilt, which is proportional to cos(angle)).

In the case of the eye, the $\cos^4$ law does not hold. While the effective pupil area decreases with distance off-axis, approximately as cos(angle), the curved shape of the retina means that the factors 2 and 3 above do not apply. The curved retina puts the image surface closer to the exit pupil, and tilts the normal to the surface in the direction of the exit pupil.

How the retinal light level depends upon peripheral angle is important in the measurement of visual fields and the calculation of the risk of the retina being damaged by hazardous radiation sources. Because of this importance, there have been a number of studies in the area (Drasdo and Fowler, 1974; Bedell and Katz, 1982; Kooijman, 1983; Kooijman and Witmer, 1986; Charman, 1989).

Using Figure 13.1, we examine this situation with a simple model of the eye looking at a plane Lambertian source of infinite subtense and of luminance L. Let us consider

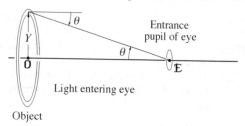

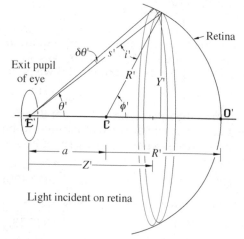

Figure 13.1. Geometry for calculating the retinal illuminance for peripheral large area sources. See text for details.

an annular zone of this source as shown in Figure 13.1. The luminous flux entering the pupil of the eye is given by the equation

$$Flux = 2\pi L A(\theta)_p \sin(\theta) \, \delta\theta \qquad (13.9)$$

where $A(\theta)_p$ is the projected or apparent area of the circular pupil in the direction of the source. This equation shows that the luminous flux incident on the pupil depends only upon the solid angle of the annulus, and not on its distance and shape.

If we now assume that this annular light source is focused on the retina, it is imaged as an annular zone on the retina as shown in the figure. The area of this zone is given by the equation

$$Area = s'\delta\theta'2\pi Y'/\cos(i') \qquad (13.10)$$

where the internal and external angles are connected by some function $\theta' = f(\theta)$. For small angles, paraxial theory predicts that

$$\tan(\overline{\theta}') = \overline{m} \tan(\theta) \qquad (13.11)$$

where $\overline{m}$ has a value of about 0.82 (Chapter 5). For larger angles, we should use a more accurate analysis (e.g. ray trace through a finite schematic eye) to determine the relationship, but we will leave this calculation for Chapters 15 and 16.

The retinal illuminance E' is the ratio of flux to illuminated area and thus is given by the equation

$$E' = \frac{LA(\theta)_p \sin(\theta)\cos(i')}{s'Y'(\delta\theta'/\delta\theta)} \qquad (13.12)$$

In order to calculate values for this equation, we need to relate s', Y' and i' to θ. We can do this as follows. First, from the figure we have

$$Y' = Z' \tan(\theta') \qquad (13.13a)$$

We can find the intersection (Y', Z') of this line with the retina, which we will assume to be circular in cross-section and described by the equation

$$Y'^2 + (Z' - a)^2 = R'^2 \qquad (13.13b)$$

and then we have

$$s' = \surd\,(Y'^2 + Z'^2) \qquad (13.13c)$$

$$\tan(\phi') = Y'/(Z' - a) \qquad (13.13d)$$

and

$$i' = \phi' - \theta' \qquad (13.13e)$$

and equation (13.11) gives

$$\delta\theta'/\delta\theta = \overline{m}\sec^2(\theta)/\sec^2(\theta') \qquad (13.14)$$

Figure 13.2 shows estimates of the relative retinal illuminance as a function of off-axis angle for a spherical retina ($R' = 12$ mm) and the distance $a = 8$ mm for a projected pupil area $A(\theta)_p$ falling off as $\cos(\theta)$. The relative retinal illuminance assuming the $\cos^4$ law is shown for comparison.

Figure 13.2 predicts that, as an object moves off-axis, the retinal illuminance decreases, although not as rapidly as predicted by the $\cos^4$ law. The simple model neglects a number of important factors:

1. The retina is not spherical.
2. The effective pupil of the eye is slightly larger at peripheral angles than that predicted by the simple cosine reduction (Chapter 3).
3. The exact relationship between the external angle θ and internal angle θ'. Equation (13.11) is only accurate for small angles. For larger angles, the aberrations affect the relationship between θ and θ'.

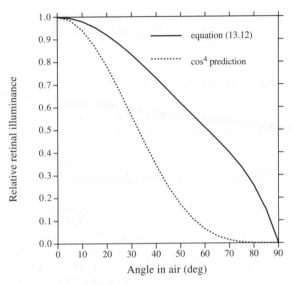

Figure 13.2. Variation of retinal illuminance with peripheral angle for a large area source, predicted from paraxial raytracing with a simple model eye.

4. Variation of ocular transmittance with peripheral angle. We expect the transmittance to decrease as peripheral angle increases because of the increase in path length within the lens.
5. Aberrations of the eye increase with increase in peripheral angle, and this will affect the illuminance distribution for small sources.

Kooijman and Witmer (1986) found that the light level in excised eyes reduces more slowly with increase in peripheral angle than given by the above theoretical predictions (Figure 13.2). In Chapter 16 we use more realistic models of the eye, with more accurate estimates of apparent pupil area $A(\theta)_p$ and of the relationship between external and internal angles θ and θ'.

Retinal illuminance: scattered light

As discussed in the previous chapter, a significant amount of light entering the eye is scattered forward, but out of the image-forming beam. In this section, we examine the light distribution due to scatter from a point source of light. This can be considered in terms of the retinal illuminance or an equivalent luminance of the image. Because we do not yet have accurate models of the complex nature of scatter, and because the light level on the retina is too low to be measured directly, the only determinations that can be made of the scattered light distribution are subjective measurements.

Several investigators have measured the light level at the retina due to scatter from a glare source in terms of the **equivalent veiling luminance**. In the presence of a glare source, the threshold luminance of a small patch of light was determined. The glare source was then turned off and the luminance L_v of a uniform background determined, which gave the same threshold for the small patch of light. This equivalent veiling luminance was fitted at the fovea $L_v(\theta)$ by equations of the form

$$L_v(\theta) = KE/\theta^n \tag{13.15}$$

where E is the illuminance in the plane of the eye of the glare source, θ is the off-axis angle in degrees of the glare source, and K and n are constants depending upon the particular investigation and the range of values of θ. Setting n to 2, this equation is well known as the Stiles–Holliday relationship. Some specific equations are as follows:

$$L_v(\theta) = 9.2\,E/\theta^2 \qquad 2.5° \le \theta \le 25°$$
$$\text{Holladay (1927)} \tag{13.16a}$$

$$L_v(\theta) = 4.16\,E/\theta^{1.5} \qquad 1° \le \theta \le 10°$$
$$\text{Stiles (1929)} \tag{13.16b}$$

$$L_v(\theta) = 29\,E/\theta^{2.8} \qquad 1° < \theta < 8°$$
$$\text{Vos and Bouman (1959)} \tag{13.16c}$$

$$L_v(\theta) = 29\,E/(\theta + 0.13)^{2.8} \qquad 0.15° < \theta < 8°$$
$$\text{Walraven (1973)} \tag{13.16d}$$

with $L_v(\theta)$ in cd/m^2, E in lux and θ in degrees.

Vos (1984) showed that, in young subjects, the equivalent veiling luminance is produced in approximately equal proportions by the cornea, lens and fundus. Scatter by the cornea and lens is discussed in Chapter 12, and scatter by the fundus is discussed in Chapter 14.

Various attempts at modelling the equivalent veiling luminance have been made. For example, Fry (1954) used a reduced schematic eye with a refractive index n' (1.333) and axial length t (20 mm), and derived the theoretical equation

$$L_v(\theta) = (2/3)tR\,E[\cot(\theta/n') - \cos(\theta/n')]/n'^2 \tag{13.17}$$

where R is a constant. If E is given a value of 1 and R is given a value of 3.39, this equation gives the same value of $L_v(\theta)$ at $5°$ as equations (13.16a) and (13.16b).

Effect of position in the lens of a scattering centre

It is often observed that the effect of a scattering centre is strongly dependent upon its position. For example, posterior polar cataracts have more severe effects on vision than cataracts of similar size that are situated more anteriorly. This has often been explained by the proximity of the scattering centre to the nodal points of the eye, but there is no optical reason why this should affect the scatter properties.

Measurement of angular distribution of scattered light

The light distribution of the image of a point source is known as the point spread function. The shape and width of the point spread function depend upon the levels of diffraction, aberrations and scatter, and upon the shape of the pupil. The effects of diffraction and aberration are discussed in Chapter 18, where it is shown that diffraction and aberrations produce a point spread function that has a half-width of a few minutes of arc. On the other hand, scatter causes light to be directed over much wider angles. Therefore, the light in the periphery of the point spread function is easily identified as scattered light. Close to the centre of the point spread function, most of the light is from both diffraction and aberrations, and it is difficult to extract the scattered component. For this reason, some investigators of scattered light (e.g. van den Berg, 1995) looked only at that component of light scattered through an angle greater than 1°.

Various methods have been developed to measure the angular distribution of scattered light. All of these methods assume that the scattering source has a very small angular subtense, and can therefore be regarded as a point source of light. Two subjective methods are described below.

Conventional threshold method

The essence of this method was given near the start of this section. The threshold luminance of a small patch of light is determined in the presence of a glare source. With the glare source turned off, the luminance of a uniform background is determined that produces the same threshold for the small patch of light. This luminance is the equivalent veiling luminance, and it is determined for a range of off-axis angles of the glare source.

Flicker method (e.g. van den Berg and IJspeert, 1992)

The glare source, which consists of annuli of various angular sizes, flickers at about 8 Hz. One of the annuli is illuminated. If the test patch in the middle of the annuli is very dim, the subject sees the test patch flicker because light is scattered onto the subject's fovea. The subject increases the luminance of the test patch, which flickers in counterphase to the glare source. When no flicker is apparent, the amount of luminance modulation of the test patch equals the amount of light scattered. This is determined for all the annuli of the glare source.

Photon density levels

Sometimes there is a need to express the light level at the retina in terms of photon or quantal density (e.g. photons/m^2/s), rather than in terms of lux or trolands. We can find an equation for this quantity by proceeding as follows.

Let us suppose that the spectral irradiance at the retina is $E'_r(\lambda)\Delta\lambda$ in the bandwidth $\Delta\lambda$. The corresponding number $N(\lambda)\Delta\lambda$ of

photons/m^2/s in the same bandwidth is given by the equation

$$N(\lambda)\Delta\lambda = \frac{E'_r(\lambda)\Delta\lambda}{h\upsilon} = \frac{E'_r(\lambda)\lambda\Delta\lambda}{hc} \qquad (13.18)$$

where h is Planck's constant (6.62620×10^{-34} J.s), c is the speed of light (2.99792×10^8 m/s), and υ is the frequency in Hertz. Weighting the photon density by a weighting function $W(\lambda)$ over the entire spectrum, we have

$$N_{tot} = \int \frac{E'_r(\lambda)W(\lambda)\lambda}{hc} \, d\lambda \qquad (13.19)$$

where $W(\lambda)$ may be the photopic or scotopic relative luminous efficiency functions, i.e. $V(\lambda)$ or $V'(\lambda)$. Now from equation (13.2a), for an extended source

$$E'_r(\lambda) = \tau\pi L_r(\lambda)D^2F^2/4 \qquad (13.20)$$

where $L_r(\lambda)$ is the corresponding spectral radiance of the source in W/(st. m^3). Equation (13.19) can now be written in the form

$$N_{tot} = \frac{\tau\pi D^2F^2}{4hc} \int L_r(\lambda)W(\lambda)\lambda d\lambda \text{ photons/m}^2/\text{s}$$
$$(13.21)$$

Black body source

The form of $L_r(\lambda)$ in the previous equation depends upon the nature of the source. One type of source of particular interest is the black body source. For a black body source of known temperature T Kelvin, the spectral radiance $L_r(\lambda)$ from Planck's law is

$$L_r(\lambda) = \frac{c_1}{\pi\lambda^5[e^{c_2/(\lambda T)} - 1]} \text{ W/(st. m}^3) \qquad (13.22)$$

where

$c_1 = 3.7418 \times 10^{-6}$ W.m^2 and
$c_2 = 1.4388 \times 10^{-2}$ m.K.

Real sources

For real sources, the amount of radiation emitted is always less than that of the black body, and the ratio of the emittances is the emissivity ε. That is

$$\varepsilon = \frac{\text{output of real source}}{\text{output of the black body at the same temperature}} \qquad (13.23)$$

This is usually a function of wavelength and temperature. However, for approximate calculations a constant value can be assumed, and values for various materials can be found in the *Handbook of Chemistry and Physics* (1975).

Maxwellian view

In many visual optical instruments, a small light source **S** provides a uniform field-of-view. If the entrance pupil of the eye coincides with the image **S'** of the source, the field-of-view has maximum width and maximum uniformity of luminance. This arrangement is called Maxwellian view (Figure 13.3). The exit pupil of the instrument at **E'** is uniformly illuminated, and subtends an angular radius α' to the eye. The eye is focused approximately on this exit pupil. If **S'** is much smaller than the entrance pupil of the eye, pupil fluctuations and small eye movements do not affect retinal illuminance.

Illumination and viewing with Maxwellian view is optically very different from conventional viewing. For example, the fact that the effective pupil may be much smaller than the normal pupil places limits on expected visual acuity. The illumination may no longer be completely incoherent, so that conventional incoherent image quality criteria such as the point spread and modulation transfer functions may no longer be valid (Westheimer, 1966). Here, only the light levels are considered.

Equivalent luminance of a Lambertian source

Based on equation (13.1), the light in the exit pupil of the instrument produces an illumi-nance E_1 at the plane of the entrance pupil of the eye, given by

$$E_1 = \pi L \sin^2(\alpha') \tag{13.24}$$

where L is the luminance of the instrument's exit pupil, and this exit pupil subtends an angular radius α' to the entrance pupil of the eye (Figure 13.3). If the image **S'** of the source **S** has an area A'_s, the luminous flux $Flux_1$ falling on the plane of the entrance pupil of the eye is given by

$$Flux_1 = E_1 A'_s = \pi L \sin^2(\alpha') A'_s \tag{13.25}$$

If **S'** is smaller than the entrance pupil of the eye, all of this flux falls on the retina, and the exit pupil appears to have a luminance L'.

If the observed bright field of the instrument exit pupil is replaced by a Lambertian source of the same luminance L', the illuminance E_2 in the plane of the entrance pupil of the eye is

$$E_2 = \pi L' \sin^2(\alpha') \tag{13.26}$$

Since the new source is Lambertian, light from it fills the pupil of the eye completely. If the entrance pupil of the eye has area A_p, the luminous flux $Flux_2$ falling on the plane of the entrance pupil of the eye is given by

$$Flux_2 = E_2 A_p = \pi L' \sin^2(\alpha') A_p \tag{13.27}$$

The illuminated area of the retina is the same in the cases given by equations (13.25) and (13.27), and therefore the ratio of retinal illuminances and hence luminances is the ratio of the fluxes entering the eye. Since the two luminances are equal, the fluxes are equal, and

$$\pi L' \sin^2(\alpha') A_p = \pi L \sin^2(\alpha') A'_s$$

Therefore

$$L' = L A'_s / A_p \tag{13.28}$$

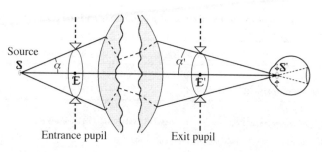

Figure 13.3. Maxwellian view.

As an example, if the area of the Maxwellian image is 2 mm^2, the area of the entrance pupil of the eye is 10 mm^2 and the luminance at the instrument exit pupil is 100 cd/m^2, the equivalent luminance of a Lambertian source is $100 \times 2/10 = 20$ cd/m^2.

Adapting pupil size

If the pupil is fully illuminated, pupil size affects retinal illuminance, which in turn controls pupil size. This feedback system cannot operate in Maxwellian view, where the source image is usually smaller than the smallest pupil size. Palmer (1966) found that, provided the source image in Maxwellian view is smaller than the natural pupil, the natural pupil is larger than is the case for the same light flux entering the eye in normal viewing.

The Stiles–Crawford effect

Stiles and Crawford (1933) discovered that the luminous efficiency of a beam of light entering the eye and incident on the fovea depends upon the entry point in the pupil. This phenomenon is known as the Stiles–Crawford effect of the first kind, but more generally as the Stiles–Crawford effect. Later, Stiles (1937) reported that varying the entry of the beam also altered the perceived saturation and hue of the light. This colour effect, called the Stiles–Crawford effect of the second kind, is not discussed further here.

The Stiles–Crawford effect is important to visual photometry and retinal image quality. It can be considered both as a neural and as an optical phenomenon, as it is retinal in origin and is explained as a consequence of the wave-guide properties of the photoreceptors. It is predominantly a cone phenomenon, and hence predominantly a photopic phenomenon. A good review of the Stiles–Crawford effect is given by Enoch and Lakshminarayanan (1991).

A number of different mathematical functions have been used to describe the Stiles–Crawford effect, with the most popular one being a Gaussian distribution as first used by Stiles (1937). This function is usually an excellent fit to experimental data out to 3 mm from the peak of the function, and has the addition virtue of simplicity. We describe the

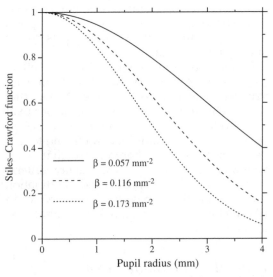

Figure 13.4. The Stiles–Crawford function for β values of 0.057, 0.116 and 0.173, which are 2.5 per cent, 50 per cent and 97.5 per cent population limits, respectively (Applegate and Lakshminarayanan, 1993).

Table 13.1. Some published values of the Stiles–Crawford β parameter and the position of the peak of the Stiles–Crawford function[a].

Investigation	No. subjects/eyes	$\beta \pm 1$ sd (mm^{-2})	peak ± 1 sd (mm)
Dunnewold (1964)[b]	29/47	–	0.37 ± 0.78 n, 0.29 ± 0.80 s[c]
Applegate and Lakshminarayanan (1993)[d]	49/49	0.116 ± 0.029[e]	0.47 ± 0.68 n, 0.20 ± 0.64 s

n – nasal; s – superior
[a]The β_{10} values in Applegate and Lakshminarayanan (1993) have been converted to β values using equation (13.29b).
[b]Relative to centre of pupil.
[c]Determined by Applegate and Lakshminarayanan (1993) from figure 45 of Dunnewold (1964).
[d]Relative to first Purkinje image.
[e]Mean of horizontal and vertical values.

Stiles–Crawford effect function $L_e(r)$ as

$$L_e(r) = \exp(-\beta r^2) \tag{13.29}$$

where r is the distance in the pupil from the peak of the function. The function is normalized to have a value of 1 at the peak. The Stiles–Crawford co-efficient β describes the steepness of the function, and is assumed to reflect the directionality (variation in alignment) of the photoreceptor population being tested. It may not have the same value for measurements in different meridians, particularly in eyes affected by retinal pathology. Measured β co-efficients for the large-scale study of Applegate and Lakshminarayanan (1993) are given in Table 13.1, and Figure 13.4 shows the Stiles–Crawford effect function for different β co-efficients. Combining the data across many studies gives a mean value of 0.12 (Applegate and Lakshminarayanan, 1993).

In many papers, the Stiles–Crawford effect function is given by equations similar to

$$L_e(r) = 10^{-\beta_{10} r^2} \tag{13.29a}$$

The co-efficients in equations (13.29) and (13.29a) are related by

$$\beta = \ln(10)\beta_{10} = 2.3026\beta_{10} \tag{13.29b}$$

Peak of the Stiles–Crawford effect

The position of the peak does not usually correspond to the centre of the pupil (which itself varies with pupil size), and it also varies between individuals. Its position is considered to reflect the overall alignment in the pupil of the photoreceptor population being tested. The ray distance r in the pupil should be measured from the peak. Measured values of the peak from two large-scale studies are given in Table 13.1. Combining the data across many studies gives mean values of ≈ 0.4 mm nasal and ≈ 0.2 mm superior relative to the pupil reference, whether this be the pupil centre or the pupillary axis (Applegate and Lakshminarayanan, 1993).

Photometric efficiency and reduced aperture model

Photometric efficiency

Although the Stiles–Crawford effect is a retinal phenomenon, the pupil of an eye with a Stiles–Crawford effect can be treated as being less efficient at transmitting light than a pupil of the same diameter when there is no Stiles–Crawford effect. We can quantify this using the concept of photometric efficiency. Following Martin (1961), we denote it as $S(\bar{\rho})$ and define it as

$$S(\bar{\rho}) = \frac{\text{Effective light collected by a pupil of radius } (\bar{\rho})}{\text{Actual light collected by the same pupil}} \tag{13.30}$$

We can write this as

$$S(\bar{\rho}) = \frac{\int_0^{\bar{\rho}} 2\pi L_e(r) r \, dr}{\pi \bar{\rho}^2} \tag{13.31}$$

If we use equation (13.29) for $L_e(r)$, the integral is easily solved to give

$$S(\bar{\rho}) = \frac{1 - \exp(-\beta\bar{\rho}^2)}{\beta\bar{\rho}^2} \tag{13.32a}$$

In terms of the entrance pupil diameter D, the photometric efficiency $S(D)$ is

$$S(D) = \frac{4[1 - \exp(-\beta D^2/4)]}{\beta D^2} \tag{13.32b}$$

Hence, if we express the luminance of an image in terms of the pupil area, we should multiply the latter by the appropriate factor $S(\bar{\rho})$ or $S(D)$.

Reduced aperture model

Sometimes we may want to know the diameter D^* of the equivalent, but smaller, pupil that would collect the same luminous flux if there was no Stiles–Crawford effect. The relationship is simply

$$D^* = D\sqrt{[S(\bar{\rho})]} \text{ or } D^* = D\sqrt{[S(D)]} \tag{13.33}$$

Figure 13.5 shows D^* as a function of D for various values of β.

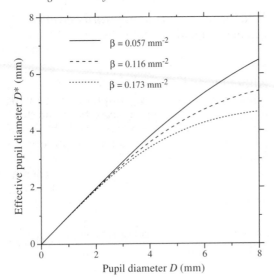

Figure 13.5. The photometric equivalent pupil diameter D^* as a function of pupil diameter D for β values of 0.057, 0.116 and 0.173.

Some factors influencing the Stiles–Crawford effect

Wavelength

The Stiles–Crawford effect varies with wavelength. For the fovea, it shows a minimum in the green and larger effects at both the short and long ends of the visible spectrum (Stiles, 1937 and 1939; Enoch and Stiles, 1961; Wijngaard and van Kruysbergen, 1975). Parafoveally (5° from the fovea) measured functions are minimal for blue and green regions of the spectrum, and increase only for the long wavelengths (Stiles, 1939). As an example, Stiles (1937) found for his own eye (foveal vision) that β varied between 0.13 and 0.17 over the visible spectrum. If allowance is made for lens absorption, estimates of the Stiles–Crawford effect increase, particularly at wavelengths less than 450 nm (Weale, 1961; Mellerio, 1971).

Eccentricity

Under photopic conditions, the Stiles–Crawford effect increases from the foveal centre out to approximately 2–3° eccentricity, where the value of β may have doubled, after which it declines slowly to reach foveal levels in the mid-periphery of the visual field (Enoch and Lakshminarayanan, 1991).

Luminance

The Stiles–Crawford effect exists also under scotopic conditions, but is small compared with the effect found under photopic conditions (Crawford, 1937; van Loo and Enoch, 1975). The magnitude of the effect makes a gradual change over the mesopic range.

Accommodation

Blank *et al.* (1975) reported that the peak of the Stiles–Crawford effect shifted between 0.4 mm and 1.0 mm nasally in three subjects with a 9 D increase in accommodative stimulus. They attributed this to retinal stretch during accommodation.

Theory

Since the discovery of the Stiles–Crawford effect, a number of explanations have been offered for it. Most theories are based around the assumption that the photoreceptors act as wave-guides.

O'Brien's (1946) geometric optical theory of the Stiles–Crawford effect considered that the cones act as wave-guides, using total internal reflection to channel the light to the photopigment. As the ray position in the pupil increases away from the centre, the rays enter the cones at a larger angle to increase the angle of incidence on the internal wall of the cones and hence increase the probability of light loss through the walls. His theory does not explain the influence of wavelength adequately. A comprehensive theory was presented by Snyder and Pask (1973). They modified the wave-guide model by using a physical optical approach, which better predicts the Stiles–Crawford effect, including the effect of wavelength.

Measurement

The Stiles–Crawford effect has been measured by a number of subjective and objective techniques (Enoch and Lakshminarayanan,

1991). The values of β and the peak position mentioned in this section are from subjective methods. Subjective techniques include flicker photometry and photometric matching. Objective methods include fundus reflectometry, consensual pupillary response, the electroretinogram, and the visual evoked response.

Role of the Stiles–Crawford effect

As mentioned at the start of this section, the Stiles–Crawford effect is important in visual photometry and retinal image quality. Concerning visual photometry, it reduces the effective retinal illuminance at photopic lighting levels. As discussed earlier, and as given by equations (13.32) and (13.33), this is equivalent to having a smaller effective pupil size.

The Stiles–Crawford effect reduces the detrimental effects of scattered light on retinal image quality at photopic lighting levels, although the extent to which this improves visual performance is not known (Enoch, 1972). In a similar fashion, it reduces the effects of defocus and aberrations on retinal image quality and thus reduces their influence on visual performance. The Stiles–Crawford effect can be included in optical modelling of the eye as an **apodization**, which means that it can be treated as an optical filter of variable density placed at the pupil. Its influence in this respect, as discussed further in Chapter 18, seems to be small.

Summary of main symbols

General

A	area of the pupil in square metres
A_{mm}	area of the pupil in square millimetres
D	pupil diameter in metres
D_{mm}	pupil diameter in millimetres
E'	retinal illuminance in lux
F	equivalent power of the eye in dioptres (i.e. m^{-1})
L	luminance of an extended source in cd/m^2
r	ray height in pupil
τ	mean luminous transmittance of ocular media of the eye

Retinal illuminance: directly transmitted light

E'_T	retinal illuminance in trolands
I	luminous intensity of a point source in cd

Retinal illuminance: scattered light

E	illuminance in plane of eye
$L_v(\theta)$	equivalent veiling luminance in a direction θ

Photon density levels

$N(\lambda)\Delta\lambda$	photon density in photons/m^2/s

Maxwellian view

A_p	area of pupil of eye
A'_s	area of image of light source, imaged in the pupil plane of the eye
L'	apparent luminance of field

Stiles–Crawford effect

$L_e(r)$	luminous efficiency for a ray entering pupil at a height r
β	Stiles–Crawford co-efficient
$S(\bar{\rho})$	photometric efficiency for pupil radius $\bar{\rho}$
$S(D)$	photometric efficiency for pupil diameter D
D^*	diameter of equivalent pupil

References

Applegate, R. A. and Lakshminarayanan, V. (1993). Parametric representation of Stiles–Crawford functions: normal variation of peak location and directionality. *J. Opt. Soc. Am. A*, **10**, 1611–23.

Bedell, H. E. and Katz, L. M. (1982). On the necessity of correcting peripheral target luminance for pupillary area. *Am. J. Optom. Physiol. Opt.*, **59**, 767–9.

Blank, K., Provine, R. P. and Enoch, J. M. (1975). Shift in the peak of the photopic Stiles–Crawford function with marked accommodation. *Vision Res.*, **15**, 499–507.

Campbell, C. (1994). Calculation method for retinal irradiance from extended sources. *Ophthal. Physiol. Opt.*, **14**, 326–9.

Charman, W. N. (1989). Light on the peripheral retina. *Ophthal. Physiol. Opt.*, **9**, 91–2.

Crawford, B. H. (1937). The luminous efficiency of light rays entering the eye pupil at different points and its relation to brightness threshold measurements. *Proc. R. Soc. B.*, **124**, 81–96.

Drasdo, N. and Fowler, C. W. (1974). Non-linear projection of the retinal image in a wide-angle schematic eye. *Br. J. Ophthal.*, **58**, 709–14.

Dunnewold, C. J. (1964). *On the Campbell and Stiles–Crawford effects and their Clinical Importance.*

Institute for Perception. The Netherlands National Defence Research Organisation RVOTNO.

Enoch, J. M. (1972). Retinal receptor orientation and the role of fiber optics in vision. *Am. J. Optom. Arch. Am. Acad. Optom.*, **49**, 455–71.

Enoch, J. M. and Lakshminarayanan, V. (1991). Retinal fibre optics. In *Visual Optics and Instrumentation*, vol. 1 of Cronly-Dillon, J. R. *Vision and Visual Dysfunction* (W. N. Charman, ed.). Macmillan Press.

Enoch, J. M. and Stiles, W. S. (1961). The colour change of monochromatic light with retinal angle of incidence. *Optica Acta*, **8**, 329–58.

Fry, G. A. (1954). A re-evaluation of the scattering theory of glare. *Illuminating Engineering*, **49**, 98–102.

Handbook of Chemistry and Physics (1975). Weast, R. C. (ed.). 56th edn. CRC Press.

Holladay, L. L. (1927). Action of a light-source in the field of view in lowering visibility. *J. Opt. Soc. Am.*, **14**, 1–15.

Kooijman, A. C. (1983). Light distribution on the retina of a wide-angle theoretical eye. *J. Opt. Soc. Am.*, **73**, 1544–50.

Kooijman, A. C. and Witmer, F. K. (1986). Ganzfeld light distribution on the retina of human and rabbit eyes: calculations and *in vitro* measurements. *J. Opt. Soc. Am. A*, **3**, 2116–20.

Martin, L. C. (1961). *Technical Optics Vol II*, pp. 247–8. Pitman and Sons.

Mellerio, J. (1971). Light absorption and scatter in the human lens. *Vision Res.*, **11**, 129–41.

O'Brien, B. (1946). A theory of the Stiles and Crawford effect. *J. Opt. Soc. Am.*, **36**, 506–9.

Palmer, D. A. (1966). The size of the human pupil in viewing through optical instruments. *Vision Res.*, **6**, 471–7.

Smith, G. and Atchison, D. A. (1997). *The Eye and Visual Optical Instruments*, pp. 286, 308, 547. Cambridge University Press.

Snyder, A. W. and Pask, C. (1973). The Stiles–Crawford effect – explanation and consequences. *Vision Res.*, **13**, 1115–37.

Stiles, W. S. (1929). The effect of glare in the brightness difference threshold. *Proc. R. Soc. B.*, **104**, 322–51.

Stiles, W. S. (1937). The luminous efficiency of monochromatic rays entering the eye pupil at different points and a new colour effect. *Proc. R. Soc. B.*, **123**, 90–118.

Stiles, W. S. (1939). The directional sensitivity of the retina and the spectral sensitivities of the rods and cones. *Proc. R. Soc. B.*, **127**, 64–105.

Stiles, W. S. and Crawford, B. H. (1933). The luminous efficiency of rays entering the eye pupil at different points. *Proc. R. Soc. B.*, **112**, 428–50.

van den Berg, T. J. J. P. (1995). Analysis of intraocular straylight, especially in relation to age. *Optom. Vis. Sci.*, **72**, 52–9.

van den Berg, T. J. T. P. and IJspeert, J. K. (1992). Clinical assessment of intraocular stray light. *Applied Optics*, **31**, 3694–6.

Van Loo, J. A. and Enoch, J. M. (1975). The scotopic Stiles–Crawford effect. *Vision Res.*, **15**, 1005–9.

Vos, J.J. (1984). Disability glare – a state of the art report. *CIE-J*, **3**(2), 39–53.

Vos, J. J. and Bouman, M. A. (1959). Disability glare; theory and practice. *Proc. CIE*, Brussels 1959, 298–306.

Walraven, J. (1973). Spatial characteristics of chromatic induction; the segregation of lateral effects from straylight artefacts. *Vision Res.*, **13**, 1739–53.

Weale, R. A. (1961). Notes on the photometric significance of the human crystalline lens. *Vision Res.*, **1**, 183–91.

Westheimer, G. (1966). The Maxwellian View. *Vision Res.*, **6**, 669–82.

Wijngaard, W. and van Kruysbergen, J. (1975). The function of the non-guided light in some explanations of the Stiles–Crawford effects. In *Photoreceptor Optics* (A. H. Snyder and R. Menzel, eds), pp. 175–83. Springer-Verlag.

14

Light interaction with the fundus

Introduction

As well as the absorption of light by the retinal photoreceptors, which initiates the neural processes of vision, other interactions of light with the **fundus** of the eye (a term that generally includes the retina, choroid and sclera) are important. Light from the fundus that passes out of the eye is essential for the diagnosis of ocular disease in ophthalmoscopy. Light from the fundus passing out of the eye is also important for determination of refractive error by retinoscopy and other objective techniques (Chapter 8). The spectral absorption by the fundus is important for understanding the processes of retinal damage by excessive light levels. In this chapter, we examine the specular reflection, scatter and absorption of light at the fundus.

These properties are affected by the optical properties of the fundus layers (see Figure 1.3). Of particular importance are four absorbing pigments: macular pigment in the retina, visual pigments in the photoreceptors, melanin mainly in the pigment epithelium, and haemoglobin mainly in the choroid. There are individual and racial differences in the amount of the pigments, particularly melanin (Hammond *et al.*, 1997). We will consider specular reflection, scatter and absorption at the layers along a typical ray path.

Inner limiting membrane to photoreceptors (six layers)

Light is first incident on the retina at the inner limiting membrane, and there will be some specular reflection at this boundary. The six layers between this boundary and the photoreceptors are highly transparent, but the regular array of the fibres in the nerve fibre layer has some effect on polarized light. There is a yellow pigment called xanthophyll in the macula (the macula pigment), and the amount of this pigment varies greatly between individuals (Ruddock, 1963; Bone and Sparrock, 1971).

The photoreceptors

Some light is then absorbed by the visual pigments in the photoreceptors. There is little data available on the proportion of light incident on the retina which is absorbed by the visual pigments and, therefore, contributes to visual perception, but the proportion will vary with state of light adaptation, retinal location and spectral light distribution. Rodieck (1998) made some estimations of the proportion of light which stimulates vision for a large pupil (≈ 7mm diameter) when looking directly at a star. Ninety-two per cent of the light incident at the inner limiting membrane reaches the cones after absorption by the macular pigment. Of this amount, 53% reaches the cone outer segments which contain the visual pigments. Of this amount, 38% is absorbed by visual pigment. Finally, 67% of this amount results in a photochemical reaction. Combining these proportions gives a retinal 'efficiency' of 12%. Combining this 12% with the 54% of the light incident on the cornea which reaches the retina, approximately 7% of the light incident at the cornea is responsible for initiating the neural responses in the retina and beyond. Rodieck made estimations at 15° eccentricity to obtain a similar overall result for the rods of the dark adapted retina.

The pigment epithelium

The remaining light passes into the pigment epithelium, where there is strong absorption and scatter by melanin granules. Some light passes through the pigment epithelium and enters the choroid.

The choroid

The thin (350–450 μm) choroid is highly vascularized, but contains some melanin. Thirty to sixty per cent of the choroid is blood (Delori and Pflibsen, 1989). This contains haemoglobin, which is mainly oxygenated and strongly absorbs short wavelength light and back-scatters longer wavelengths. A small amount of light penetrates the choroid to reach the sclera.

The sclera

This dense, whitish tissue back-scatters light strongly, so that most light reaching the sclera passes back through the retina.

Fundus reflectance

The term fundus reflectance refers to the light specularly reflected and scattered at the fundus and which eventually passes back out of the eye. Fundus reflectance can be measured by illuminating the fundus with a light source and analysing the spectrum of light emerging from the eye. However, this is complicated by a number of factors:

1. *In vivo* spectral reflectance measurements involve the passage of light through the ocular media twice. We know from Chapter 12 that the ocular media absorb light, and that this absorption is not spectrally neutral. The effect of the spectral absorption of the ocular media is thus doubled.
2. *In vivo* results are contaminated by specular reflections from the refracting surfaces.
3. Reflectance measurements must use a reference baseline, which is often taken to be a white tile of high, diffuse reflectance, such as one based upon magnesium oxide.
4. Pigment absorption by the photoreceptors depends upon the level of bleaching and hence their immediate previous light exposure.

Measured values of fundus reflectance are shown in Figure 14.1. Reflectance is low at short wavelengths, and gradually increases with increase in wavelength. The high reflectance at the longer wavelengths is attributed to the blood in the choroid.

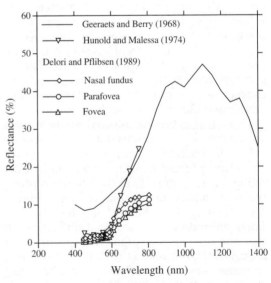

Figure 14.1. Spectral reflectance of the fundus from Geeraets and Berry (1968) – reflectance of pigment epithelium and choroid, Hunold and Malessa (1974) – derived from their extinction values, and Delori and Pflibsen (1989) – *in vivo* measurements on 10 normal subjects at different retinal locations.

Polarized light

Some early workers in ocular polarization concluded that most polarized light incident upon the fundus is depolarized upon return out of the eye. This was because conversion of linear polarized light into elliptical polarized light was mistaken as depolarization (van Blokland, 1985). More recent studies have found that most polarization is retained, although the orientation of polarization may change (birefringence). Van Blokland (1985) found about 90 per cent retention (fovea, 514 nm) and Dreher *et al.* (1992) found 50–80 per cent retention (close to the optic disc, 633 nm). Van Blokland and van Norren (1986) found that the retained polarization at the fovea decreases with increase in wavelength ($\approx$ 90 per cent at 488 nm and $\approx$ 40 per cent at 647 nm).

Guided and unguided light

Some of the light incident on the retinal pigment epithelium is returned within the outer segments of photoreceptors, and can be considered to be guided or directed (van Blokland and van Norren, 1986). The rest of the returned light may be considered to be unguided. Burns *et al.* (1995 and 1997) developed and used an objective instrument for measuring cone photoreceptor alignment by measuring the distribution of light returning from the retina corresponding to different positions of a small light source at the pupil. The distribution is affected by the guiding of light along the photoreceptors. For bleached retinas, this produced functions with peak pupil positions that match those obtained by psychophysical measurements of the Stiles–Crawford effect (see Chapter 13, *The Stiles–Crawford effect*).

Layers responsible for the fundus reflectance

On the basis that different components of reflectance (polarized versus unpolarized, and guided versus unguided) showed similar dependencies on wavelength, van Blokland and van Norren proposed a simple model in which one layer is mainly responsible for the fundus reflectance. Because the wavelength dependence of the fundus reflectance was similar to that of the retinal pigment epithelium, they suggested that the retinal pigment epithelium is this layer. This argument was supported by the fact that the guided component increased with increased bleaching of retinal pigment, an effect that would not occur if the responsible layer was in front of the receptors. More sophisticated models have been developed since with van de Kraats *et al.* (1996) proposing that the outer aspects of the cones are responsible for the guided component of reflectance.

Veiling glare

Some of the light scattered by the fundus will contribute to veiling glare, because light that is scattered sideways (**halation**) and backwards can illuminate photoreceptors, some a long way from the original site of incidence. The Stiles–Crawford effect may reduce the luminous efficiency of this scattered light. Veiling glare is reduced for people with dark irides compared with people with light irides, and this has been attributed largely to the level of fundus pigmentation (IJspeert *et al.*, 1990; van den Berg, 1995).

Absorption

Light that is not specularly reflected or scattered back out of the eye from the fundus is either absorbed or scattered in other directions within the eye. Since scattered light has the potential to excite photoreceptors in other parts of the fundus, one would expect the fundus to preferentially absorb rather than scatter. The layers of the retina in front of the cones and rods are highly transparent. Absorption is due mainly to visual pigments in the photoreceptors, melanin in the pigment epithelium, and haemoglobin in the choroid.

Figure 14.2a shows spectral absorption of the pigment epithelium and choroid (Geeraets and Berry, 1968). Figure 14.2b shows spectral absorption of oxygenated hemoglobin (van Assendelft, 1970), and Figure

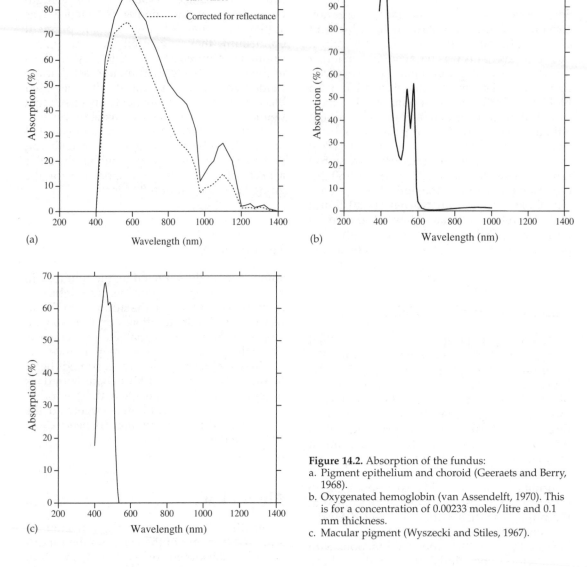

Figure 14.2. Absorption of the fundus:
a. Pigment epithelium and choroid (Geeraets and Berry, 1968).
b. Oxygenated hemoglobin (van Assendelft, 1970). This is for a concentration of 0.00233 moles/litre and 0.1 mm thickness.
c. Macular pigment (Wyszecki and Stiles, 1967).

14.2c shows spectral absorption of the macular pigment (Wyszecki and Stiles, 1967).

Birefringence

Birefringence has been discussed in Chapter 12 (*Birefringence*) with regard to the media of the eye. In birefringent materials, refractive index depends upon the direction of the light beam and upon the direction of the electric vector. The retinal nerve fibre layer exhibits birefringence because of the structure of the nerve fibres and their regular arrangement (Dreher *et al.*, 1992). The nerve fibres form a radial pattern centred on the optic disc but, because over short distances neighbouring fibres can be regarded as parallel, the nerve fibres can be regarded as a layer of long parallel cylinders perpendicular to the retinal surface. Such an arrangement acts as a uniaxial crystal, with its optic axis being parallel to the axis of the cylinders and perpendicular to the incident light. The refractive index will be at minimum for the electric vector perpendicular to the nerve fibre direction and maximum for the electric vector parallel to the nerve fibres. The arrangement of nerve fibres is similar to the fibril layers in the cornea (Chapter 12, *Scatter*), but whereas the corneal fibril diameters are smaller than the wavelength of light, the nerve fibre diameters in the retina are about the same size or larger than the incident wavelengths (0.6–2.0 μm, Hogan *et al.*, 1971).

There have been several *in vivo* studies of retinal birefringence, for example, van Blokland (1985) and Dreher *et al.* (1992). Measurements of retinal birefringence must take into account or eliminate any birefringence from the cornea.

Birefringence of the nerve fibre layer has an application in scanning laser polarimetry (Dreher *et al.*, 1992; Weinreb *et al.*, 1995), which estimates nerve fibre loss due to diseases such as glaucoma. Red or near infrared light from a laser, initially linearly polarized, passes into the retina. It is scattered from the deeper retinal layers and the choroid to pass back out of the eye. The plane of polarization is changed by its passage (twice) through the nerve fibre layer. The degree of polarization change is used to estimate nerve fibre layer thickness, and the thickness is determined at the retinal area of interest.

References

Bone, R. A. and Sparrock, J. M. B. (1971). Comparison of macular pigment densities in human eyes. *Vision Res.*, **11**, 1057–64.

Burns, S. A., Wu, S., Delori, F. and Elsner, A. E. (1995). Direct measurement of human-cone photoreceptor alignment. *J. Opt. Soc. Am. A.*, **12**, 2329–38.

Burns, S. A., Wu, S., He, J. C. and Elsner, A. E. (1997). Variations in photoreceptor directionality across the central retina. *J. Opt. Soc. Am. A*, **14**, 2033–40.

Delori, F. C. and Pflibsen, K. P. (1989). Spectral reflectance of the human ocular fundus. *Appl. Optics*, **28**, 1061–77.

Dreher, A. W., Reifer, K. and Weinreb, R. M. (1992). Spatially resolved birefringence of the retinal nerve fiber layer assessed with a retinal laser ellipsometer. *Appl. Optics*, **31**, 3730–35.

Geeraets, W. J. and Berry, E. R. (1968). Ocular spectral characteristics as related to hazards from lasers and other light sources. *Am. J. Ophthal.*, **66**, 15–20.

Hammond, B. R., Wooten, B. R. and Snodderly, D. M. (1997). Individual variations in the spatial profile of human macular pigment. *J. Opt. Soc. Am. A*, **14**, 1187–96.

Hogan, M. J., Alvarado, J. A. and Weddell, J. E. (1971). *Histology of the Human Eye*, p. 483. W. B. Saunders and Co.

Hunold, W. and Malessa, P. (1974). Spectrophotometric determination of the melanin pigmentation of the human fundus *in vivo*. *Ophthal. Res.*, **6**, 355–62.

Ijspeert, J. K., de Waard, P. W. T., van den Berg, T. J. J. P. and de Jong, P. T. V. M. (1990). The intraocular straylight function in 129 healthy volunteers; dependence on angle, age and pigmentation. *Vision Res.*, **30**, 699–707.

Rodieck, R. W. (1998). Chapters 4 and 6. *The first steps in seeing*. Sinauer, pp. 68–87, 122–33.

Ruddock, K. H. (1963). Evidence for macular pigmentation from colour matching data. *Vision Res.*, **3**, 417–29.

van Assendelft, O. W. (1970). *Spectrophotometry of Haemoglobin Derivatives*. Royal VanGorcum.

van Blokland, G. J. (1985). Ellipsometry of the human retina *in vivo*: preservation of polarization. *J. Opt. Soc. Am. A*, **2**, 72–5.

van Blokland, G. J. and van Norren, D. (1986). Intensity and polarization of light scattered at small angles from the human fovea. *Vision Res.*, **26**, 485–94.

van de Kraats, J., Berendschot, T. T. J. M. and van Norren, D. (1996). The pathways of light measured in fundus reflectometry. *Vision Res.*, **36**, 2229–47.

van den Berg, T. J. J. P. (1995). Analysis of intraocular straylight, especially in relation to age. *Optom. Vis. Sci.*, **72**, 52–9.

Weinreb, R. N., Shakiba, S. and Zangwill, L. (1995). Scanning laser polarimetry to measure the nerve fiber layer of normal and glaucomatous eyes. *Am. J. Ophthal.*, **119**, 627–36.

Wyszecki, G. and Stiles, W. S (1967). *Color Science. Concepts and Methods, Quantitative Data and Formulas*, pp. 218–19. John Wiley and Sons.

Section 4:

Aberrations and retinal image quality

15

Monochromatic aberrations

Introduction

Like defocus, aberrations reduce the image quality of optical systems such as the eye. When an eye is corrected by ophthalmic lenses, we are mainly correcting defocus but are actually finding a balance between defocus and aberrations. Defocus is the most important optical defect of eyes, and it should be appreciated that aberrations are usually only of consequence for an eye well-corrected for defocus.

The representation of aberrations of optical systems depends on what is most convenient in the particular circumstances. These representations include the following (Figure 15.1a):

1. Wave aberration. This is departure of the wavefront from the ideal waveform, as measured at the exit pupil.
2. Transverse aberration. This is the departure of a ray from its ideal position at the image surface.
3. Longitudinal aberration. The departure of the intersection, where this occurs, of a ray with a reference axis (i.e. the pupil ray) from its ideal intersection.

Because we cannot easily measure the aberrations on the image side of the eye's optical system, the aberrations of the eye are usually measured in object space (Figure 15.1b). All but one method of measuring aberrations of the eye described in this chapter work in this fashion. Provided that

the aberration and defocus levels are not unduly high, these 'object' aberrations are similar to 'image' aberrations. When the aberrations are large, such as in the case of peripheral vision, this is no longer the case.

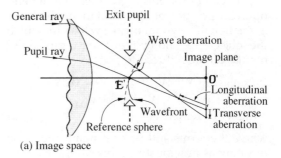

(a) Image space

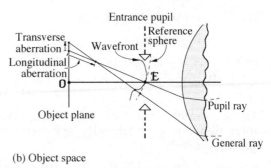

(b) Object space

Figure 15.1. Wave, transverse and longitudinal aberrations:
a. For a general optical system.
b. For the eye, when these must be determined in object space.
Note that longitudinal aberration occurs for a ray only when it intersects the reference ray (i.e. pupil ray).

The aberrations of a general optical system with a point object can be represented by a wave aberration polynomial (or function) of the form

$$W(X,Y) = W_1X + W_2Y + W_3X^2 + W_4XY$$
$$+ W_5Y^2 + W_6X^3 + W_7X^2Y + W_8XY^2 + W_9Y^3$$
$$+ W_{10}X^4 + W_{11}X^3Y + W_{12}X^2Y^2 + W_{13}XY^3$$
$$+ W_{14}Y^4 + \text{higher order terms} \tag{15.1}$$

where X and Y are co-ordinates in the entrance pupil. The co-efficients can be described as follows:

W_1 and W_2	tilt (prismatic or distortion) co-efficients
W_3, W_4 and W_5	defocus and astigmatism co-efficients
W_6, W_7, W_8 and W_9	'coma-like' co-efficients
W_{10}, W_{11}, W_{12}, W_{13} and W_{14}	'spherical aberration-like' co-efficients

The values of these co-efficients depend upon the position of the object in the field. For a rotationally symmetrical system in which the object lies along the Y-axis, this polynomial can be reduced to

$$W(X,Y) = W_2Y + W_3X^2 + W_5Y^2 + W_7X^2Y$$
$$+ W_9Y^3 + W_{10}X^4 + W_{12}X^2Y^2 + W_{14}Y^4$$
$$+ \text{higher order terms} \tag{15.2}$$

where the terms still present retain the same meaning as previously. In this case,

$$W_7 = W_9 \text{ and } W_{10} = W_{14} = 0.5 \, W_{12}$$

so we can now write

$$W(X,Y) = W_2Y + W_3X^2 + W_5Y^2 + W_7Y(X^2$$
$$+ Y^2) + W_{10}(X^2 + Y^2)^2 + \text{higher order terms} \tag{15.3}$$

An alternative way of expressing the aberrations of a rotationally symmetrical optical system is

$$W(\eta;X,Y) = {}_0W_{4,0}(X^2 + Y^2)^2 + {}_1W_{3,1}\eta(X^2 + Y^2)Y$$
$$+ {}_2W_{2,0}\eta^2(X^2 + Y^2) + {}_2W_{2,2}\eta^2Y^2 + {}_3W_{1,1}\eta^3Y$$
$$+ \text{higher order terms} \tag{15.4}$$

where η indicates dependence on the position of the object in the field. The first five terms in this expansion are known as mono-

chromatic **primary aberrations** or **third order aberrations**, and the co-efficients are as follows:

${}_0W_{4,0}$	spherical aberration co-efficient	${}_1W_{3,1}$	coma co-efficient
${}_2W_{2,0}$	field curvature co-efficient	${}_2W_{2,2}$	astigmatism co-efficient
${}_3W_{1,1}$	distortion co-efficient		

The significance of the term 'primary' is explained in Appendix 2, where general aberration theory is discussed. Of these five monochromatic aberrations, only spherical aberration occurs on-axis for a rotationally symmetric system. The other four occur only off-axis for a rotationally symmetric system, and generally worsen with increase in distance off-axis. There are two other primary aberrations called chromatic aberrations, which become manifest when more than one wavelength is imaged by an optical system. We will leave the chromatic aberrations until Chapter 17.

Eyes are not rotationally symmetric about an appropriate reference axis such as the line-of-sight or the visual axis. Consequently, ocular aberrations are not described well by equations such as equations (15.2), (15.3) and (15.4), but require the use of an equation such as equation (15.1). Contributors to this lack of rotational symmetry are the difference between the best-fit optical axis and the line-of-sight (because of component tilts and displacements), the lack of rotational symmetry of refracting surfaces, and possibly a lack of rotational symmetry of the lens refractive index.

Methods of measuring monochromatic aberrations

Aberrations of the eye have been noted and measured since at least the time of Thomas Young (1801). Some methods have measured the tranverse aberration and others longitudinal aberration, usually in the form of the refraction required. Other aberration forms, for example the wave aberration, can usually be derived from these values.

Subjective methods

Vernier alignment

Transverse aberrations are measured in this technique. The technique is closely related to the coincidence technique for refraction described in *Subjective/objective refraction techniques* in Chapter 8. Light from a reference target passes through a reference part of the pupil, and light from a test target passes through another pupil location. If there is no aberration of the ray bundle associated with the second pupil location, the targets appear aligned when they have the same location in space. If there is aberration of the ray bundle, the targets do not appear aligned. The linear or transverse movement of one target necessary to achieve apparent alignment is then a measure of tranverse aberration. Typically the two targets are thin lines, to take advantage of the visual system's ability to make precise vernier alignments.

There have been many variations of the technique – for example, Ames and Proctor (1921), Ivanoff (1953), Smirnov (1962), Jenkins (1963a), Schober *et al.* (1968), Campbell *et al.* (1990), Woods *et al.* (1996), Cui and Lakshminarayanan (1998), and He *et al.* (1998). One variation by Woods *et al.* (1996) of the technique is shown in Figure 15.2. The subject aligns a laser spot projected onto a diffuse reflector with the gap between a co-linear pair of lines displayed on a computer monitor. The vertical lines are visible through the entire pupil, while the spot is visible only through a 0.75 mm diameter aperture in a polaroid filter. The aperture is translated horizontally across the pupil in steps, and the subject adjusts the location of the vertical lines until these are aligned subjectively with the spot. Woods and colleagues fitted the tranverse aberrations to a polynomial up to the fifth power of the form

$$TA(X) = A_0 + A_1X + A_2X^2 + A_3X^3 + A_4X^4 + A_5X^5 \tag{15.5}$$

where $TA(X)$ is the transverse ray aberration at the computer monitor, X is the horizontal ray location in the entrance pupil, and A_0 to A_5 are co-efficients. Figure 15.3 shows the results for one subject.

Transverse ray aberration measurements along a meridian can be converted into longitudinal aberrations LA (X). If the distance from the eye's entrance pupil to the targets is l_0 and the distance from the entrance pupil to where the test ray intersects the reference axis is l, from similar triangles in Figure 15.4

$$TA(X)/X = (l - l_0)/l$$

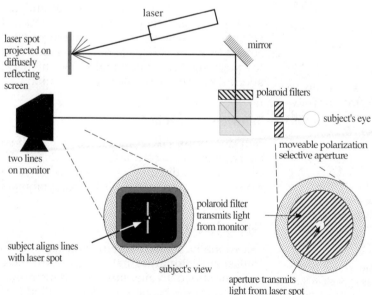

two lines on monitor

subject aligns lines with laser spot

laser

laser spot projected on diffusely reflecting screen

mirror

polaroid filters

subject's eye

moveable polarization selective aperture

polaroid filter transmits light from monitor

subject's view

aperture transmits light from laser spot

Figure 15.2. Vernier alignment apparatus for measuring transverse aberration. The optical arrangement uses a mirror and a cube beam-splitter, so that the subject sees a bright laser spot aligned horizontally with the gap between two vertical lines. The subject controls the lines' horizontal movement so that the spot is aligned in the gap. Modified from Figure 2 of Woods *et al.* (1996), with kind permission of Elsevier Press.

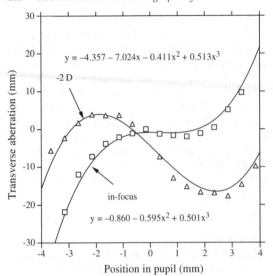

Figure 15.3. Transverse aberration for one subject at two levels of defocus in the study of Woods *et al.* (1996). Object distance 4 m. Modified from Figure 5a of Woods *et al.* (1996), with kind permission of Elsevier Press.

which can be arranged to

$$l - l_o = TA(X)l/X \tag{15.6}$$

Note that $TA(X)$ has the opposite sign to X in the figure. The longitudinal aberration $LA(X)$ is given, as a difference of vergences, by

$$LA(X) = 1/l - 1/l_o$$

or

$$LA(X) = -(l - l_o)/(ll_o) \tag{15.7}$$

Substituting the right-hand side of equation (15.6) for $(l - l_o)$ into equation (15.7) gives

$$LA(X) = -TA(X)/(Xl_o) \tag{15.8}$$

The transverse aberration polynomial can be altered also into a wave aberration polynomial $W(X)$ by using the relationship (Smith and Atchison, 1997, equation (33.76))

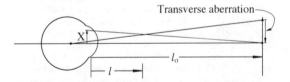

Figure 15.4. The determination of longitudinal aberration from transverse aberration, as applied to the study of Woods *et al.* (1996).

$$TA(X) = -l_o dW(X)/dX \tag{15.9}$$

where $dW(X)/dX$ is the derivative of $W(X)$ with respect to X. From this equation,

$$W(X) = -(A_0 X + A_1 X^2/2 + A_2 X^3/3 + A_3 X^4/4 + \text{higher order terms})/l_o \tag{15.10}$$

This is a one-dimensional equivalent of equation (15.1).

The vernier alignment method is slow compared with recent objective techniques, and most studies have considered only one or a few meridians. With improvements in design and in computer-aided data collection and processing, it is possible to measure a large number of points across the whole pupil in a few minutes (He *et al.*, 1988). In this case, the equations to derive aberration polynomials from the transverse aberration data will be more complex than indicated above.

Scheiner disc and annulus methods

Von Bahr (1945) used the Scheiner principle (Chapter 8, *Subjective/objective refraction techniques*) to measure the subjective refraction (longitudinal aberration) corresponding to different diameters in the pupil, in both vertical and horizontal meridians.

For the annulus method, the Scheiner discs are replaced in front of the eye by apertures consisting of annuli of various radii. The object can be moved, or correcting ophthalmic lenses are placed in front of the eye. Koomen *et al.* (1949) kept the area of all annuli the same. Like most other subjective techniques, it is only applicable for foveal vision. Because it considers all meridians at once, it is only able to measure the rotationally symmetrical aberration known as spherical aberration.

Telescope focusing

Van den Brink (1962) measured longitudinal aberrations by isolating small parts of the pupil and adjusting the eyepiece of a telescope for optimum focusing for a target.

Refraction in the periphery

Occasionally, subjective refraction techniques (measuring longitudinal aberration) have been modified to measure astigmatism and field curvature in the periphery (Millodot *et al.*, 1975; Wang *et al.*, 1995). These are very slow.

Objective tests

Knife-edge tests

The basic principles of retinoscopy were discussed in Chapter 8, *Objective-only refraction techniques*. Retinoscopy was used in some of the earliest attempts to measure longitudinal monochromatic aberrations associated with foveal vision, by comparing the state of refraction through various regions of the pupil (Jackson, 1888; Pi, 1925; Stine, 1930; Jenkins, 1963a). These studies showed that, for the relaxed eye, peripheral pupil regions require usually more negative correction (i.e. are more myopic) than the central part of the pupil. Retinoscopy has also been used for determining the peripheral refraction of the eye, taking the whole of the pupil into account, and hence determining field curvature and oblique astigmatism (see, for example, Rempt *et al.*, 1971; Millodot *et al.*, 1975). Here retinoscopy can be considered to be a longitudinal aberration measure, because it determines the lens power required to correct the aberrations of the eye.

Berny (1969) and Berny and Slansky (1970) developed a technique based on the Foucault test. Light returning from the retina of the eye was intercepted by a knife edge near the focal plane. The image of the pupil was photographed and its intensity pattern analysed to determine transverse aberrations, which were then transformed to give the corresponding wave aberrations.

Aberroscope technique

A possible set up of the aberroscope is shown in Figure 15.5. The method employs a distant light source and an aberroscope placed close to the eye. The aberroscope consists of a square (or nearly square) grid sandwiched between positive and negative plano-cylindrical lenses of equal power (typically 5 D), with the cylindrical axes perpendicular and at 45° to the vertical. Additional correcting lenses are added as required to place the retinal shadow of the grid midway between

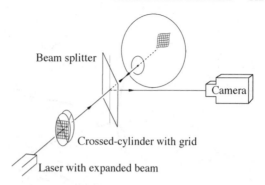

Figure 15.5. A setup for the aberroscope technique, showing the retinal image of a 7×7 grid in the presence of primary spherical aberration.

the two focal lines produced by the cylindrical lenses. Without the lenses, the grid shadow intersection points would be too close to resolve. Aberrations are revealed by distortions away from a square shadow pattern. For grid intersection separations of 1 mm and for an 8 mm pupil, the grid shadow subtends an angle at the nodal point of approximately 2°. The central part of the grid shadow is used to determine intersection points that the whole grid shadow would have if it were aberration-free. The departures of the actual intersection points from the aberration-free points are transverse ray aberrations. From the transverse ray aberrations, a wave aberration polynomial is derived of the form of equation (15.1). Figure 15.6 shows the variation in wave aberration across the pupil of one eye.

The original aberroscope technique involved subjects drawing the grid image. Later, Walsh *et al.* (1984) and Walsh and Charman (1985) made the technique objective by photographing the grid shadow. Further advances in imaging methods were described by Atchison *et al.* (1995) and Walsh and Cox (1995). It may be thought that this is now a 'double pass' technique, in which the aberrations of the eye are involved for the passage of light both into and out of the eye. However, it is only for the passage of light into the eye that each grid intersection point is 'distorted' in the image by a small part of the pupil. For the passage out of the eye, light from each intersection point passes through the whole pupil – the aberrations of the eye for this direction serve only to blur the final image rather than to distort it.

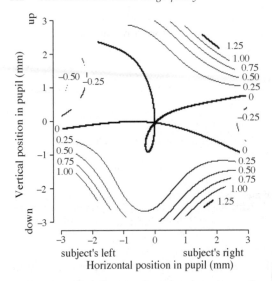

Figure 15.6. Example of the wave aberration across the pupil of a subject's right eye, as determined with the aberroscope technique. Contour intervals are in units of 10^{-3} mm. Data kindly provided by Michael Cox.

The original aberroscope grid was 'pre-distorted', with the intention that its projection onto the entrance pupil would be square so that orthogonal fitting techniques could be used to derive the aberrations. Smith *et al.* (1996) showed that this pre-distortion is unnecessary if a least squares fitting technique is used.

This method is distinct from most other methods described here in that it is effectively a ray trace from a point object into the eye, rather than a ray trace from a retinal point out of the eye (however, note that Navarro and colleagues (Navarro and Losada, 1997; Navarro *et al.*, 1998) have recently described a technique in which a laser beam is projected into the eye through different points on the pupil and the aerial image of the retinal spot is recorded). There are a number of calibration issues with the aberroscope technique, which are discussed by Smith *et al.* (1998). The level of defocus must be within approximately ± 0.5 D. Highly aberrated eyes and those with higher degrees of ametropia are very difficult to measure (Collins *et al.*, 1995), and it is necessary to use a coarser grid for such eyes, thereby yielding less information. The sampling rate across the pupil is relatively low, usually of the order of one sample per 1 mm. This suggests that high order contri-

butions to the aberration cannot be determined. Williams *et al.* (1994) and Liang and Williams (1997) suggested that the low sampling density leads to an apparent over-estimation of the image quality for this method compared with some other methods (see Chapter 18, *Retinal image quality*).

Wave-front sensor (Liang *et al.*, 1994; Liang and Williams, 1997)

A narrow beam (e.g. 1 mm wide) from a point light source is imaged by the eye, and the light passed back from the fundus travels through a wave-front sensor consisting of an array of micro-lenses (typically of the order of 0.5 mm diameter) and onto the array of a CCD camera. Each micro-lens isolates a small bundle of light passing through a small region of the pupil. The transverse ray aberration associated with each microlens can be determined from the departure of the centroid of its corresponding image from the ideal image position. Using an adaptive mirror, this technique has been used to correct the aberrations of the eye (Liang *et al.*, 1997).

Objective optometers

Objective optometers have been used to measure longitudinal peripheral aberrations of astigmatism and field curvature – see, for example, Ferree *et al.* (1931, 1932 and 1933), Millodot (1981) and Smith *et al.* (1988).

Choice of reference point and/or axis

With all methods, there is a problem of choice of the reference point and axis in the pupil that will be designated as aberration free. This point and axis are critical to the determined aberrations. In conventional optical systems, this is usually the pupil ray. Koomen *et al.* (1956) showed the effect of a different choice of the reference axis on asymmetries of measured aberrations. The reference point and/or axis do not appear to have been well defined or well monitored in many early studies. The most obvious choices are the centre of the entrance pupil as the reference point and the line-of-sight as the reference axis. However, this has the disadvantage that the pupil centre shifts as pupil size changes under the influence of lighting level and drugs (Walsh, 1988; Wilson *et al.*, 1992). Some investigators have used the visual axis (e.g. Ivanoff, 1953; Millodot and Sivak, 1979; Woods *et al.*, 1996) (see Chapter 4, *Axes of the eye*). This will not change with pupil size and has the added advantage of being the reference axis for describing chromatic aberrations (see Chapter 17, *Chromatic aberrations*).

Types and magnitudes of monochromatic aberrations

Early investigators noted that the monochromatic ocular aberrations were not usually rotationally symmetrical within the pupil. However, many have considered the aberration measured to be conventional spherical aberration, which is a rotationally symmetrical aberration. Because of this, care needs to be taken when interpreting their results, particularly where measurements have been made along only a single meridian. Later authors (for example, Smirnov, 1962; Howland and Howland, 1976 and 1977) emphasized the asymmetric nature of the eye's aberrations.

Spherical aberration

The effect of spherical aberration is shown in Figure 15.7a, which shows a set of rays from an axial point at **O**. Its paraxial focus is at **O'** on the retina. When spherical aberration is present, non-paraxial rays do not intersect at the paraxial focus. The further a ray is from the optical axis, the further its axial crossing point is from the paraxial focus. The figure shows the case of positive spherical aberration. For negative aberration, the rays (if projected) cross the axis beyond the retina.

The aberration for each ray may be expressed in terms of the longitudinal aberration distance $\delta l'$ as a function of the height r of the ray entering the eye. It may be

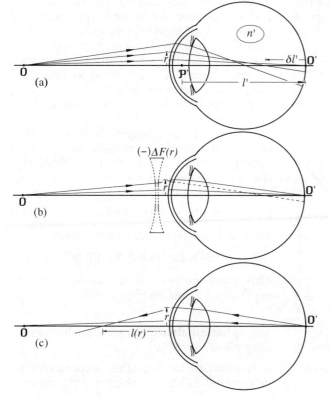

Figure 15.7. Positive spherical aberration:
a. The effect of positive spherical aberration on rays passing through the eye.
b. 'Compensation' or 'correction' of positive spherical aberration by a negative power lens $-\Delta F(r)$.
c. Determination of spherical aberration by finding the retinal conjugate for a ray. The longitudinal spherical aberration is $-L(r)$ $(= -1/l(r))$.

expressed as a power error $\Delta F(r)$, where

$$\Delta F(r) = n'/(l' + \delta l') - n'/l' \qquad (15.11)$$

where n' is the refractive index of the vitreous and l' is the distance from the back principal plane of the eye at $\mathbf{P'}$ to the paraxial image at $\mathbf{O'}$.

In object space, the longitudinal spherical aberration may be expressed as the power of a correcting lens $-\Delta F(r)$ placed in front of the eye, but only covering a narrow region of the pupil at a distance r from the centre, as shown in Figure 15.7b. This lens will alter the path of the ray so that it crosses the axis at the retina. The power of this lens will depend upon vertex distance. The longitudinal spherical aberration may be expressed also in terms of the object vergence

$$-\Delta F(r) = L(r) = 1/l(r) \qquad (15.12)$$

of the retinal conjugate for a ray, as shown in Figure 15.7c. If the excess power is positive, as it usually is for the unaccommodated eye, the correcting lens will have a negative power.

The power error $\Delta F(r)$ is an image space quantity that should be similar to the object space quantities of the correcting lens and change in object vergence $L(r)$, except for the change of sign. We usually define the sign of

the spherical aberration as the sign of the power error, and not that of the correcting lens. Discrepancies will arise when the correcting lens is not placed at the first principal plane of the eye but at a short distance in front of it, and if the object vergence is not referenced to the first principal plane. Also, increasing discrepancies result as aberration levels become very high, as noted by Thibos *et al.* (1997).

The mean results of some investigations are plotted in Figure 15.8 in terms of the power error. All of these investigations found mean spherical aberration was positive for the relaxed eye.

Aberration theory predicts that, for a rotationally symmetric optical system, the power error can be expressed as an even order power function in ray height r, and can thus be expressed in the form

$$\Delta F(r) = br^2 + \text{terms of order } r^4 \text{ and higher} \qquad (15.13)$$

If the eye contains only primary aberration, all the terms can be neglected except the first so that the power error is quadratic in ray height r in the pupil. Some investigators have assumed that this rule can be applied to the real eye, at least out to some specified pupil diameter (e.g. van Meeteren, 1974; Charman *et al.*, 1978). The b values determined from some published values of spherical aberration shown in Figure 15.8 are listed in Table 15.1. Following re-analysis of data, the values are slightly different from those given in Table 35.2 of Smith and Atchison (1997). These values of b show a large variation, which is due partly to the variation in spherical aberration between subjects. From Table 15.1, the mean weighted value of b (for non-aberroscopic studies) is

$$b = 0.076 \times 10^{-3} \pm 0.035 \times 10^{-3} \text{ mm}^{-3} \qquad (15.14)$$

Thus, we can write equation (15.13) as

$$\Delta F(r) = 0.076 \times 10^{-3} (\pm 0.035 \times 10^{-3})r^2 \qquad (15.15)$$

This equation is plotted, as well as the experimental data, in Figure 15.8.

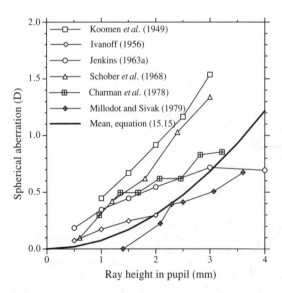

Figure 15.8. Some experimental measures of spherical aberration of the relaxed eye. The thick curve is the weighted mean fitted by a quadratic function of the form of equation (15.15).

The spherical aberration term in the wave aberration function

If we wish to use this experimentally determined value of spherical aberration to

Table 15.1. Values of the co-efficients b of r^2 and $W_{4,0}$ calculated from experimentally determined spherical aberration from various sources.

	b (mm^{-3})	Sample size	$W_{4,0}$ (mm^{-3})
Studies not using the aberroscope technique			
Koomen *et al.* (1949)	0.188×10^{-3}	3	
Ivanoff (1956)	0.0876×10^{-3}	10	
Jenkins (1963a)	0.0589×10^{-3}	12	
Schober *et al.* (1968)	0.163×10^{-3}	1	
Charman *et al.* (1978)*	0.104×10^{-3}	2	
Millodot and Sivak (1979)	0.0552×10^{-3}	20	
Mean (weighted)	$0.076 \times 10^{-3} \pm 0.035 \times 10^{-3}$		$0.019 \pm 0.009 \times 10^{-3}$
Studies using the aberroscope technique			
Walsh and Charman (1985)		11	$0.0084 \times 10^{-3} \pm 0.0134 \times 10^{-3}$
Walsh and Cox (1995)		10	$0.0091 \times 10^{-3} \pm 0.0127 \times 10^{-3}$

*Charman *et al.* quoted an approximate value of 0.12×10^{-3}.

further examine its effect on retinal image quality, using criteria such as the point spread or optical transfer functions, we need to know the value of the corresponding wave spherical aberration co-efficient. In equation (15.4), this co-efficient is denoted as $_0W_{4,0}$, which is only the axial term. However, the fovea is off-axis, and therefore measured values of spherical aberration include field dependent values, which would be summed. We denote this sum by a single co-efficient $W_{4,0}$. This is related to b by the equation

$$W_{4,0} = b/4 \qquad (15.16)$$

Using the value of b given by equation (15.14), we have

$$W_{4,0} = 0.019 \times 10^{-3}(\pm 0.009 \times 10^{-3}) \text{ mm}^{-3} \qquad (15.17)$$

Studies of the aberrations using the aberroscope technique (see *Methods of measuring monochromatic aberrations*, this chapter) have used an equation of the form of equation (15.1), with truncation of the series at the W_{14} term. We refer to the co-efficients W_{10} to W_{14} as 'spherical aberration-like' terms. If the aberration present were purely spherical aberration, we would have

$$W_{10} = W_{14} = W_{12}/2 = W_{4,0} \qquad (15.18)$$

with all of the other co-efficients equal to zero. However, because of the asymmetrical nature of the aberrations, this does not occur in real eyes. Howland and Howland (1997) showed

that, in these cases, the spherical aberration can still be derived. Using their equations and those of Atchison (1995), we can obtain

$$W_{4,0} = (3W_{10} + W_{12} + 3W_{14})/8 \qquad (15.19)$$

Applying this equation to the data of Walsh and Charman (1985) gives

$$W_{4,0} = 0.0084 \times 10^{-3}(\pm 0.0134 \times 10^{-3}) \text{ mm}^{-3} \qquad (15.20a)$$

and applying the equation to the Walsh and Cox (1995) data gives

$$W_{4,0} = 0.0091 \times 10^{-3}(\pm 0.0127 \times 10^{-3}) \text{ mm}^{-3} \qquad (15.20b)$$

The mean value of the spherical aberration for the above two sets of results is

$$W_{4,0} = 0.0088 \times 10^{-3} (\pm 0.0131 \times 10^{-3}) \text{ mm}^{-3} \qquad (15.21)$$

Substituting this mean value into equation (15.16), we have a predicted b value of

$$b = 0.035(\pm 0.052) \text{ mm}^{-3} \qquad (15.22)$$

and hence, from equation (15.13), the power error at the edge of an 8 mm diameter pupil is

$$\Delta F(r = 4 \text{ mm}) = 0.56(\pm 0.84) \text{ D} \qquad (15.23)$$

The value of $W_{4,0}$ in equation (15.21) is about half the value predicted from combining the previous studies and given by equation (15.17), but they are probably not statistically significantly different because of the large standard deviations.

Effect of accommodation

Most eyes are considered to suffer from positive spherical aberration when unaccommodated, with a trend to negative spherical aberration being observed upon accommodation (e.g. Koomen *et al.*, 1949; Ivanoff, 1956; Jenkins, 1963a; Schober *et al.*, 1968; Berny, 1969; Atchison *et al.*, 1995; Collins *et al.*, 1995; He *et al.*, 1999). Koomen and colleagues (1949) found that the aberration reduced considerably for two of their three subjects by about 2.5 D of accommodation stimulus, and was clearly negative for one of those subjects at 3.7 D of accommodation stimulus. Ivanoff (1956) and Jenkins (1963a) found the mean aberration was approximately zero by about 3 D and 1.5 D accommodation stimulus, respectively, but with the actual value depending upon the subject and ray position in the pupil. Atchison *et al.* (1995) and He *et al.* (1999) found that the mean aberration became approximately zero by 2 D and 3 D, respectively, of accommodation response.

Coma

In a rotationally symmetric system, coma is an off-axis aberration. Figure 15.9 shows the effect of coma on the image of an off-axis point, providing no other aberrations are present. The image has a straightened-out comma shape, with the pointed end facing either towards or away from the optical axis. The light distribution is not uniform across

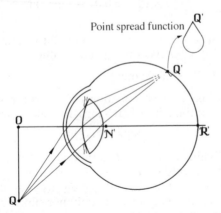

Figure 15.9. The retinal image of a point object produced by coma.

this patch, but is highest at the pointed end. The complex details of the ray pattern are not shown.

In real eyes, 'coma-like' aberrations are present at the fovea because of the lack of symmetry of the eye about an appropriate reference axis. The terms W_6 to W_9 in equation (15.1) are these coma-like terms. The values of these co-efficients in Walsh and Charman's (1985) study varied from −0.128 to +0.108 mm^{-2}, which is much greater than the range of −0.030 to +0.075 mm^{-3} for the 'spherical aberration-like' terms W_{10} to W_{14}. Changes in accommodation produce changes in the coma-like aberrations as well as in spherical aberration (Howland and Buettner, 1989; Lu *et al.*, 1993).

Coma estimated from measured spherical aberration and a pupil decentration factor

Coma can arise on-axis in an otherwise rotationally symmetric system if the pupil is decentred, and the amount of induced coma can be predicted as follows. For a rotationally symmetric system containing only the $W_{4,0}$ spherical aberration term, from equation (15.4), the wave aberration $W(X,Y)$ can be written as

$$W(X,Y) = W_{4,0}(X^2 + Y^2)^2 \qquad (15.24)$$

If the pupil is decentred to the point $X = X_o$, the wave aberration becomes

$$W(X,Y) = W_{4,0}[(X - X_o)^2 + Y^2]^2 \qquad (15.25)$$

Expanding the brackets and re-grouping the terms

$$W(X,Y) = W_{4,0}(X^2 + Y^2)^2 - 4W_{4,0}X_o(X^2 + Y^2)X + \text{other terms} \qquad (15.26)$$

The 'other terms' correspond to field curvature, astigmatism, a lateral shift of focus and a constant term. These have no application at this point. However, the second term corresponds to coma lying along the X-axis direction, with a wave aberration co-efficient

$$W_{3,1} = -4W_{4,0}X_o \text{ mm}^{-2} \qquad (15.27)$$

Once again, we have dropped the digit in front of the $_1W_{3,1}$, because we are now considering all field dependent coma terms.

It is clear from this equation that, if the pupil is decentred by only 0.25 mm, the induced coma co-efficient $W_{3,1}$ has the same magnitude as the spherical aberration co-efficient $W_{4,0}$, providing the wave aberration and pupil co-ordinates are both in millimetres.

If we take a pupil decentration (X_o) of 0.5 mm and the value of $W_{4,0}$ from equation (15.17), we have

$$W_{3,1} = 0.038 \times 10^{-3} \, (\pm 0.018 \times 10^{-3}) \text{ mm}^{-2}$$
$$(15.28)$$

This is twice the value of the spherical aberration co-efficient $W_{4,0}$.

We should note that the values of these co-efficients are also the values of aberration for a point in the pupil 1 mm from the pupil centre. At other points in the pupil, the amounts of coma and spherical aberration will be different and the spherical aberration will increase more rapidly than coma with increase in ray height.

Astigmatism and peripheral power errors

Astigmatism can occur in central vision, due again to the lack of a rotational symmetry about an appropriate reference axis. Usually the cause is lack of rotational symmetry of at least one surface, most frequently the anterior cornea. This central astigmatism is conventionally corrected by ophthalmic lenses. In the aberroscope technique, residual astigmatic effects in foveal vision contribute to the terms W_3 to W_5 in equation (15.1).

Here we consider the additional astigmatism that arises in the periphery of the visual field. Its effect on the image of a point source is shown in Figure 15.10a. When astigmatism only is present, a beam of light entering the eye from a point source will be focused down to two mutually perpendicular and distinct focal lines at different positions inside the eye. Vertical sections (or fans) of rays in the beam (i.e. parallel to the plane of the page) focus to points along a focal line at **T**. Sections of rays perpendicular to the plane of the page focus to points along a focal line at **S**. The focal line at **T** is perpendicular to the page (i.e. horizontal), and the focal line at **S** is perpendicular to the **T** focal line. The letters **T** and **S** have been used because these foci are called the **tangential** and **sagittal** foci,

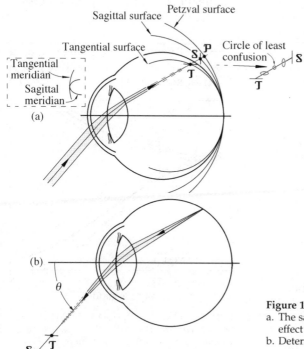

Figure 15.10. Sagittal, tangential and field curvature errors.
a. The sagittal, tangential and field curvature errors and their effect on the point spread function.
b. Determining the magnitude of the sagittal and tangential power errors in object space.

respectively. As the direction of the incoming incident beam changes, the sagittal and tangential foci move over surfaces called the sagittal and tangential surfaces.

The aberration effect can be measured in two ways:

1. In terms of sagittal and tangential power errors. The principal powers of the eye, corresponding to the sagittal and tangential foci, are called the sagittal and tangential powers. The corresponding power errors are the differences in the powers from that required to image the focal lines on the retina. As in the case of spherical aberration, sagittal and tangential imagery is usually measured in object space by the correcting lens powers. These lens powers are the same as lens powers found by conventional refraction, but are functions of the off-axis angle. This approach is the same as finding the sagittal and tangential vergences of the beam exiting the eye from a point on the retina, as shown in Figure 15.10b. The **T** and **S** correcting lens powers are not the same as the image power errors, even with a change of sign, with the discrepancies increasing as the angle increases (Atchison, 1998). In the rest of this chapter and in the next, we will use the term 'power error', but it is to be understood that this refers to the correcting lens power. Please note that this is the opposite to the convention adopted for spherical aberration.

2. Astigmatism. This is a measure of the distance between the sagittal and tangential foci, either as a distance or as a vergence, but usually the latter. When measured as an object space quantity by refraction, it is the difference in refractive errors between the sagittal and tangential sections. Astigmatism occurs in a rotationally symmetrical system because of the oblique incidence of rays at optical surfaces. The effect is the same as conventional astigmatism associated with the fovea which, as already mentioned, is commonly due to one or more surfaces not being rotationally symmetrical. To make the distinction, the astigmatism associated with peripheral vision is often called **oblique astigmatism**.

The values of the sagittal and tangential

power errors will be influenced by the presence of any foveal astigmatism and by the direction of its axis.

The mean results for a number of investigations are shown in Figure 15.11. The range of individual results within each investigation, and of the means between investigations, shows that there is significant variation in the form of the sagittal and tangential power errors. The measurements were usually made with the fixation or accommodation stimulus at a finite distance. Smith *et al.* (1988) investigated the effect of accommodation and found that, while sagittal power errors change little with accommodation, tangential power errors increase considerably. Thus, astigmatism increases with accommodation.

Charman and Jennings (1982) suggested that much of the variation in peripheral power error curves between subjects is due to variations in the shape of the retina. If refractive error is due to a variation in axial length but equatorial diameter is the same, refractive errors should converge towards the equator (angle of about 60° in air). This was demonstrated theoretically by Dunne *et al.* (1987), who modelled the retina as ellipses of varying asphericity.

For a general, rotationally symmetrical,

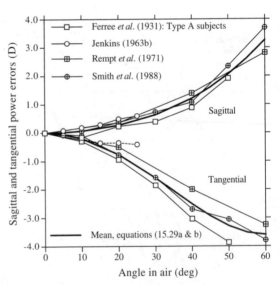

Figure 15.11. Mean values of the sagittal and tangential power errors from various sources. The solid lines are the corresponding means fitted by equations (15.29a) and (15.29b).

optical system, aberration theory predicts that the sagittal and tangential power errors denoted here as $L_s(\theta)$ and $L_t(\theta)$ can be expressed in the form of an even order polynomial in the object off-axis angle θ. We fitted such polynomials to the experimental data shown in Figure 15.11. Taking only the first two terms of the polynomials, the equations are

$$L_s(\theta) = 6.31 \times 10^{-4}\theta^2 + 7.64 \times 10^{-8}\theta^4 \quad (15.29a)$$

$$L_t(\theta) = -2.03 \times 10^{-3}\theta^2 + 2.86 \times 10^{-7}\theta^4 \quad (15.29b)$$

where θ is in degrees and L_s and L_t are in dioptres. These equations are shown in the figure (solid curve without symbols).

The astigmatism $A(\theta)$ is the difference between sagittal and tangential power errors, that is

$$A(\theta) = L_s(\theta) - L_t(\theta) \quad (15.30)$$

Substituting for $L_s(\theta)$ and $L_t(\theta)$ from equations (15.29) gives the equation

$$A(\theta) = 2.66 \times 10^{-3}\theta^2 - 2.09 \times 10^{-7}\theta^4 \quad (15.31a)$$

Lotmar and Lotmar (1974) used the data of Rempt *et al.* (1971) for 363 subjects to obtain the equation

$$A(\theta) = \theta^{1.5} \times 10^{-2} \quad (15.31b)$$

where θ is again in degrees and $A(\theta)$ is in dioptres. We should note that this form is not consistent with theory for a rotationally symmetric system, which predicts that the aberration is an even order polynomial in angle θ.

Equations (15.31a) and (15.31b), and Millodot's (1981) results for 62 eyes, separately in the nasal and temporal meridians, are plotted in Figure 15.12. Our equation (15.31a) predicts larger astigmatism than that of Lotmar and Lotmar (1974) and of Millodot (1981).

Wave aberration co-efficients $W_{2,0}$ and $W_{2,2}$

The sagittal and tangential power errors and astigmatism in a rotationally symmetric system can be converted into wave aberration co-efficients $W_{2,0}$ and $W_{2,2}$. From the theory and equations provided by Smith and Atchison (1997), we have

$$W_{2,0} = -L_s(5°)/2 \quad (15.32a)$$

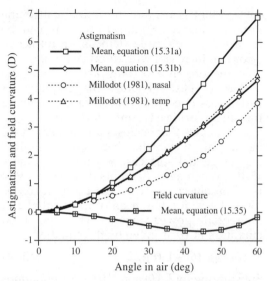

Figure 15.12. Estimates of astigmatism and field curvature from several sources. Solid lines are mean values obtained from equations (15.31a), (15.31b) and (15.35).

$$W_{2,2} = [L_s(5°) - L_t(5°)]/2 \quad (15.32b)$$

where the values of $W_{2,0}$ and $W_{2,2}$ are for 5° from the optical axis. While this angle is arbitrary, we chose it because the fovea is on average 5° from the best fit optical axis.

From equations (15.29) and (15.32), we have the following estimates of these wave aberration co-efficients, remembering that the values of L_s and L_t are in dioptres and that the wave aberration will normally be expressed in millimetres

$$W_{2,0} = -7.91 \times 10^{-6} \text{ mm}^{-1} \quad (15.33a)$$

$$W_{2,2} = 3.32 \times 10^{-5} \text{ mm}^{-1} \quad (15.33b)$$

Field curvature

This is another off-axis aberration. If field curvature is the only aberration present, the image of a point source is imaged as a point, but not on the image plane predicted by paraxial optics (the Gaussian image plane). For optical systems that are composed of mostly positive power components and form a real image (such as the eye), the image is formed in front of the Gaussian image plane. For small angles, the image point falls on a surface that is behind the retina, called the **Petzval surface** (Figure 15.10a). It can be regarded as a simple defocus or refractive error that increases with distance off-axis.

In the presence of only astigmatism, the surface of best 'general' image quality is usually assumed to be the surface containing the **circle of least confusion**. This is the smallest circle that encloses all the rays in the beam. This surface lies between the sagittal and tangential surfaces, as shown in Figure 15.10a. When measured outside the eye – that is, as an object quantity – its position can be found by taking the mean of the sagittal and tangential power errors. That is, field curvature $FC(\theta)$ is given by the equation

$$FC(\theta) = [L_s(\theta) + L_t(\theta)]/2 \qquad (15.34)$$

Substituting for $L_s(\theta)$ and $L_t(\theta)$ from equations (15.29) gives the equation

$$FC(\theta) = -7.00 \times 10^{-4}\theta^2 + 1.81 \times 10^{-7}\theta^4 \quad (15.35)$$

where θ is in degrees and $FC(\theta)$ is in dioptres. This equation is plotted in Figure 15.12. The flatness of the curve indicates that the circle of least confusion lies close to the retina.

Distortion

This is the last of the 'primary' monochromatic aberrations. It is also an off-axis aberration. It is similar to field curvature in that a point source is imaged as a point, this time in the Gaussian image plane but not at the expected position. It is formed either further away (positive distortion) or closer (negative distortion) to the optical axis. If the eye contains negative distortion, the image position of an off-axis point will be as shown schematically in Figure 15.13. The presence of distortion in a conventional optical system is best shown by imaging a square, centred on the optical axis, as shown in Figure 15.14. In the presence of distortion, the image of the square is smaller or larger than the expected Gaussian image, and the sides are bowed in or out. This conventional distortion is probably not meaningful in the eye, because of the curvature of the retina and also because the change in spatial relationship between image points, brought on by distortion, is unlikely to have an effect on vision.

Perhaps more important than distortion is the functional relationship between the actual image position at $\overline{Q}'$ as shown in Figure 15.13 and the position of the object Q in the object space (or the incident off-axis angle θ). The presence of distortion in the eye means that $\overline{Q}'$ is different from that at the position Q' expected from Gaussian optics. There are few studies of this relationship in real eyes. Ames and Proctor (1921) mentioned studies of Donders (1877), who carried out measurements on a person who had exophthalmia (protruding eyeballs), and of Drault (1898), who examined extracted eyes and two eyes of people with exophthalmia. These studies gave the external angle and the position of the retinal image from the corneal margin, and Ames and Proctor converted these retinal positions to internal angles but without giving any details. Figure 15.15 shows the results.

We can compare such image point positions with those expected from Gaussian optics. If the eye were free of distortion, then the

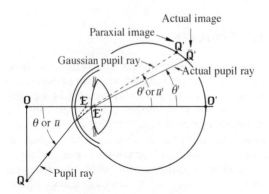

Figure 15.13. Pupil ray angles and distortion.

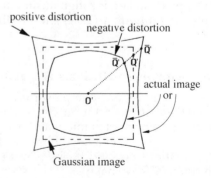

Figure 15.14. The effect of distortion on the image of a square centred on the optical axis.

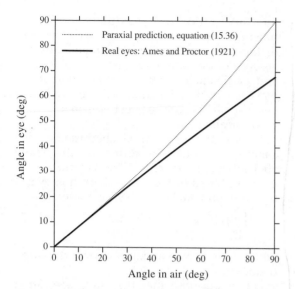

Figure 15.15. The measured values of internal and external angles, from Ames and Proctor (1921). Predicted paraxial angles are determined from equation (15.36). The Ames and Proctor data was smoothed but well fitted by the equation $\theta' = 0.823085\theta - 0.000753260\theta^2$. The co-efficient of the θ term was fixed at the value expected from the Gullstrand eye, which was used to predict the expected distortion-free values.

paraxial pupil ray angles $\bar{u}'$ and $\bar{u}'$, shown in Figure 15.13, would be related by equation (5.7), i.e.

$$\bar{u}' = \bar{m}\,\bar{u} \tag{15.36}$$

where these paraxial angles are related to real angles θ by the equations

$$\bar{u} = \tan(\theta) \text{ and } \bar{u}' = \tan(\theta') \tag{15.36a}$$

and $\bar{m}$ depends upon the actual construction of the particular eye (0.823085 for the Gullstrand exact relaxed eye). These equations have been used to plot θ' against θ as shown in Figure 15.15 and show that the actual image is closer to the axis than that predicted by Gaussian optics, indicating that there is negative distortion in the eye.

Higher order aberrations with foveal vision

In many studies of monocular aberration, the order of aberration terms has been very limited – for example, aberroscope studies have not investigated beyond the fourth

power. In equation (15.1), the terms in the wave aberration polynomial are shown only up to the fourth power in pupil co-ordinates. Using the wave-front sensor method, Liang and Williams (1997) determined aberration terms up to the 10th order. For 3 mm pupils, they found that the aberrations beyond the fourth order were small and had minimal effect on image quality. However, for large 7.3 mm pupils, the fifth to eighth orders made substantial contributions to deterioration of image quality relative to diffraction limited performance, according to different image quality criteria such as the Maráchel criterion, the Strehl intensity ratio, and the modulation transfer function (the latter two are discussed further in Chapter 18).

He *et al.* (1999) found that the overall aberrations of fifth and higher orders were at a minimum at approximately 2 D of accommodation and increased for smaller and higher accommodation levels.

Symmetry between fellow eyes

Liang and Williams (1997) found that aberrations are similar for the two eyes of the same observer.

Significance of monochromatic aberrations

Foveal vision

Spatial visual performance

For corrected vision and moderate photopic luminances, visual acuity is maximum for pupil diameters of 2–3 mm (Atchison *et al.*, 1979). For pupil diameters smaller than 2–3 mm, the decrease in visual acuity is predominantly due to diffraction, although reduced retinal illumination may have some effect. For larger pupil diameters there is a less dramatic decrease in acuity, which must be due to aberrations.

A similar influence of pupil size has been found for the contrast sensitivity function (Campbell and Green, 1965) and the retinal line spread function (Campbell and Gubisch, 1966). (These measures of visual performance are described in Chapter 18).

No one has yet demonstrated that correcting monocular aberrations of the eye will improve visual acuity, although Liang *et al.* (1997) were able to improve grating resolution using an adaptive optics method to correct aberrations. Van Heel (1946) attempted to improve visual acuity with a lens designed to correct the eye's spherical aberration. Some studies comparing contact lenses and spectacle lens attributed better performance with one or the other type of correction to different levels of aberration (Millodot, 1969; Oxenberg and Carney, 1989), but there could have been other factors such as small variations in refraction and spectacle magnification. Collins *et al.* (1992) demonstrated that it is possible to worsen visual acuity by manipulating the front surface asphericity and, consequently, aberrations of contact lenses. For large pupils, Applegate *et al.* (1998) found a negative correlation between visual performance as measured by the contrast sensitivity function (see Chapter 18) and the magnitude of corneal aberrations following refractive surgery.

The effect of aberrations on image quality will be considered further in Chapter 18.

Effect of spherical aberration on refractive error

In the presence of spherical aberration, the plane of best image quality is not the paraxial image plane. For positive spherical aberration and a positive powered optical system such as the eye, the plane of optimum image quality lies between the paraxial image plane and the optical system. The position of this best image plane depends upon the particular criterion used to assess the quality of the image, the level of the aberration (which in turn depends upon pupil size), and the particular form of the detail in the image.

When analysing image quality of conventional optical systems, a range of criteria are used, including minimizing the width of the point spread function, maximizing the Strehl intensity ratio, maximizing the modulation transfer function at set frequencies, and minimizing the variance of the wave aberration function. We do not know if the eye uses any of these for optimum focusing. Burton and Haig (1984) found that the Strehl

intensity ratio and modulation transfer function were not good measures or predictors of perceived image quality. In the absence of definitive information pointing to any particular criterion, the variance of the wave aberration function will be used here because it is the easiest to manipulate algebraically.

The variance of the wave aberration is very easy to quantify in terms of the wave aberration co-efficients. The variance V is given in terms of the wave aberration $W(r,\phi)$ by Smith and Atchison (1997, equation (34.3))

$$V = \{\int\int_{E'} [W(r,\phi) - \overline{W}]^2 \, r \, dr \, d\phi\} / A \qquad (15.37)$$

where E' indicates integration over the pupil of area A.

Let us suppose that the wave aberration $W(r)$ is purely spherical and consists of only one spherical aberration order, the spherical aberration term $W_{4,0}$. If we defocus the system, the wave aberration polynomial can be written as

$$W = W(r) = W_{2,0}r^2 + W_{4,0}r^4 \qquad (15.38)$$

where r is the ray height in the pupil and $W_{2,0}$ is the term allowing for defocus. The value of $W_{4,0}$ is constant, but the value of $W_{2,0}$ can be manipulated by refocusing to minimize the variance of the wave aberration given by equation (15.37). This value is minimized with respect to $W_{2,0}$ when

$$dV/dW_{2,0} = 0$$

Differentiating V with respect to $W_{2,0}$ and then setting the result to zero gives the optimum defocus occuring at a defocus level of

$$W_{2,0} = - W_{4,0}\bar{\rho}^2 \qquad (15.39)$$

where $\bar{\rho}$ is the pupil radius. The corresponding change in refractive error $\Delta R_x(\bar{\rho})$ is given by

$$\Delta R_x(\bar{\rho}) = 2W_{2,0} \qquad (15.40)$$

Thus

$$\Delta R_x(\bar{\rho}) = -2W_{4,0}\bar{\rho}^2 \qquad (15.41)$$

Thus the amount of refocusing depends upon the pupil radius $\bar{\rho}$. It should be remembered that this equation applies if the wave aberration function consists of only the spherical aberration term $W_{4,0}$. If more than one term exists, all terms should be included in the integration of the variance equation (15.37).

We can use equation (15.41) to predict the effect of spherical aberration on refractive error. Substituting the spherical aberration coefficients from the non-aberroscope studies and from the aberroscope studies, provided by equations (15.17) and (15.21), respectively, into equation (15.41) gives

$$\Delta R_{x}(\bar{\rho}) = -0.038 \times 10^{-3}(\pm\, 0.018 \times 10^{-3})\bar{\rho}^2\ \text{mm}^{-1}$$
$$(15.42a)$$

$$\Delta R_{x}(\bar{\rho}) = -0.0176 \times 10^{-3}(\pm\, 0.0262 \times 10^{-3})\bar{\rho}^2\ \text{mm}^{-1}$$
$$(15.42b)$$

These values indicate that a change in pupil diameter from 2 mm to 6 mm would lead to a change in focus of 0.29 D according to equation (15.42a) and of 0.14 D according to equation (15.42b).

The above results neglect the Stiles–Crawford effect, which reduces the influence of spherical aberration towards the edge of the pupil and hence reduces the defocusing prediction given by the above equations. However, its influence is likely to be small (Atchison *et al.*, 1998).

Under photopic conditions, refraction using letter targets alters little with changes in pupil size (Koomen *et al.*, 1949 and 1951; Charman *et al.*, 1978; Atchison *et al.*, 1979). For example, Charman *et al.* (1978) found less than 0.3 D variation in refraction with pupil size, even in the presence of greater than 1 D spherical aberration, while Atchison *et al.* (1979) did not observe variation in refraction across 1–8 mm pupil diameters for any of their 22 subjects (refraction interval 0.25 D). Charman *et al.* (1978) and Atchison (1984a) showed that the optimum refraction for high frequency sinusoidal targets (≥ 20 cycles/degree) should be little affected by changes in pupil size, even in the presence of substantial spherical aberration (Figure 15.16). The small variation in refraction with pupil size is thus explained by the use of small letters containing a relatively high proportion of high spatial frequency information.

When luminance is lowered, there is often a substantial negative (myopic) shift in refraction (Koomen *et al.*, 1951). A large amount of this is due to the combination of decrease in visual acuity, which means that

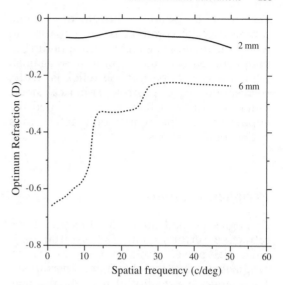

Figure 15.16. Theoretical optimum refraction as a function of spatial frequency for 2 mm and 6 mm pupil sizes. Wavelength 605 nm, with primary spherical aberration of 0.11 D and 1.0 D at the edge of 2 mm and 6 mm pupils, respectively.

high spatial frequencies are not available for determining refraction, and the natural increase in pupil size (and increase in aberrations). Green and Campbell (1965) and Charman *et al.* (1978) showed that optimal focus did not depend upon spatial frequency for small pupils, but would shift considerably for large pupils – for example, Green and Campbell found that optimum refraction for a 7 mm diameter pupil shifted approximately 0.8 D between 1.5 and 26 cycles/degree in two subjects. Charman *et al.* (1978) and Atchison (1984a) showed that this shift could be explained by the presence of spherical aberration (Figure 15.16).

Retinoscopy

This objective refraction technique was described in Chapter 8 (*Objective-only refraction techniques*), and its use in early studies of the aberrations was mentioned earlier in this chapter (*Methods of measuring monochromatic aberrations*). If an eye is aberration-free, at the reversal point the complete pupil will appear either dark or light as the light returning from the patient's pupil is scanned across the sighthole of the retinoscope. In the presence of aberration, the shadow movement is more complex. Quite common is the situation in which the retinoscope reflex corresponding to peripheral parts of the pupil moves 'against' while the central part of the reflex is 'with', corresponding to positive spherical aberration. Roorda and Bobier (1996) related the appearance of the retinoscopic reflex to a variety of aberrations.

Peripheral vision

At angles beyond about 20° the peripheral refractive errors, that is, sagittal and tangential power errors and the associated astigmatism, are the dominant aberrations. These affect the quality of the retinal image during ophthalmoscopy. Correcting peripheral refractive errors has little effect on visual acuity beyond a few degrees from the fovea (Millodot *et al.*, 1975; Rempt *et al.*, 1976), but improves peripheral detection (Leibowitz *et al.*, 1972; Wang *et al.*, 1995; Williams *et al.*, 1996). This is discussed further in Chapter 18.

Ocular component contributions

There is considerable interest in understanding the corneal and lens contributions to the aberration of the eye. This interest has increased with advances in the treatment of refractive errors by surgically manipulating the anterior corneal surface. It is important to know the best shape to make the cornea and the visual consequences of poor post-surgical shapes (Applegate and Howland, 1997; Applegate *et al.*, 1998; Martínez *et al.*, 1998).

There have been several attempts to identify the magnitude of the corneal and lenticular contributions to ocular aberrations (Jenkins, 1963a; El Hage and Berny, 1973; Millodot and Sivak, 1979; Sivak and Kreuzer, 1983). These studies suffered from problems such as inaccurate measurements of the cornea and measuring the lens *in vitro*, where its shape will be different from the natural state or its optical conjugates have been altered. The emphasis has been on spherical aberration and the cornea has often been modelled as a rotationally symmetrical sur-

face, which is a considerable over-simplification.

The approach to determining the relative contribution of the components is to measure the total aberration of the eye and determine the aberrations of either the cornea or lens. The easiest component to measure is the anterior cornea. The shape of this can be measured with corneal topographical instruments. The aberration of the cornea is given by its departure from the ideal shape, which would give no aberration about the chosen reference axis. For a distant object, the ideal cornea would have a front surface conicoid asphericity Q, independent of radius, related to the cornea's refractive index n by

$$Q = -1/n^2 \approx -1/1.376 \approx -0.53 \qquad (15.43)$$

Q was explained in Chapter 2. The corneal aberration in wave aberration terms for any ray traced through the cornea is given by

$$corneal\ aberration \approx (n-1)z \qquad (15.44)$$

where z is the departure of the anterior cornea from its ideal shape for the particular ray. The lenticular contribution is then obtained by subtracting the corneal contribution from the total aberration. In determinations such as these, the aberration contribution of the posterior cornea is ignored. This is assumed to be small because of the small refractive index difference between cornea and aqueous.

The corneas of most eyes have negative corneal asphericities, but the corneas usually contribute positive aberration because the asphericity is not high (Kiely *et al.*, 1982; Guillon *et al.*, 1986; see Chapter 2). The direction and magnitude of the aberration of lenses of eyes is still unclear, with the literature giving results of both positive and negative spherical aberration (Jenkins, 1963a; El Hage and Berny, 1973; Millodot and Sivak, 1979; Sivak and Kreuzer, 1983; Tomlinson *et al.*, 1993). There is more about this in the next chapter.

Correction of myopia by refractive surgery increases the aberrations associated with the cornea, with the fourth order (spherical aberration-like) aberrations increasing considerably relative to the third-order (coma-like) aberrations represented in equation (16.1) (Oliver *et al.*, 1997; Applegate *et al.*, 1998; Martínez *et al.*, 1998; Oshika, 1999).

Pupil aberration

Ocular aberrations affect not only the quality of the retinal image, but also the formation of the entrance pupil. The entrance pupil is the image of the aperture of the iris (the actual pupil), and ocular aberrations arising from the cornea will affect the appearance of the pupil. Of the five monocular aberrations, the aberration of most significance will be distortion, which affects the apparent size of the pupil (i.e. the position of the pupil margin).

According to Gaussian optics, the entrance pupil is about 13 per cent larger than the actual pupil (see Appendix 3). Since distortion is a non-linear magnification effect that increases with image size by at least the square of the image size, we expect pupil distortion to have a greater effect, the larger the pupil. The pupil distortion arising at the cornea is negative, and therefore as the real pupil becomes wider, distortion leads to a smaller magnification than the 13 per cent predicted from Gaussian optics.

Alexandridis and Baumann (1967) examined the effect of pupil size on the apparent pupil diameter using excised corneas. They showed that, for large pupil sizes, the pupil magnification was less than the expected Gaussian value of about 1.13. We have determined the expected magnification effect for the Gullstrand number 1 relaxed schematic eye with the anterior corneal surface aspherized with a Q value of –0.2, which is close to the means of the studies of Kiely *et al.* (1982) and Guillon *et al.* (1986). Figure 15.17 compares the experimental and theoretical results. They show similar trends, although the magnification changes more quickly for the former.

Aberrations of ophthalmic devices

Many optical instruments are used in combination with the eye, including telescopes and microscopes and clinical instruments such as optometers, keratometers and ophthalmoscopes. There are ergonomic issues relating to the way in which instruments must be used, e.g. the most appropriate alignment of the two tubes of binocular instruments so that the two eyes are not placed under undue accommodative and convergence stress when

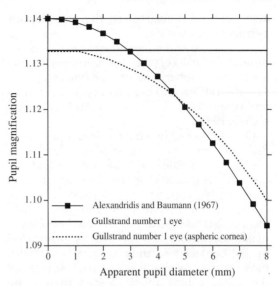

Figure 15.17. The magnification of the pupil from measurements of Alexandridis and Baumann (1967), paraxial prediction of the Gullstrand number 1 eye, and theoretical results using Gullstrand's number 1 schematic eye with an anterior corneal surface of asphericity $Q = -0.2$. The experimental measurements are the means from three excised corneas, which were positioned approximately 3.6 mm in front of a grid.

looking at close objects. The aberrations of the eye and instrument must be combined. When instruments are aberration-free or have large exit pupils relative to that of the eye, the eye limits image quality. If alignment with the eye is poor, additional aberrations will occur. These matters are covered by Smith and Atchison (1997).

The most common correcting ophthalmic devices are spectacle lenses. Optical design is concerned with ensuring that good foveal vision is maintained for various rotations of the eye for which the line of sight will not coincide with the lens optical axis. The spectacle lens is designed as a wide angle, small pupil system whose stop is at the centre of rotation of the eye (approximately 15 mm behind the corneal apex). Accordingly, the monochromatic aberrations considered to be important are the sagittal and tangential power errors of the lens (and their combinations, i.e. astigmatism and field curvature). The aberrations of the eye itself are ignored, together with spherical aberration and coma of the lens, because these are small. Aberrations associated with peripheral vision are also ignored because of the eye's poor peripheral resolution.

The sagittal and tangential power errors are minimized by varying the bending of the lenses and aspherizing one or both surfaces. The aberrations and design of spectacle lenses are covered by Jalie (1984) and Atchison (1984b, 1992).

Design issues of contact lenses are very different from those of spectacle lenses. A contact lens rotates with the eye so that the off-axis aberrations of the lens are not of considerable concern. The surfaces are very curved so that they fit well to the eye, which means that spherical aberration becomes a major aberration. The aberrations introduced by the contact lens must be combined with those of the eye. Because the back surface of the contact lens must closely match the cornea, the degree of freedom provided by altering lens bending is no longer available. The major design variable is aspherizing. The large difference between the refractive indices of the cornea and air (≈ 0.376) is replaced by a much larger difference between the refractive indices of the contact lens and air (≈ 0.45–0.49). This has a considerable effect on the combined aberrations. When rigid contact lens are placed on eyes, aberrations change to different extents in different eyes for two reasons (Atchison, 1995): (1) different eyes have different anterior corneal shapes, and (2) approximately 90 per cent of the departure of the anterior corneal surface away from a sphere is neutralized by the tear film between the lens and eye.

An artificial intraocular lens can replace the natural lens of the eye when the latter is removed, usually because of cataract. Like the contact lens, the intraocular lens moves with the eye, and its aberrations must be combined with those of the eye. Degrees of freedom are lens bending and surface aspherizing. Spherical aberration is an important aberration, but considerable sagittal and tangential power errors may result if the lenses are tilted or decentred. The aberrations and design of intraocular lenses are covered by Atchison (1990 and 1991).

Summary of main symbols

LA longitudinal aberration

TA transverse aberration

$\bar{\rho}$ entrance pupil radius

D entrance pupil diameter

r ray height in the pupil

b co-efficient in equation (15.13)

$\Delta F(r)$ spherical aberration as a power error for a ray entering the eye at a height r. Also used for correcting power to minimize wavefront variance in equation (15.41)

$W(X,Y)$ wave aberration for a ray passing through a point (X,Y) in the pupil

$W(r)$ wave aberration for an axial point in a rotationally symmetric system

W_1 etc   general wave aberration co-efficients

${}_0W_{4,0}$ primary spherical aberration wave aberration co-efficient

$W_{4,0}$ spherical aberration wave aberration co-efficient, which includes all field varying terms

${}_1W_{3,1}$ primary coma wave aberration co-efficient

$W_{3,1}$ coma wave aberration co-efficient, which includes all field varying terms

$W_{2,0}$ wave aberration polynomial co-efficient for defocus

$W_{2,2}$ wave aberration polynomial co-efficient for astigmatism

V variance of wave aberration over pupil

θ angular distance off-axis in air

$L_s(\theta)$ sagittal power error for off-axis direction θ

$L_t(\theta)$ tangential power error for off-axis direction θ

$A(\theta)$ astigmatism corresponding to $L_s(\theta)$ and $L_t(\theta)$

$FC(\theta)$ field curvature corresponding to $L_s(\theta)$ and $L_t(\theta)$

$\bar{u}, \bar{u}'$ paraxial pupil ray angles in object and image space respectively

$\bar{m}$ ratio of paraxial pupil ray angles, defined by equation (15.36)

Q asphericity

n refractive index

References

Alexandridis, E. and Baumann, C. H. (1967). Wirkliche und scheinbare Pupillenweiten des menschlichen Auges. *Optica Acta.*, **14**, 311–16.

Ames, A. and Proctor, C. A. (1921). Dioptrics of the eye. *J. Opt. Soc. Am.*, **5**, 22–84.

Applegate, R. A. and Howland, H. C. (1997). Refractive surgery, optical aberrations, and visual performance. *J. Refract. Surg.*, **13**, 295–9.

Applegate, R. A., Howland, H. C., Sharp, R. P. *et al.* (1998). Corneal aberrations and visual performance after radial keratotomy. *J. Refract. Surg.*, **14**, 397–407.

Atchison, D. A. (1984a). Visual optics in man. *Aust. J. Optom.*, **67**, 141–50.

Atchison, D. A. (1984b). Spectacle lens design – development and present state. *Aust. J. Optom.*, **67**, 97–107.

Atchison, D. A. (1990). Optical design of poly(methyl methacrylate) intraocular lenses. *J. Cataract. Refract. Surg.*, **16**, 178–87.

Atchison, D. A. (1991). Optical design of low index intraocular lenses. *J. Cat. Refract. Surg.*, **17**, 292–300.

Atchison, D. A. (1992). Spectacle lens design: a review. *Applied Opt.*, **31**, 3579–85.

Atchison, D. A. (1995). Aberrations associated with rigid contact lenses. *J. Opt. Soc. Am. A.*, **12**, 2267–73.

Atchison, D. A. (1998). Oblique astigmatism of the Indiana eye. *Optom. Vis. Sci.*, **75**, 247–8.

Atchison, D. A., Collins, M. J., Wildsoet, C. F. *et al.* (1995). Measurement of monochromatic ocular aberrations of human eyes as a function of accommodation by the Howland aberroscope technique. *Vision Res.*, **35**, 313–23.

Atchison, D. A., Smith, G. and Efron, N. (1979). The effect of pupil size on visual acuity in uncorrected and corrected myopia. *Am. J. Optom. Physiol. Opt.*, **56**, 315–23.

Atchison, D. A., Smith, G. and Joblin, A. (1998). Influence of Stiles–Crawford apodization on spatial visual performance. *J. Opt. Soc. Am. A*, **15**, 2545–51.

Berny, F. (1969). Étude de la formation des images rétiniennes et détermination de l'aberration de sphéricité de l'œil humain. *Vision Res.*, **9**, 977–90.

Berny, F. and Slansky, S. (1970). Wavefront determination resulting from Foucault test as applied to the human eye and visual instruments. In *Optical Instruments and Techniques* (J. H. Dickson, ed.), pp. 375–86. Oriel Press.

Burton, G. J. and Haig, N. D. (1984). Effects of the Seidel aberrations on visual target discrimination. *J. Opt. Soc. Am. A*, **1**, 373–85.

Campbell, F. W. and Green, D. G. (1965). Optical and retinal factors affecting visual resolution. *J. Physiol. (Lond.)*, **181**, 576–93.

Campbell, F. W. and Gubisch, R. W. (1966). Optical quality of the human eye. *J. Physiol. (Lond.)*, **186**, 558–78.

Campbell, M. C. W., Harrison, E. M. and Simonet, P. (1990). Psychophysical measurement of the blur on the retina due to optical aberrations of the eye. *Vision Res.*, **30**, 1587–1602.

Charman, W. N. and Jennings, J. A. M. (1982). Ametropia and peripheral refraction. *Am. J. Optom. Physiol. Opt.*, **59**, 922–3.

Charman, W. N., Jennings, J. A. M. and Whitefoot, H.

(1978). The refraction of the eye in relation to spherical aberration and pupil size. *Br. J. Physiol. Opt.*, **32**, 78–93.

Collins, M. J., Wildsoet, C. F. and Atchison, D. A. (1995). Monochromatic aberrations and myopia. *Vision Res.*, **35**, 1157–63.

Collins, M. J., Brown, B., Atchison, D. A. and Newman, S. D. (1992). Tolerance to spherical aberration induced by rigid contact lenses. *Ophthal. Physiol. Opt.*, **12**, 24–8.

Cui, C. and Lakshminarayanan, V. (1998). Choice of reference axis in ocular wave-front aberration measurement. *J. Opt. Soc. Am. A*, **15**, 2488–96.

Donders, F. C. (1877). Die Grenzen des Gesichtsfeldes in Beziehung zu denen der Netzhaut. *v. Graefes Arch. Ophthalmol.*, **23**, 255–80. Cited by Ames and Proctor (1921).

Drault, A. (1898). Note sur la situation des images rétiennes formées par les rayons très obliques sur l'axe optique (1). *Arch. D'Ophtalmol.*, **18**, 685–92. Cited by Ames and Proctor (1921).

Dunne, M. C. M., Barnes, D. A. and Clement, R. A. (1987). A model for retinal shape changes in ametropia. *Ophthal. Physiol. Opt.*, **7**, 159–60.

El Hage, S. G. and Berny, F. (1973). Contribution of the crystalline lens to the spherical aberration of the eye. *J. Opt. Soc. Am.*, **63**, 205–11.

Ferree, L. E. and Rand, G. (1933). Interpretation of refractive conditions in the peripheral field of vision. *Arch. Ophthal.*, **9**, 925–38.

Ferree, C. E., Rand, G. and Hardy, C. (1931). Refraction for the peripheral field of vision. *Arch. Ophthal.*, **5**, 717–31.

Ferree, C. E., Rand, G. and Hardy, C. (1932). Refractive asymmetry in the temporal and nasal halves of the visual field. *Am. J. Ophthal.*, **15**, 513–22.

Green, D. G. and Campbell, F. W. (1965). Effect of focus on the visual response to a sinusoidally modulated spatial stimulus. *J. Opt. Soc. Am.*, **55**, 1154–7.

Guillon, M., Lydon, D. P. M. and Wilson, C. (1986). Corneal topography: a clinical model. *Ophthal. Physiol. Opt.*, **6**, 47–56.

He, J. C., Burns, S. A. and Marcos, S. (1999). Monochromatic aberrations in the accommodated human eye. *Vision Res.*, **40**, 41–8.

He, J. C., Marcos, S., Webb, R. H. and Burns, S. A. (1998). Measurement of the wave-front aberration of the eye by a fast psychophysical procedure. *J. Opt. Soc. Am. A*, **15**, 2449–56.

Howland, H. C. and Buettner, J. (1989). Computing high-order wave aberration co-efficients from variations of best focus for small artificial pupils. *Vision Res.*, **29**, 979–83.

Howland, B. and Howland, H. C. (1976). Subjective measurement of high-order aberration of the eye. *Science*, **193**, 580–82.

Howland, H. C. and Howland, B. (1977). A subjective method for the measurement of monochromatic aberrations of the eye. *J. Opt. Soc. Am.*, **67**, 1508–18.

Ivanoff, A. (1953). *Les aberrations de l'oeil*. Éditions de la Revue d'Optique Théoretique et Instrumentale, Paris.

Ivanoff, A. (1956). About the spherical aberration of the eye. *J. Opt. Soc. Am.*, **46,** 901–3.

Jackson, E. (1888). Symmetrical aberration of the eye. *Trans. Am. Ophthal. Soc.*, **5**, 141–50.

Jalie, M. (1984). *Principles of Ophthalmic Lenses*, 4th edn, chapters 18 and 21. The Association of Dispensing Opticians.

Jenkins, T. C. A. (1963a). Aberrations of the eye and their effects on vision: Part 1. *Br. J. Physiol. Opt.*, **20**, 59–91.

Jenkins, T. C. A. (1963b). Aberrations of the eye and their effects on vision: Part 2. *Br. J. Physiol. Opt.*, **20**, 161–201.

Kiely, P. M., Smith, G. and Carney, L. G. (1982). The mean shape of the human cornea. *Optica Acta.*, **29**, 1027–40.

Koomen, M., Scolnik, R. and Tousey, R. (1951). A study of night myopia. *J. Opt. Soc. Am.*, **41**, 80–90.

Koomen, M., Scolnik, R. and Tousey, R. (1956). Spherical aberration of the eye and the choice of axis. *J. Opt. Soc. Am.*, **46**, 903–4.

Koomen, M., Tousey, R. and Scolnik, R. (1949). The spherical aberration of the eye. *J. Opt. Soc. Am.*, **39**, 370–76.

Leibowitz, H. W., Johnson, C. A. and Isabelle, E. (1972). Peripheral motion detection and refractive error. *Science*, **177**, 1207–8.

Liang, J. and Williams, D. R. (1997). Aberrations and retinal image quality of the normal human eye. *J. Opt. Soc. Am. A.*, **14**, 2873–83.

Liang, J., Williams, D. R. and Miller, D. T. (1997). Supernormal vision and high-resolution retinal imaging through adaptive optics. *J. Opt. Soc. Am. A.*, **14**, 2884–92.

Liang, J., Grimm, B., Goelz, S. and Bille, J. F. (1994). Objective measurement of wave aberrations of the human eye with the use of a Hartmann-Shack wavefront sensor. *J. Opt. Soc. Am. A.*, **11**, 1949–57.

Lotmar, W. and Lotmar, T. (1974). Peripheral astigmatism in the human eye: experimental data and theoretical model prediction. *J. Opt. Soc. Am.*, **64**, 510–13.

Lu, C., Munger, R. and Campbell, M. C. W. (1993). Monochromatic aberrations in accommodated eyes. In Technical Digest Series, vol. 3, *Ophthalmic and Visual Optics*, pp. 160–63. Optical Society of America.

Martínez, C. E., Applegate, R. A., Klyce, S. D. *et al.* (1998). Effect of pupillary dilation on corneal optical aberrations after photorefractive keratectomy. *Arch. Ophthal.*, **116**, 1053–62.

Millodot, M. (1969).Variation of visual acuity with contact lenses. *Arch. Ophthal.*, **82**, 461–5.

Millodot, M. (1981). Effect of ametropia on peripheral refraction. *Am. J. Optom. Physiol. Opt.*, **58**, 691–5.

Millodot, M. and Sivak, J. (1979). Contribution of the cornea and lens to spherical aberration of the eye. *Vision Res.*, **19**, 685–7.

Millodot, M., Johnson, C. A., Lamont, A. and Leibowitz, H. W. (1975). Effect of dioptrics on peripheral visual acuity. *Vision Res.*, **15**, 1357–62.

Navarro, R. and Losada, M. A. (1997). Aberrations and relative efficiency of ray pencils in the living human eye. *Optom. Vis. Sci.*, **74**, 540–47.

Navarro, R., Moreno, E. and Dorronsoro, C. (1998). Monochromatic aberrations and point-spread functions of the human eye across the visual field. *J. Opt. Soc. Am. A*, **15**, 2522–9.

Oliver, K. M., Hemenger, R. P., Corbett, M. C. *et al.* (1997). Corneal optical aberrations induced by photorefractive keratectomy. *J. Refract. Surg.*, **13**, 246–54.

Oshika, T., Klyce, S. D., Applegate, R. A., Howland, H. C. *et al.* (1999). Comparison of corneal wavefront aberrations after photorefractive keratectomy and laser in situ keratomileusis. *Am. J. Ophthal.*, **127**, 1–7.

Oxenberg, L. D. and Carney, L. G. (1989). Visual performance with aspheric rigid contact lenses. *Optom. Vis. Sci.*, **66**, 818–21.

Pi, H. T. (1925). The total peripheral aberration of the eye. *Trans. Ophthal. Soc. U.K.*, **45**, 393–9.

Rempt, F., Hoogerheide, J. and Hoogenboom, W. P. H. (1971). Peripheral retinoscopy and the skiagram. *Ophthalmologica*, **162**, 1–10.

Rempt, F., Hoogerheide, J. and Hoogenboom, W. P. H. (1976). Influence of correction of peripheral refractive errors on peripheral static vision. *Ophthalmologica*, **173**, 128–35.

Roorda, A. and Bobier, W. R. (1996). Geometrical technique to determine the influence of monochromatic aberrations on retinoscopy. *J. Opt. Soc. Am. A.*, **13**, 3–11.

Schober, H., Munker, H. and Zolleis, F. (1968). Die Aberration des menschlichen Auges und ihre Messung. *Optica Acta*, **15**, 47–57.

Sivak, J. and Kreuzer, R. O. (1983). Spherical aberration of the crystalline lens. *Vision Res.*, **23**, 59–70.

Smirnov, H. S. (1962). Measurement of wave aberration of the human eye. *Biophysics*, **6**, 776–95.

Smith, G. and Atchison, D. A. (1997). *The Eye and Visual Optical Instruments*, Chapters 33, 34 and 35. Cambridge University Press.

Smith, G., Applegate, R. and Atchison, D. A. (1998). An assessment of the accuracy of the crossed-cylinder aberroscope technique. *J. Opt. Soc. Am. A.*, **14**, 2477–87.

Smith, G., Applegate, R. and Howland, H. (1996). The crossed-cylinder aberroscope: An alternative method of calculation of the aberrations. *Ophthal. Physiol. Opt.*, **16**, 222–9.

Smith, G., Millodot, M. and McBrien, N. (1988). The effect of accommodation on oblique astigmatism and field curvature of the human eye. *Clin. Exp. Optom.*, **71**, 119–25.

Stine, G. H. (1930). Variations in refraction of the visual and extra-visual pupillary zones. *Am. J. Ophthal.*, **13**, 101–12.

Thibos, L. N., Ye, M., Zhang, X. and Bradley, A. (1997). Spherical aberration of the reduced schematic eye with elliptical refracting surface. *Optom. Vis. Sci.*, **74**, 548–56.

Tomlinson, A., Hemenger, R. P. and Garriott, R. (1993). Method for estimating the spheric aberration of the human crystalline lens *in vivo*. *Invest. Ophthal. Vis. Sci.*, **34**, 621–9.

van den Brink, G. (1962). Measurements of the geometrical aberration of the eye. *Vision Res.*, **2**, 233–44.

van Heel, A. C. S. (1946). Correcting the spherical and chromatic aberrations of the eye. *J. Opt. Soc. Am.*, **36**, 237–9.

van Meeteren, A. (1974). Calculations on the optical modulation transfer function of the human eye for white light. *Optica Acta.*, **21**, 395–412.

von Bahr, G. (1945). Investigations into the spherical and chromatic aberrations of the eye, and their influence on its refraction. *Acta Ophthal.*, **23**, 1–47.

Walsh, G. (1988). The effect of mydriasis on pupillary centration of the human eye. *Ophthal. Physiol. Opt.*, **8**, 178–82.

Walsh, G. and Charman, W. N. (1985). Measurement of the axial wavefront aberration of the human eye. *Ophthal. Physiol. Opt.*, **5**, 23–31.

Walsh, G. and Cox, M. J. (1995). A new computerized video-aberroscope for the determination of the aberration of the human eye. *Ophthal. Physiol. Opt.*, **15**, 403–8.

Walsh, G., Charman, W. N. and Howland, H. C. (1984).

Objective technique for the determination of monochromatic aberrations of the human eye. *J. Opt. Soc. Am. A.*, **1**, 987–92.

Wang, Y.-Z., Thibos, L. N., Lopez, N. *et al.* (1996). Subjective refraction of the peripheral field using contrast detection acuity. *J. Amer. Optom. Assoc.*, **67**, 584–9.

Williams, D. R., Brainard, D. H., McMahon, M. J. and Navarro, R. (1994). Double pass and interferometric measures of the optical quality of the eye. *J. Opt. Soc. Am. A.*, **11**, 3123–35.

Williams, D. R., Artal, P., Navarro, R. *et al.* (1996). Off-axis optical quality and retinal sampling in the human eye. *Vision Res.*, **36**, 1103–14.

Wilson, M. A., Campbell, M. C. W. and Simonet, P. (1992). Change of pupil centration with change of illumination and pupil size. *Optom. Vis. Sci.*, **69**, 129–36.

Woods, R. L., Bradley, A. and Atchison, D. A. (1996). Monocular diplopia caused by ocular aberrations and hyperopic defocus. *Vision Res.*, **36**, 3597–606.

Young, T. (1801). The Bakerian Lecture. On the mechanism of the eye. *Phil. Trans. R. Soc. Lond.*, **91**, 23–88 (and plates).

16

Monochromatic aberrations of schematic eyes

Introduction

The monochromatic aberrations of schematic eyes are considered in this chapter. We begin with paraxial model eyes, which were introduced in Chapter 5, and show that these models predict ocular aberrations poorly. The construction of more accurate schematic eyes, known as **finite** or **wide angle** schematic eyes, will then be considered. These models have useful applications, such as predicting retinal image sizes (Drasdo and Fowler, 1974), predicting light levels on the retina (Kooijman, 1983), and predicting the effects of changes in any ocular structure on ocular aberrations and hence image quality. The last of these is particularly relevant now that corneal shapes are being surgically modified to reduce refractive errors.

Aberrations of schematic eyes have been the subject of many investigations. Simple equations do not exist for their exact calculation from the system parameters. Useful, although approximate, equations exist in the form of Seidel aberration equations, and these will be used in this chapter, as well as determining exact aberrations. Seidel equations increase in accuracy with decrease in pupil and field size; that is, as aberration levels decrease. Seidel aberration equations provide surface contributions to the total aberrations. The equations indicate how these surface contributions depend upon the position of the aperture stop and surface asphericity, factors that will be explored when

finite schematic eyes are discussed. Many of the Seidel aberration equations that appear in this chapter were explained in detail by Smith and Atchison (1997a).

The aberrations of the Gullstrand number 1 eye are representative of those of the Le Grand full theoretical, Gullstrand–Emsley and Bennett and Rabbetts eyes, at least in the case of the relaxed (unaccommodated) versions (Appendix 3). Thus in this chapter, the aberrations of the Gullstrand number 1 relaxed eye are compared with those of finite schematic eyes and real eyes.

Note on notation for the wave aberration polynomial co-efficients

In Chapter 15, we dropped the field dependent sub-prefix before the 'W' of the wave aberration co-efficients. The reason for this was that, since the aberrations of real eyes are measured at the fovea (which is about 5° off axis), the sum of all field dependent terms is actually being measured. In this chapter, where we use Seidel aberration theory to predict the corresponding wave aberration co-efficients, we must retain the field dependent prefixes.

Aberrations of paraxial schematic eyes

Spherical aberration

For an object at infinity, a positive power spherical surface or a positive power single lens with spherical surfaces has positive spherical aberration, and the aberration level increases with the power. Since paraxial schematic eyes have spherical surfaces and the powers of all surfaces except the posterior cornea are positive, it may be expected that relaxed paraxial schematic eyes have positive spherical aberration that will increase with increase in accommodation. While the back surface of the cornea has negative power and is therefore expected to have negative spherical aberration, it has the lowest of the surface powers of the eyes and therefore cannot cancel the positive aberration of the other surfaces. These predictions are confirmed by Seidel aberration results in Appendix 3.

The exact spherical aberration can be calculated as a power error $\Delta F(r)$ by finite (exact) ray-tracing. This is done by tracing rays from the axial point on the retina, through and out of the eye into air, and determining the vergence of these rays at the front principal plane. Such a ray is shown in Figure 15.7c. Apart from the sign, the vergence of this ray at the front principal plane is the power error $\Delta F(r)$.

Aberration theory predicts that the power error $(F(r)$ can be expressed as an even power polynomial in ray height r at the eye. That is,

$$\Delta F(r) = br^2 + cr^4 + dr^6 + er^8 + fr^{10} \quad (16.1)$$

In Chapter 15, we assumed for the real eye that $c = d = e = f = 0$. Fitting this polynomial to the Gullstrand number 1 schematic eye's power error values gives

$b = 0.355 \times 10^{-3}$ mm^{-3},
$c = 0.0128 \times 10^{-3}$ mm^{-5},
$d = -0.00166 \times 10^{-3}$ mm^{-7},
$e = 0.000242 \times 10^{-3}$ mm^{-9},
$f = -0.00000857 \times 10^{-3}$ mm^{-11} \quad (16.1a)

The value of b can be used to calculate the primary wave aberration co-efficient $_0W_{4,0}$ by the simple equation (15.16). Alternatively, if the value of $_0W_{4,0}$ is known, this can be used to predict the value of b, using the same

equation. The value of $_0W_{4,0}$ can be found from either a finite ray trace or from the Seidel spherical aberration S_1 using equation (A2.14a). Values of S_1 are given in Appendix 3 for a number of schematic eyes. The value of b predicted by Seidel theory for the Gullstrand number 1 eye is 0.000359 mm^{-3}, which is close to the value derived from the finite ray trace.

It follows from equations (15.13) and (15.16) that

$$\Delta F(r) \approx br^2 = 4_0W_{4,0}r^2 \quad (16.2)$$

This equation and variants have appeared in the literature several times – for example, Charman *et al.* (1978). For the Gullstrand number 1 schematic eye,

$$\Delta F(r) \approx 0.000359\, r^2 \quad (16.2a)$$

Equation (16.2) is approximate because the higher order terms in equation (16.1) have been neglected. Such an approximation can be called a **Seidel approximation**. The error induced by ignoring the higher order terms will become less important as the ray height r decreases.

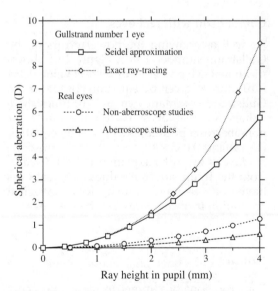

Figure 16.1. Spherical aberration of the Gullstrand number 1 schematic eye and of real eyes. Power errors of the Gullstrand eye were calculated both from the values in equation (16.1a) derived from finite ray-tracing, and by using the value of b in equation (16.2a) derived from the Seidel approximation. Power errors of real eyes were derived from non-aberroscope studies as given by equation (15.14), and by aberroscope studies as given by equation (15.22).

Figure 16.1 shows the power errors of the Gullstrand number 1 eye, with exact power errors derived from the values in equation (16.1a) after finite ray-tracing, and approximate power errors derived from equation (16.2a). The Seidel approximation is in error by –8 per cent at a ray height of 2 mm.

Surface contributions

Although the Seidel approximation is not accurate for the larger ray heights (Figure 16.1), the Seidel equations indicate the relative surface contributions to the spherical aberration. In the Gullstrand number 1 eye, the anterior corneal surface provides most of the Seidel spherical aberration (≈ 60 per cent) with the posterior surface of the lens being the next largest contributor (≈ 30 per cent) (Appendix 3). The accommodated version of the Gullstrand number 1 eye has about 3 times the spherical aberration of that of the relaxed eye, with the increase being due mainly to a 4.6 times increase in the aberration of the lens.

Comparison with real eyes

As well as showing the power errors of the Gullstrand number 1 eye, Figure 16.1 shows mean real eye power errors. The b value 0.354 $\times 10^{-3}$ mm^{-3}, given by equation (16.1a) for the Gullstrand schematic eye, is 5–10 times the b values for real eyes: 0.076×10^{-3} mm^{-3} for non-aberroscope studies as given by equation (15.14) and 0.035×10^{-3} mm^{-3} for aberroscope studies as given by equation (15.22). Clearly from the figure and the values of b, real eyes have on average much less spherical aberration than the paraxial schematic eyes.

Coma

For a rotationally symmetric eye, coma occurs only off-axis and increases with distance off-axis. It will be calculated at the fovea, assuming this to be 5° from the optical axis, and with the pupil centred on the optical axis. The exact amount of coma in a schematic eye can be determined by tracing two finite rays in the tangential section of the pupil, calculating the wave aberrations of each, and taking the difference. If we trace a finite ray at a height of 1 mm in the upper and lower tangential sections of the pupil and denote these aberrations as $W(1,0°)$ and $W(1,180°)$, respectively, providing there are no other odd off-axis aberrations present, the coma wave aberration co-efficient $W_{3,1}$ (including all field dependent terms) will be

$$W_{3,1} = [W(1, 0°) - W(1, 180°)]/2 \qquad (16.3)$$

For the Gullstrand number 1 schematic eye, $W(1, \ 0°) = 0.000300$ mm and $W(1,180°) = 0.000194$ mm. Thus,

$$W_{3,1} = +0.0000530 \text{ mm}^{-2} \qquad (16.4a)$$

Since this value is positive, the coma flare is on the axis side of the image point $\mathbf{Q'}$ as shown in Figure 15.9.

The Seidel coma S_2 is given in Appendix 3, and the corresponding primary wave aberration co-efficient $_1W_{3,1}$ is related to it by equation (A2.14b) to give

$$_1W_{3,1} = 0.0000573 \text{ mm}^{-2} \qquad (16.4b)$$

The coma co-efficients in equations (16.4a) and (16.4b) are similar, showing that Seidel theory predicts accurately the level of exact coma for a ray height of 1 mm and at the fovea of a schematic eye. This is probably because the higher order terms are not significant at a 5° off-axis angle.

Comparison with real eyes

There are measures of coma-like aberration terms from aberroscope studies. Walsh and Charman's (1985) determined values of $\mathbf{W}_6$ to $\mathbf{W}_9$ co-efficients, as given in equation (15.1), in the range -0.000128 mm^{-2} to $+0.000108$ mm^{-2}. The above estimates for the Gullstrand number 1 schematic eye lie within this range, and therefore it is possible that the coma of real eyes is greater than expected from schematic eyes.

Some of the coma found in the aberroscope studies may be because of inaccurate pupil centre location (Smith *et al.*, 1998), and because the pupil is probably decentred from the best fit optical axis. In Chapter 15 we determined the amount of coma arising from pupil decentration in the presence of spherical aberration. For a transverse pupil shift ΔX, we can rewrite equation (15.27), giving the change in coma $\Delta W_{3,1}$ as

$$\Delta W_{3,1} = -4 \; \Delta X \; W_{4,0} \tag{16.5}$$

If the pupil shifts longitudinally from the nodal point by the distance **EN** and the pupil ray is inclined at an angle θ to the optical axis, the centre of the pupil is transversely shifted by a distance ΔX given by the equation

$$\Delta X = \theta \mathbf{EN} \tag{16.6}$$

for small angles. Substituting this value of ΔX into equation (16.5) gives the expected change $\Delta W_{3,1}$ in coma of

$$\Delta W_{3,1} = -4\theta \mathbf{EN} \; W_{4,0} \tag{16.7}$$

Guidarelli (1972) argued that the eye is almost 'homocentric', because the centres of curvature of the corneal surfaces and the retina lie almost on the nodal points. If the aperture stop was also at the nodal points, the eye would have no off-axis aberrations. If the aperture stop was not at the nodal points, the value of $\Delta W_{3,1}$ in equation (16.7) would be the absolute value of coma, not merely a change. van Meeteren (1974) relied on Guidarelli's argument that the eye is homocentric to

predict the level of coma in real eyes from measured values of spherical aberration and the above equation.

If we are to rely on this argument for predictions of coma, we need to confirm whether equation (16.7) predicts accurately the level of coma in the eye. While the centres of curvatures of the corneal surfaces do lie near the nodal points, those of the lens and retina do not. The primary coma co-efficient $_1W_{3,1}$ of the Gullstrand number 1 eye is plotted against aperture stop position in Figure 16.2. This eye has zero coma if the aperture stop is 1.5 mm in front of the front nodal point, with the corresponding entrance pupil position 3.8 mm from the corneal vertex instead of the usual 3.05 mm. Therefore, placing the aperture stop at the front or back nodal point does not eliminate coma, and the parameters of Gullstrand number 1 schematic eye do not support Guidarelli's hypothesis of homocentricity.

Astigmatism and peripheral power errors

Sagittal and tangential power errors

If we trace thin beams of light (pencils) rays into a schematic eye as shown in Figure 15.10a, the fans in the sagittal and tangential sections focus on the sagittal and tangential image surfaces, respectively. In general, the sagittal image surface is behind the retina and the tangential surface is in front of the retina. For real eyes, we measure the vergences in object space of the sagittal and tangential foci conjugate with the retina (Figure 15.10b), so peripheral power errors in a schematic eye are calculated by tracing finite or exact rays out of the eye. Figure 16.3 shows exact power errors $L_s(\theta)$ and $L_t(\theta)$ of the Gullstrand number 1 eye as measured from the corneal vertex plane. The results depend upon the shape of the retina, which has been assumed to be spherical with a radius of curvature of −12 mm.

We can investigate the effect of the retinal radius of curvature using Seidel aberration theory. According to Seidel theory, the sagittal and tangential image surfaces shown in Figure 15.10a are spherical, and the radii of curvature can be calculated from equations

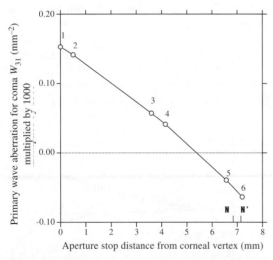

Figure 16.2. Primary wave coma co-efficient of the Gullstrand number 1 eye for different positions of the aperture stop relative to the corneal vertex (off-axis angle 5°). The nodal points **N** and **N'** are also indicated. The numbers represent the positions of surfaces: 1 – anterior cornea; 2 – posterior cornea; 3 – anterior lens; 4 – anterior lens core; 5 – posterior lens core; 6 – posterior lens.

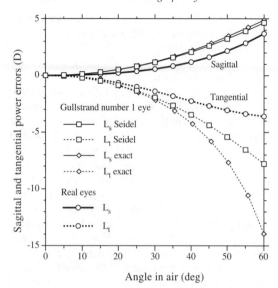

Figure 16.3. The sagittal and tangential power errors of the Gullstrand number 1 eye and of real eyes.

(A2.15) and the Seidel data given in Appendix 3. For the Gullstrand number 1 eye, the sagittal radius r_s and tangential radius r_t have the values

$$r_s = -13.89 \text{ mm and } r_t = -9.77 \text{ mm} \qquad (16.8)$$

These values were used to plot the sagittal and tangential surfaces shown in Figure 15.10a and so predict the astigmatism. The power errors can be expressed in terms of the object space field angle θ and the sagittal and tangential surface radii of curvature using equations (A2.19), which are Seidel equations (A2.16) modified to take into account the curvature of the retina. These equations are:

$$L_s(\theta) \approx \frac{\theta^2}{2n_{\text{vit}}} [\frac{1}{r_s} - \frac{1}{r_R}] \qquad (16.9a)$$

$$L_t(\theta) \approx \frac{\theta^2}{2n_{\text{vit}}} [\frac{1}{r_t} - \frac{1}{r_R}] \qquad (16.9b)$$

where r_R is the radius of curvature of the retina, θ is the off-axis angle in radians, and n_{vit} is the refractive index of the vitreous.

Figure 16.3 compares the power errors obtained from these equations with the exact power errors for the Gullstrand number 1 eye. The Seidel equations are reasonably accurate within about 15–20° from the optical axis.

Comparison with real eyes

As well as showing the power errors of the Gullstrand number 1 eye, Figure 16.3 shows mean real eye power errors. The sagittal power errors of the schematic eye are similar to those of real eyes. However, the tangential power errors of the schematic eye are much larger than those of real eyes.

Astigmatism

As in Chapter 15, astigmatism $A(\theta)$ is quantified as the difference between the sagittal $L_s(\theta)$ and tangential $L_t(\theta)$ power errors. Recalling equation (15.30),

$$A(\theta) = L_s(\theta) - L_t(\theta) \qquad (16.10)$$

Figure 16.4 shows exact astigmatism for the Gullstrand number 1 eye from the data shown in Figure 16.3. Combining equations (16.9a and b) and equation (16.10), the Seidel approximation for astigmatism is

$$A(\theta) \approx \frac{\theta^2}{2n_{\text{vit}}} [\frac{1}{r_s} - \frac{1}{r_t}] \qquad (16.11)$$

This equation shows that, within the Seidel approximation, astigmatism is independent of the value of the radius of curvature r_R of the retina. For the Gullstrand relaxed eye,

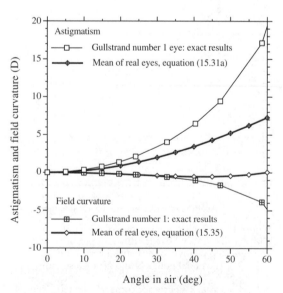

Figure 16.4. Astigmatism and field curvature of the Gullstrand number 1 eye and of real eyes.

equation (16.11) predicts that the astigmatism varies with field angle as

$$A(\theta_{deg}) \approx 0.198 \; \theta^2_{deg} \; D \qquad (16.11a)$$

where θ_{deg} is now the off-axis angle in degrees.

Equations (A2.17) can be used to predict the expected value of the two wave aberration coefficients $W_{2,0}$ and $W_{2,2}$. Using the data in Figure 16.3, for 5° off-axis,

$$W_{2,0} = -1.61 \times 10^{-5} \; mm^{-1} \qquad (16.12a)$$

and

$$W_{2,2} = 4.33 \times 10^{-5} \; mm^{-1} \qquad (16.12b)$$

At 5°, the exact and Seidel values are the same to three significant figures.

Comparison with real eyes

As well as showing the astigmatism of the Gullstrand number 1 eye, Figure 16.4 shows the mean astigmatism of real eyes as taken from equation (15.31a). Once again, the schematic eye has worse aberration than real eyes.

Petzval and field curvature

In equation (15.34), **field curvature** was defined as the mean of the sagittal and tangential power errors

$$\text{Field curvature}(\theta) = [L_s(\theta) + L_t(\theta)]/2 \qquad (16.13)$$

If astigmatism is zero, the sagittal and tangential surfaces coincide. In Seidel theory, this surface is called the **Petzval surface** (Figure 15.10a). The radius of curvature r_p of the Petzval surface is related to the value of the Seidel aberration S_4 by equation (A2.15c) and, using the data given in Appendix 3, for the relaxed Gullstrand number 1 eye:

$$r_p = -17.85 \; mm \qquad (16.14)$$

which is considerably larger than the retinal radius of curvature, assumed here to be −12 mm.

Using the definition of field curvature given by equation (16.13) and the expressions for $L_s(\theta)$ and $L_t(\theta)$ given by equations (16.9a and b), the Seidel estimate of field curvature is

given by

$$\text{Field curvature } (\theta) \approx \frac{\theta^2}{2n_{vit}} \left[\frac{1}{r_s} + \frac{1}{r_t} - \frac{2}{r_R} \right]$$

$$(16.15)$$

which shows that field curvature is dependent upon the shape of the retina. For the Gullstrand number 1 schematic eye, this equation reduces to

$$\text{Field curvature}(\theta) \approx -8.73 \times 10^{-4} \; \theta^2_{deg} \; D$$

$$(16.15a)$$

Comparison with real eyes

As well as values of astigmatism, Figure 16.4 shows exact values of field curvature of the Gullstrand number 1 schematic eye and the mean field curvature of real eyes. The schematic eye values are similar to those of real eyes to about 30°, but at higher angles the schematic eye values are greater.

Distortion

As discussed in Chapter 15 (*Types and magnitudes of monochromatic aberrations*), distortion has little meaning for the eye because of the curvature of the retina. Of

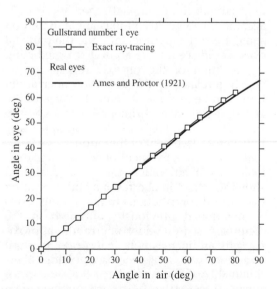

Figure 16.5. Internal and external angles for the pupil ray of the Gullstrand number 1 eye and of the 'real eye' results of Ames and Proctor (1921).

importance is the relationship between the angles of the pupil ray θ' inside the eye and that θ outside the eye. We can calculate the exact relationship by tracing exact rays. The results for the Gullstrand number 1 schematic eye from exact ray-tracing are shown in Figure 16.5, together with the data of Ames and Proctor (1921), which have been replotted from Figure 15.15. The two curves are similar, suggesting that paraxial schematic eyes can predict retinal image positions accurately, even for large off-axis angles.

Summary

The reader is reminded that there are considerable inter-individual variations in aberrations of real eyes, and the comparisons given here are based on the authors' estimations of mean levels of aberrations for real eyes.

Paraxial schematic eyes do not predict accurately the spherical aberration of real eyes, with the predictions being 5–10 times that occurring in real eyes. The paraxial schematic eyes do better at predicting the off-axis sagittal and tangential power errors, with the sagittal power error prediction being much better than tangential power error. The astigmatism of paraxial schematic eyes is approximately twice that of real eyes, and the field curvature of paraxial schematic eyes is accurate to about 30° off-axis angle. Based on some indirect experimental data, the paraxial eyes would seem to be accurate in predicting the position of the off-axis retinal image, which is related to the distortion aberration. Little can be said about coma, because of the lack of definitive experimental data, except to state that its value will depend upon any transverse placement of the pupil.

We have already mentioned that approximate Seidel aberration theory is useful in showing trends in aberrations and indicating the surface contributions to aberrations. Also as mentioned previously, although in the reciprocal sense, Seidel aberration approximations are increasingly inaccurate as pupil size or off-axis angle increases. Seidel aberration theory underestimates the amount of spherical aberration in the schematic eye, by about a factor of two at a ray height of 4 mm. In the case of sagittal and tangential power

errors, the Seidel aberrations are reasonably accurate to about 15–20° from the optical axis, after which the Seidel astigmatism becomes too large, particularly for the tangential errors. This leads to over-estimations of both astigmatism and field curvature.

Modelling surface shapes

Having shown that paraxial schematic eyes predict some of the aberrations of real eyes poorly, particularly spherical aberration, we will investigate the ways in which the paraxial models can be improved to more accurately represent real eyes. The properties of aspheric surfaces, the ways of representing the gradient refractive index of the lens, and how these affect the aberrations, will be considered. In this section, surface asphericity is considered.

All paraxial schematic eyes have spherical surfaces, but surfaces of real eyes are non-spherical. More accurate model eyes should include aspheric refracting surfaces. As the word 'aspheric' simply means 'non-spherical', there is an infinite range of aspheric surfaces. However, we will restrict this range to rotationally symmetric aspheric smooth surfaces. In conventional optics, the aspherical surface most frequently found to be useful is the conicoid.

Conicoid surfaces

Equation (2.4) gives the form of a conicoid surface as

$$h^2 + (1 + Q)Z^2 - 2ZR = 0 \qquad (16.16)$$

where

the Z axis is the optical axis
$h^2 = X^2 + Y^2$
R is the vertex radius of curvature and
Q is the surface asphericity where
    $Q < 0$ surface flattens away from its vertex
    $Q = 0$ specifies a sphere
    $Q > 0$ surface steepens away from its vertex.

The effect of the value and sign of Q on surface shape is shown in Figure 2.2. Asphericity is sometimes expressed in terms of a quantity p called the **shape factor**, which is related to Q by the equation

$$p = 1 + Q \tag{16.17a}$$

Another quantity which has often been used is the eccentricity e. This is related to Q by the equation

$$Q = -e^2 \tag{16.17b}$$

but while e^2 is always positive, e by itself only has meaning if Q is negative. For ellipses (ellipsoids in one section only), the following equation is also popular

$$(Z - a)^2/a^2 + Y^2/b^2 = 1 \tag{16.18}$$

where a and b are the ellipse axes semi-lengths. The vertex radius of curvature R is related to a and b by the equation

$$R = +b^2/a \tag{16.19}$$

and the asphericity Q is related to a and b by

$$Q = b^2/a^2 - 1 \tag{16.20}$$

Effect of conicoid asphericity on Seidel aberrations

Hopkins (1950) and Welford (1986) defined a surface aspheric aberration contribution factor k, which is

$$k = C^2 h^4 FQ \tag{16.21}$$

where C is the surface curvature, h is the paraxial marginal ray height at the surface, and F is the surface power. In terms of this factor k, aspherizing produces the following changes in the Seidel aberrations:

$$\Delta S_1 = k, \ \Delta S_2 = Ek, \ \Delta S_3 = E^2 k \text{ and } \Delta S_5 = E^3 k \tag{16.22}$$

where E is the stop shift factor defined as $\overline{h}/h$, h is the marginal ray height at the surface, and $\overline{h}$ is the height of the paraxial pupil ray at the surface.

Equations (16.21) and (16.22) show that aberrations are likely to change more quickly with asphericity as surface power increases – e.g. asphericity is likely to have its greatest influence at the anterior corneal surface. However, for off-axis aberrations this is dependent on the stop shift factor E such that aspherizing is more effective the further a surface is away from the aperture stop. Aberrations such as astigmatism will not be affected by aspherizing the lens anterior surface where E has a value of zero.

Figured conicoid surfaces

Another type of aspheric surface is given by the polynomial

$$Z = v_1 h^2 + v_2 h^4 + v_3 h^6 + \dots \tag{16.23}$$

A conicoid can always be expressed in this form, but not all polynomials of this form are conicoids. A conicoid can be expressed in this form by firstly solving equation (16.16) as a quadratic equation in Z to give

$$Z = \frac{R - \sqrt{[R^2 - (1 + Q)h^2]}}{(1 + Q)} \tag{16.24a}$$

and then using the binomial theorem to expand the square root term to express this equation for Z in polynomial form. However, equation (16.24a) is not useful for a flat surface (i.e. $R = \infty$) or paraboloids ($Q = -1$), and an alternative form is

$$Z = \frac{h^2}{R + \sqrt{[R^2 - (1 + Q)h^2]}} \tag{16.24b}$$

which is solvable for all values of the parameters.

Some non-conicoid surfaces can be approximated by a conicoid and a small surface adjustment. These surfaces are called figured conicoids, and can be described by the equation

$$Z = Z_{\text{conicoid}} + f_4 h^4 + f_6 h^6 + f_8 h^8 + \text{etc.} \tag{16.25}$$

where Z_{conicoid} is the value of Z given by equation (16.24a or b) and the co-efficients f_4, f_6, etc are called figuring co-efficients. The values of the figuring co-efficients depend upon the aspheric surface being modelled. If the surface curvature is not zero, the term f_4 can be omitted provided that the value of Q and all other figuring co-efficients are changed appropriately.

Usually, an exact representation of a non-conicoid aspheric in equation (16.25) requires an infinite number of figuring terms. In practice, the figuring power series is terminated at a finite number of terms, leaving a residual error. The required number of figuring co-efficients depends upon the permissible error.

Modelling the anterior corneal surface

There is considerable published data on the anterior corneal asphericity. Many investigators fitted their corneal shape data to either a conic in certain sections or to conicoids using three-dimensional data. They expressed the results in terms of the asphericity Q, shape factor p or the eccentricity e. Some results, all in terms of Q, are given in Table 2.3. The mean values obtained by the larger scale studies are very similar, being in the approximate range –0.2 to –0.3. The effect of the value of Q on corneal shape is shown in Figure 2.3 for corneas with a vertex radius of curvature of 7.8 mm. Equations (16.21) and (16.22) show that negative values of Q will reduce spherical aberration.

Other types of equations have been used to describe corneal shape, e.g. those of Bonnet and Cochet (1962) and Bonnet (1964).

Modelling the posterior corneal surface

In contrast with the anterior corneal surface, the posterior corneal surface has not attracted a great deal of attention. It is neglected in simplified eye models (Chapter 5). This is usually justified on the grounds that it has much less power than the anterior surface (about one-tenth of the power).

It is difficult to measure accurately the shape of this surface, because it is so close to the anterior surface and its apparent shape is influenced by the shape of the anterior surface. As mentioned in Chapter 2, Patel *et al.* (1993) measured the shape of the anterior surface and the corneal thickness, and then deduced the posterior surface from that data. They found a mean posterior surface asphericity Q value of –0.42. However, their results must be viewed with caution because their anterior mean asphericity was –0.03, which is very different from most other values shown in Table 2.3.

Equations (16.21) and (16.22) show that the above negative values of Q would increase positive spherical aberration, but since the power of this surface is small, the effect would be small.

Modelling the lenticular surfaces

Attempts to extract asphericity Q values from the *in vitro* data of Howcroft and Parker (1977) are given in Table 2.5, together with Q values derived from the data of Brown (1974) by Liou and Brennan (1997). Probably there is a wide variation in values due to a combination of the difficulty in accurate measurement of asphericity and of inter-individual variations in asphericity values (Smith *et al.*, 1991).

Modelling the lenticular refractive index distribution

The refractive index of all ocular media except the lens can be regarded as uniform, and thus only the lens needs special treatment. It has been known for well over a hundred years that the lens has a varying refractive index, and Gullstrand's (1909) representation of the refractive index is given in equation (2.12).

In modelling the internal structure of the lens, two types of lens models have been used. These are a multiple layered shell structure (e.g. Gullstrand, 1909; Pomerantzeff *et al.*, 1984; Raasch and Lakshminarayanan, 1989; Mutti *et al.*, 1995) and a continuously varying index (e.g. Gullstrand, 1909; Blaker, 1980 and 1991; Smith *et al.*, 1991). The advantage of the shell model is that it allows conventional paraxial ray-tracing procedures to be used to examine powers, but has the disadvantage that it is more difficult to analyze its aberrations, because conventional Seidel theory and finite ray-tracing routines cannot be used with such shell structures. By contrast, while ray-tracing through a gradient refractive index and aberration analysis is much more complex, routines for performing these calculations are well established. We will look at both these models, beginning with the continuous refractive index model.

Continuous refractive index model

A general mathematical form for representing the refractive index distribution $N(Y,Z)$ in the Y–Z section, assuming rotational symmetry about the optical (Z) axis, is

$$N(Y,Z) = N_0(Z) + N_1(Z)Y^2 + N_2(Z)Y^4 \dots \quad (16.26)$$

where

$$N_0(Z) = N_{0,0} + N_{0,1}Z + N_{0,2}Z^2 \ldots$$
$$N_1(Z) = N_{1,0} + N_{1,1}Z + N_{1,2}Z^2 \ldots$$
$$N_2(Z) = N_{2,0} + N_{2,1}Z + N_{2,2}Z^2 \ldots$$
$$\text{etc.} \ldots \tag{16.26a}$$

The values of the $N_{i,j}$ co-efficients set the refractive index distribution within the lens.

Smith *et al.* (1991) presented a gradient index model of the lens in which the index along any line from the centre of the lens to the edge and at a relative distance r from the lens centre can be described by

$$N(r) = c_0 + c_1 r^2 + c_2 r^4 + c_3 r^6 \tag{16.27}$$

They divided the refractive index distribution into two half ellipses (Figure 16.6). The front ellipse has a semi-axis a_1 along the optical axis and a semi-axis b along the equatorial meridian. The back ellipse has a semi-axis a_2 along the optical axis and semi-axis b along the equatorial meridian. For the front half of the ellipse, some of the $N_{i,j}$ co-efficients are given by

$$N_{0,0} = c_0 + c_1 + c_2 + c_3$$
$$N_{0,1} = (-2c_1 - 4c_2 - 6c_3)/a_1$$
$$N_{0,2} = (c_1 + 6c_2 + 15c_3)/a_1^2$$
$$N_{1,0} = (c_1 + 2c_2 + 3c_3)/b^2 \tag{16.28a}$$

For the back half of the ellipse, some of the $N_{i,j}$ co-efficients are given by

$$N_{0,0} = c_0$$
$$N_{0,1} = 0$$
$$N_{0,2} = c_1/a_2^2$$
$$N_{1,0} = c_1/b^2 \tag{16.28b}$$

A full set of co-efficients was given by Smith *et al.* (1991).

The refractive index distribution has been investigated in many vertebrate lenses and has been often fitted by a parabolic form of equation (16.27) in which c_2 and c_3 are set to zero. However, Pierscionek and Chan's (1989) results with human lenses indicate that the distribution is more complex and may require a higher order polynomial description.

The power of the lens

The power of the lens can be divided into two components: (a) one arising from the front and back surfaces, and (b) one arising from the gradient index alone.

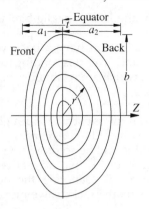

Figure 16.6. The gradient index of the lens modelled as two half ellipses joined at the equator. Some iso-incidal lines are shown.

Surface powers

The power of the surfaces can be found from the equation

$$F = (n' - n)/R \tag{16.29}$$

where R is the radius of curvature of a surface and n and n' are refractive indices on either side of the surface.

The gradient index power

We can study the gradient index contribution to the total refractive power of the lens by regarding the lens bulk as a slab as shown in Figure 16.7. The slab of gradient index material has thickness t and is immersed in a medium of refractive index μ. We can find an approximate equation for the power of this slab by tracing the ray **AA'**, assuming it is a paraxial ray and that the change of height of

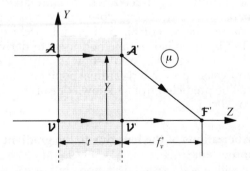

Figure 16.7. The power of the gradient index of the lens modelled as a 'slab' lens.

this ray in the lens is negligible, and finding where this ray crosses the optical axis at $\mathbf{F'}$. This lens will then have a back vertex focal length f'_v and a corresponding back vertex power F'_v, which are related by the equation

$$F'_v = \mu/f'_v \qquad (16.30)$$

The paraxial ray must pass through the point $\mathbf{F'}$ for all ray heights Y. According to Fermat's principle, this will be so providing the optical path lengths for the two ray paths $\mathbf{VV'F'}$ and $\mathbf{AA'F'}$ are equal. Denoting the optical path length by square brackets, we must have

$$[\mathbf{VV'}] + \mu f'_v = [\mathbf{AA'}] + \mu\sqrt{(Y^2 + f'^2_v)}$$

Atchison and Smith (1995) have shown that this equation reduces to

$$\begin{aligned} F'_v \approx -2(&N_{1,0}t + N_{1,1}t^2/2 + N_{1,2}t^3/3 + N_{1,3}t^4/4 \\ &+ N_{1,4}t^5/5 + \ldots) \end{aligned} \qquad (16.31)$$

Within the approximation, this equation shows that this power is dependent only upon the co-efficients $\{N_{1,j}, j = 0, 1\ldots\}$ which are the co-efficients of Y^2 in the refractive index function $N(Y,Z)$ given by equations (16.26). Therefore, the power does not depend on terms of higher order than Y^2 in the $N(Y,Z)$ function. These higher order terms are, in effect, aberration terms.

Total lens power and positions of the cardinal points

Equation (16.31) does not give the equivalent power or any information that allows us to calculate the positions of the cardinal points. If the equivalent power and cardinal point positions are needed, a paraxial ray trace suitable for gradient index media can be used, such as those of Moore (1971) or Doric (1984), or a finite ray traced which simulates a paraxial ray by being close to the axis e.g. Sharma *et al.* (1982). Smith and Atchison (1997b) extended the method used to derive equation (16.31), and showed that the equivalent power and cardinal point positions can be predicted from a knowledge of the $N_{i,j}$ co-efficients.

Aberrations of the lens due to the gradient index lens

Sands (1970) presented a set of equations for determining the Seidel aberrations of gradient index media. To make these equations consistent with the Seidel aberrations of Hopkins (1950) and Welford (1986), Sands' aberration values must be multiplied by a factor of two and the signs changed. The modified equations are given in Appendix 2. As argued in the appendix, these equations show that $N_{2,j}$ terms are likely to be the main contributors to the Seidel or primary spherical aberration, with a smaller contribution from the $N_{0,j}$ and $N_{1,j}$ terms. The spherical aberration has the opposite sign to that of the $N_{2,j}$ terms, so the sign of these co-efficients must be positive to reduce the spherical aberration of the eye.

The shell model

While the lens has a continuous gradient index structure, the refractive index has often been represented by a shell structure, with the refractive index in each shell kept constant, but varying from shell to shell. In the construction of such a model, it is necessary to decide the number of shells, how the refractive index varies from shell to shell, and the value of the curvatures of the surface of each shell.

Once the shell structure is established, paraxial ray-tracing can determine the lens power. Gullstrand (1909) presented a model of the lens with only two shells, but if it is intended to represent accurately the continuously varying index by such a shell structure, a larger number of shells should be taken. For example, Mutti *et al.* (1995) used 10 shells and Pomerantzeff *et al.* (1984) used 200 shells.

The power of the lens

The advantage of the shell model over the gradient index model is that conventional paraxial ray-tracing can be used to find the lens equivalent and vertex powers. Given a shell structure with a large number of shells, Atchison and Smith (1995) derived an equation for the power of the bulk medium, according to the same principles that they used to derive equation (16.31). They showed that the back vertex power F'_v is given by the equation

$$F'_v \approx \int N'(Z)C(Z) \, dZ \qquad (16.32)$$

where $N'(Z)$ is the derivative of the refractive index with respect to the distance Z along the optical axis and $C(Z)$ is the shell curvature as a function of Z. This equation shows that the shell model will have some power providing $N(Z)$ is not constant and $C(Z)$ is not zero.

Aberrations of the lens

As stated above, aberration analysis of shell structures is not possible with conventional Seidel theory or conventional ray-tracing, and the authors are not aware of any procedures for such calculations.

Modelling the retina

Compared with many other ocular parameters, the shape of the retina has not been extensively studied because of its inaccessability. Some schematic eye values are listed in Table 16.1. The retina is not necessarily spherical.

Usually, Seidel theory assumes that the image surface is flat. For analysing the sagittal and tangential power errors, we took into account the curved nature of the retina by modifying the respective aberrations, as given by equations (16.9a and b).

Survey of finite eye models

Comprehensive details of the more anatomically accurate schematic eyes are given in Appendix 3. Most of the finite model eyes are based upon established paraxial schematic eyes, improved by aspherizing one or more of the refracting surfaces, but one includes a lens

Table 16.1. Schematic eye values of retinal radius of curvature.

Source	Radius of retina (mm)
Stine (1934)	−11.06
Drasdo and Fowler (1974)	−12
Lotmar (1971)	−12.3
Kooijman (1983)	−10.8
(ellipsoidal with $Q = 0.346$)	−14.1

gradient index (Liou and Brennan, 1997). Schematic eyes of Pomerantzeff *et al.* (1971, 1972 and 1984) and Wang *et al.* (1983) are not discussed further because they did not provide full constructional details.

Many finite eye models have been developed for a restricted set of conditions. For example, the eye of Liou and Brennan was designed to give realistic spherical aberration, and off-axis monochromatic aberrations were not considered. It is unfair to be critical of a model if it does not predict quantities accurately that are outside the scope of its purpose.

Lotmar (1971)

Lotmar (1971) modified the Le Grand full theoretical eye, a four surface schematic eye. He aspherized the anterior surface of the cornea using the data of Bonnet and Cochet (1962) and Bonnet (1964), who used a special type of function that was not readily suitable for ray-tracing. Lotmar represented the front surface of the cornea by equation (16.23) up to the sixth power. This function can be interpreted as a figured paraboloid, that is with $Q = -1$, and figuring co-efficients of f_4 and f_6. Smith and Atchison (1983) showed that the f_4 term can be eliminated, providing the value of Q and all the other figuring co-efficients are adjusted suitably. If this transformation is done for the Lotmar cornea, we have $Q = -0.286$ and new figuring co-efficients as given in Appendix 3. There are two advantages of using this ellipsoid model. First, calculations show that this ellipsoid gives a better fit than the paraboloid to Lotmar's full polynomial form. Second, it allows a comparison with the data of other investigators, who fitted ellipsoids or ellipses to the cornea and found similar values of Q (Table 2.3). Lotmar also modified the lens by replacing the posterior spherical surface by a paraboloid.

This schematic eye is not an accurate representation of real eyes. While the corneal asphericity is close to that of real eyes, the lens is not accurately modelled. Lotmar ignored the aspheric nature of the anterior lens surface, and as yet there is no firm evidence that the posterior surface is parabolic.

Lotmar determined the spherical aberration and astigmatism of his model. He claimed that the spherical aberration was of the same order as found experimentally, but did not show any comparison. Lotmar also claimed that the astigmatism was in good agreement with experimental data from Ferree *et al.* (1931) and Rempt *et al.* (1971).

Drasdo and Fowler (1974)

This is a modified form of a schematic eye attributed by Stine (1934) to Cowan (1927), which is the same as the Gullstrand–Emsley simplified eye except that it uses 1.336 for the refractive index of the aqueous and vitreous and 1.43 for the refractive index of the lens. Stine added a retinal radius of curvature of −11.06 mm. The corneal surface has a radius of curvature of 7.8 mm and an asphericity of $Q = -0.25$, obtained from published data of Prechtel and Wesley (1970) and Mandell and St Helen (1971).

The purpose of this model was to determine retinal projection from the visual field. While Drasdo and Fowler (1974) acknowledged that real crystalline lenses have aspherical surfaces, they argued that the level of asphericity would make little difference to the path of principal rays, and therefore used a simplified lens with spherical surfaces. This argument is supported by the data in Figure 16.5.

Kooijman (1983)

Kooijman modified the Le Grand full theoretical eye model for the purpose of predicting retinal illumination. Both corneal surfaces have a Q value of −0.25, with the value of the anterior corneal surface taken from Mandell and St Helen (1971). The anterior lens surface is hyperbolic with a Q value of −3.06, taken from Howcroft and Parker (1977). The posterior lens surface is parabolic ($Q = -1$), again taken from Howcroft and Parker (1977). Two forms of the retinal shape were obtained from Krause (Helmholtz, 1909). One is spherical with a radius of curvature of −10.8 mm and the other is elliptical with a radius of curvature of −14.1 mm and an asphericity of $Q = +0.346$. The aberration results presented in the next section and in Appendix 3 were obtained with the spherical retina.

Navarro, Santamaría and Bescós (1985)

Navarro *et al.* (1985) used a variable accommodating model, in which the crystalline lens parameters and the distance between the cornea and lens are expressed as functions of the level of accommodation. Two paraxial variable accommodating eyes have been discussed already in Chapter 5.

The base paraxial model is the Le Grand schematic eye, except for a slightly different anterior corneal radius and corneal index. The anterior corneal surface and the lenticular surfaces are conicoids. The lens surface curvatures and asphericities, the lens thickness, the anterior chamber depth and the lens refractive index vary as functions of accommodation, most in a logarithmic manner. The combination of parameters lead to spherical aberration decreasing with accommodation, as in real eyes (see Chapter 15, *Types and magnitudes of monochromatic aberrations*), and it is approximately zero at an accommodation level of 5 D out to approximately 2 mm pupil height.

Escudero-Sanz and Navarro (1999) added a spherical retina of −12 mm radius of curvature. The aberration results presented in the next section were obtained with this retina.

Liou and Brennan (1997)

This model includes conicoid corneal and lenticular surfaces and a gradient index lens. Liou and Brennan selected, where possible, anatomical values based on 45-year-old eyes. The primary purpose of this schematic eye was to model the spherical aberration of real eyes, and it has a level of 1.0 D longitudinal spherical aberration at a ray height of 4 mm. It was also intended that the model should have normal levels of chromatic aberration; however all the chromatic aberration of the model occurs at the anterior corneal surface and its range of chromatic difference of refraction is only 1.1 D (400–700 nm), which is about half the normal level (see Chapter 17). The lenticular gradient index was based on the model of Smith *et al.* (1991) as described by equations (16.27), (16.28a) and (16.28b). Liou and Brennan used a parabolic gradient in which $c_0 = 1.407$, $c_1 = -0.039$ and c_2 and c_3 are set to zero in equation (16.27). To obtain the $N_{i,j}$ co-efficients of the front and back halves of the lens, the values of a_1, a_2 and b are 1.59 mm, 2.43 mm and 4.4404 mm, respectively, in equations (16.28a) and (16.28b).

The aperture stop is displaced 0.5 mm from the optical axis to the nasal side and the angle between the line of sight and the optical axis in object space is 5° (also the angle between visual axis and optical axis).

The model does not specify a retinal shape. The aberration results presented in the next section were obtained with a spherical retina of –12 mm radius of curvature.

Reduced eye models of Thibos and colleagues

Unlike the above eye models, there is no intention of anatomical accuracy in these models. However, they are included because they demonstrate features of real eyes such as axes and aberration levels.

Thibos *et al.* (1992) developed their 'Chromatic' eye based on Emsley's reduced eye, with an aspheric surface of $Q = -0.56$ in order to correct spherical aberration. This eye contains an aperture stop 1.91 mm from the cornea so that the entrance pupil is a similar distance from the nodal point as that in more sophisticated models. It has longitudinal chromatic aberration similar to that of real eyes (see Chapter 17). The Chromatic eye is not a rotationally symmetrical eye, but has a number of axes with no fixed relationship between them.

Thibos *et al.* (1997) developed a second schematic eye called the 'Indiana' eye. The asymmetries of the Chromatic eye were removed. The asphericity of the eye is variable, but they selected $Q = -0.4$ as giving the best fit to experimental results of longitudinal spherical aberration. This asphericity gives $\approx +1.2$ D aberration at a ray height of 2.5 mm.

By moving the stop further towards the nodal point, Wang and Thibos (1997) claimed that it was possible to obtain reasonable levels of both spherical aberration and peripheral astigmatism, for example with $Q = -0.4$ and the stop 2.55 mm inside the eye. However, this allows no control over coma, or over the sagittal and tangential powers. Atchison (1998) pointed out that their results for astigmatism are not comparable with experimental results at larger angles because they calculated the astigmatism inside the eye rather than outside. If $Q = -0.4$, the aperture stop is moved from 2.55 mm to 2.9 mm inside the eye, and the retinal radius of curvature is changed from its value of –11 mm to –13.25 mm, then the sagittal and tangential power errors and astigmatism better match the mean experimental values used by Wang and Thibos.

The aberration results presented in the next section were obtained with the Indiana eye with $Q = -0.4$ and a –11 mm retinal radius of curvature.

Performance of finite eye models

Seidel aberrations of finite schematic eyes

The Seidel aberrations were calculated for each of the above models. These values were transformed to wave aberration co-efficients using equations (A2.14) and (A2.20), and the results are listed in Table 16.2, along with mean values for real eyes in the case of spherical aberration, astigmatism and field curvature.

Spherical aberration

The spherical aberrations of the finite eyes are, apart from the Drasdo and Fowler eye, considerably smaller than those of paraxial eyes. However, only the Liou and Brennan eye has a level similar to that of real eyes. The high level of the Drasdo and Fowler eye may seem surprising, since the anterior cornea is asperized at the level expected in real eyes. However, the rear lenticular surface of the Drasdo and Fowler eye has more aberration than the rear two surfaces of the Gullstrand eye.

Coma

Coma is similar for both paraxial and finite eyes, except that the Thibos *et al.* eyes have extremely high levels and the Liou and Brennan eye has extremely low levels.

Table 16.2. The mean wave aberration co-efficients of real eyes and the wave aberration co-efficients of unaccommodated schematic eyes. The latter were determined using Seidel theory. All off-axis co-efficients are for 5° off-axis.

	$W_{4,0}$ (mm^{-3})	$W_{3,1}$ (mm^{-2})	$W_{2,0}$ (mm^{-1})	$^{a}W_{2,0}$ (mm^{-1})	$W_{2,2}$ (mm^{-1})
Real eyes	$^{b}1.89 \times 10^{-5}$ $^{c}8.8 \times 10^{-6}$	–	–	-7.91×10^{-6}	3.32×10^{-5}
Paraxial schematic eyes for reference					
Gullstrand No. 1	8.96×10^{-5}	5.73×10^{-5}	1.031×10^{-4}	-1.57×10^{-5}	4.34×10^{-5}
Le Grand Full theoretical	9.01×10^{-5}	5.76×10^{-5}	1.038×10^{-4}	-1.56×10^{-5}	4.14×10^{-5}
Finite schematic eyes					
Lotmar (1971)	4.67×10^{-5}	6.54×10^{-5}	9.56×10^{-5}	-2.08×10^{-5}	2.50×10^{-5}
Drasdo and Fowler (1974)	7.99×10^{-5}	7.38×10^{-5}	1.06×10^{-4}	-1.34×10^{-5}	3.84×10^{-5}
Kooijman (1983)	3.63×10^{-5}	5.78×10^{-5}	9.65×10^{-5}	-3.61×10^{-5}	2.69×10^{-5}
Navarro *et al.* (1985)	3.19×10^{-5}	6.50×10^{-5}	9.64×10^{-5}	-2.24×10^{-5}	2.52×10^{-5}
Liou and Brennan (1997)	1.70×10^{-5}	1.54×10^{-5}	8.76×10^{-5}	-3.11×10^{-5}	3.99×10^{-5}
Thibos *et al.* (1997)^{d}	3.96×10^{-5}	2.45×10^{-4}	1.16×10^{-4}	-3.78×10^{-6}	5.92×10^{-5}
Thibos *et al.* (1997)^{e}	3.96×10^{-5}	2.36×10^{-4}	1.03×10^{-4}	-1.63×10^{-5}	3.43×10^{-5}

[a] For real eyes, the measured values. For schematic eyes, adjusted $W_{2,0}$, taking into account the radius of the retina using equation (A2.20).
[b] Non-aberroscope studies, equation (15.14).
[c] Aberroscope data studies, equation (15.22).
[d] Aperture stop 1.91 mm inside eye.
[e] Aperture stop 2.55 mm inside eye.

Astigmatism and field curvature

Astigmatism is a similar level for real, paraxial and finite eyes, with a $W_{2,2}$ co-efficient range of 2.5×10^{-5} mm^{-1} to 5.9×10^{-5} mm^{-1}. The change in the aperture stop position of 0.64 mm of the Thibos *et al.* eye alters the astigmatism by a factor of two. The $W_{2,0}$ (sagittal) co-efficient is 1.6–5 times higher for the schematic eyes than for real eyes.

Exact aberrations of finite schematic eyes

Aberrations of the models, apart from the reduced eye of Thibos *et al.*, are shown in Figures 16.8 to 16.11.

Spherical aberration

Figure 16.8 shows spherical aberration. Comparing this figure with Figure 16.1 shows that, with the exception of the Drasdo and Fowler model, the finite schematic eyes perform much better than the Gullstrand schematic eye. The Liou and Brennan schematic eye has the lowest level of spherical aberration, which is close to mean real eye values. The Kooijman, Navarro *et al.* and Lotmar models all have similar levels of aberration.

Sagittal and tangential power errors

Figure 16.9 shows sagittal and tangential power errors. Sagittal and tangential power errors are sensitive to retinal shape, and the spread of the plots is partly because of the different retinal radii specified for the eyes. Comparing Figure 16.9 with Figure 16.3 shows that the finite models are generally

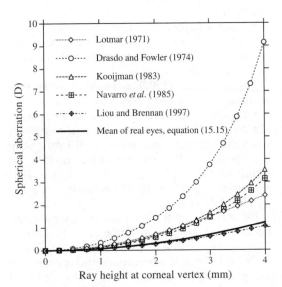

Figure 16.8. Spherical aberration of finite schematic eyes and of real eyes.

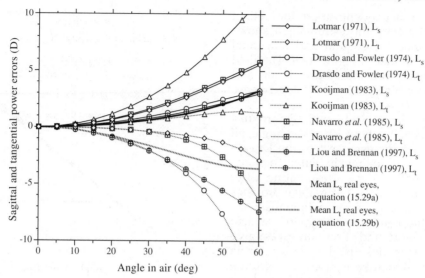

Figure 16.9. Sagittal and tangential power errors of finite schematic eyes and of real eyes.

much better than the Gullstrand number 1 eye for estimating mean tangential power errors, but not for estimating mean sagittal power errors. The Lotmar, Navarro *et al.* and Liou and Brennan eyes have reasonable estimations of both these errors. The Drasdo and Fowler eye estimates sagittal power errors well, but is inaccurate for the tangential power errors beyond approximately 40°. The Kooijman eye values for both sagittal and

tangential power errors are much too positive. If the flatter retina proposed by Kooijman is used, the estimations with his eye improve considerably to be similar to those of the Liou and Brennan eye.

Astigmatism and field curvature

Figure 16.10 shows astigmatism and field curvature. The astigmatism, at least for small

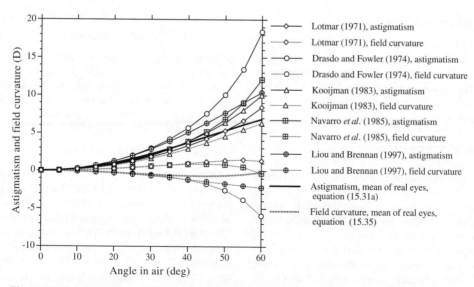

Figure 16.10. Astigmatism and field curvature of finite schematic eyes and of real eyes.

angles, is not dependent upon the retinal shape and therefore the astigmatism shows less spread than the sagittal and tangential power errors shown in Figure 16.9. The field curvature curves are more spread out, and this is explained in part by their dependence upon retinal shape.

Comparing Figure 16.10 with Figure 16.4 shows that, beyond about 30° object angle, all the finite schematic eyes, except the Drasdo and Fowler eye, are much better than the Gullstrand number 1 eye at estimating astigmatism of real eyes. The Lotmar eye provides excellent estimation of the astigmatism (as claimed by him), and the Kooijman, Navarro *et al.*, and Liou and Brennan eyes give reasonable estimates. If the flatter retina proposed by Kooijman is used, the estimations with his eye are worse beyond 40° object angle.

Improvement in predictions of field curvature of the majority of finite schematic eyes, compared with the Gullstrand number 1 eye, are only apparent beyond about 50°. Field curvature estimation is reasonable for the Lotmar, Navarro *et al.* and Liou and Brennan eyes. The Drasdo and Fowler eye has reasonable estimates, except beyond about 40° object angle. The Kooijman eye estimates the field curvature poorly, but if the flatter retina proposed by Kooijman is used, the estimations improve considerably to be similar to those of the Liou and Brennan eye.

Retinal image position

Figure 16.11 shows the relationship between internal and external angles of the pupil ray for the Gullstrand number 1 eye, four finite schematic eyes and 'real' eyes. This relationship is similar for all these eyes.

Retinal illuminance

Close to the optical axis and for small pupils, paraxial schematic eyes give an accurate estimate of retinal illuminance. For large pupils and point sources, the effect of aberrations must be included.

For off-axis points, we must consider the influences of distortion, retinal shape, and the size of the oblique pupil. In Chapter 13 (*Retinal illuminance: directly transmitted light*),

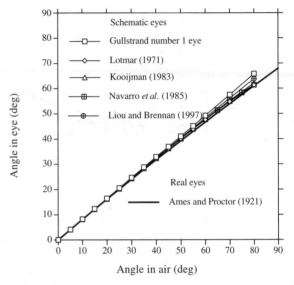

Figure 16.11. Internal and external angles of the pupil ray for the Gullstrand number 1 eye, some finite schematic eyes and 'real eyes'.

we estimated the relative retinal illuminance as a function of off-axis angle using paraxial data, a spherical retina and equation (13.12). The estimations were smaller than measurements with excised eyes (Figure 13.2). More accurate estimates require accurate estimates of the apparent pupil area $A(\theta)_p$ and the quantity $\delta\theta'/\delta\theta$ used in equation (13.12).

An accurate estimate of the apparent pupil area was given by equation (3.5b), which is

$$A(\theta)_p = A(0)_p (1 - 1.0947 \times 10^{-4}\, \theta^2 + 1.8698 \times 10^{-9}\, \theta^4)\ (\theta\ \text{in degrees})... \quad (16.33)$$

where $A(0)_p$ is the on-axis pupil area. Accurate estimates of $\delta\theta'/\delta\theta$ can be found by exact ray-tracing through finite schematic eyes (Figure 16.11). For the Liou and Brennan (1997) eye, ray trace results were fitted to a second order polynomial giving

$$\theta' = 0.82219\theta - 2.8689 \times 10^{-4}\theta^2 \quad (16.34)$$

Estimates of retinal illuminance for this model eye are shown in Figure 16.12, using the derivative of equation (16.34) together with results using the approximate model in Chapter 13 and measurements of Kooijman and Witmer (1986). The model eye shows higher values of retinal illuminance than given by both the approximate model and the experimental data.

The quantity $\delta\theta'/\delta\theta$ is sensitive to small changes in the relationship between θ and θ' (see Figure 16.11), and will vary between the different eye models. Kooijman (1983) showed that retinal illuminance depends upon the retinal shape, i.e. its radius of curvature and asphericity. The effect of retinal asphericity has not been included in the equations that affect some of the parameters in equation (13.12), but a more sophisticated analysis should take this into account.

Summary

The reader is again reminded to take into account the purpose of a schematic eye before criticizing it for failure for accurate estimation in other areas. The majority of schematic eyes that were surveyed give better estimations than a representative paraxial schematic eye of mean levels of spherical aberration, tangential power errors, astigmatism and retinal illuminance. The retinal shape of these eyes could be modified to make some improvement in estimations of the sagittal and tangential power errors, astigmatism and field curvature. Despite being intended only for the estimation of spherical aberration,

Liou and Brennan's (1997) model (with a retina having a -12 mm radius of curvature) appears to give the best overall estimations of average monochromatic aberrations of real eyes.

Summary of main symbols

n_{vit}	refractive index of the vitreous humour
h	ray height in pupil (say in millimetres)
θ	direction of a point in the object field

Seidel aberrations

S_1	spherical aberration
S_2	coma
S_3	astigmatism
S_4	Petzval curvature
S_5	distortion
$L_s(\theta), L_t(\theta)$	sagittal and tangential power errors at off-axis angle θ
$A(\theta)$	astigmatism at off-axis angle θ
r_s, r_t, r_p, r_R	radii of sagittal, tangential, Petzval and retinal surfaces
$W(r)$	wave aberration for ray passing through the pupil at a height r
$_0W_{4,0}$ etc.	wave aberration co-efficients (for the wave aberration in millimetres)
n	refractive indices
R	radius of curvature
C	surface curvature $(= 1/R)$
e	eccentricity of an aspheric surface
Q	surface asphericity $(= -e^2)$
p	surface asphericity $(= 1 + Q)$
ΔF	power error measure of spherical aberration
a, b	elliptical parameters

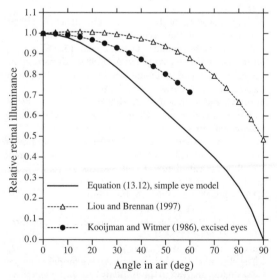

Figure 16.12. Retinal illuminance obtained from paraxial calculations with a simple eye model (shown also in Figure 13.2), exact ray-tracing calculations with the Liou and Brennan eye, and experimental results of Kooijman and Witmer (1986).

References

Ames, A. and Proctor, C. A. (1921). Dioptrics of the eye. *J. Opt. Soc. Am.*, **5**, 22–84.

Atchison, D. A. (1998). Oblique astigmatism of the Indiana eye. *Optom. Vis. Sci.*, **75**, 247–8.

Atchison, D. A. and Smith, G. (1995). Continuous gradient index and shell models of the human lens. *Vision Res.*, **35**, 2529–38.

Blaker, J. W. (1980). Toward an adaptive model of the human eye. *J. Opt. Soc. Am.*, **70**, 220–23.

Blaker, J. W. (1991). A comprehensive model of the aging, accommodative adult eye. In *Technical Digest on Ophthalmic and Visual Optics*, vol. 2, pp. 28–31. Optical Society of America.

Bonnet, R. (1964). *La Topographie Cornéenne* (cited by Lotmar, 1971). Desroches.

Bonnet, R. and Cochet, P. (1962). New method of topographic ophthalmometry – its theoretical and clinical applications (translated by E. Eagle) *Am. J. Optom. Arch. Am. Acad. Optom.*, **39**, 227–51.

Brown, N. P. (1974). The change in lens curvature with age. *Exp. Eye Res.*, **19**, 175–83.

Charman, W. N., Jennings, J. A. M. and Whitefoot, H. (1978). The refraction of the eye in relation to spherical aberration and pupil size. *Br. J. Physiol. Opt.*, **32**, 78–93.

Cowan, A. (1927). *An Introductory Course in Ophthalmic Optics.* F. A. Davis Co.

Doric, S. (1984). Paraxial ray trace for rotationally symmetric homogeneous and inhomogeneous media. *J. Opt. Soc. Am. A.*, **1**, 818–21.

Drasdo, N. and Fowler, C. W. (1974). Non-linear projection of the retinal image in a wide-angle schematic eye. *Br. J. Ophthal.*, **58**, 709–14.

Escudero-Sanz, I. and Navarro, R. (1999). Off-axis aberrations of a wide-angle schematic eye model. *J. Opt. Soc. Am. A.*, **16**, 1881–91.

Ferree, C. E., Rand, G. and Hardy, C. (1931). Refraction for the peripheral field of vision. *Arch. Ophthal.*, **5**, 717–31.

Guidarelli, S. (1972). Off-axis imaging in the human eye. *Atti. Fond. Giorgio Ronchi*, **27**, 449–60.

Gullstrand, A. (1909). Appendix II in von Helmholtz's *Handbuch der Physiologischen Optik*, volume 1, 3rd edn (English translation edited by J. P. Southall, Optical Society of America, 1924).

Helmholtz, H. von (1909). *Handbuch der Physiologischen Optik*, vol 1, 3rd edn (English translation edited by J. P. Southall, Optical Society of America, 1924.)

Hopkins, H. H. (1950). *The Wave Theory of Aberrations.* Clarendon Press.

Howcroft, M. J. and Parker, J. A. (1977). Aspheric curvatures for the human lens. *Vision Res.*, **17**, 1217–23.

Kooijman, A. C. (1983). Light distribution on the retina of a wide-angle theoretical eye. *J. Opt. Soc. Am.*, **73**, 1544–50.

Kooijman, A. C. and Witmer, F. K. (1986). Ganzfeld light distribution on the retina of human and rabbit eyes: calculations and *in vitro* measurements. *J. Opt. Soc. Am. A.*, **3**, 2116–20.

Liou, H.-L. and Brennan, N. A. (1997). Anatomically accurate, finite model eye for optical modeling. *J. Opt. Soc. Am. A.*, **14**, 1684–95.

Lotmar, W. (1971). Theoretical eye model with aspheric surfaces. *J. Opt. Soc. Am.*, **61**, 1522–9.

Mandell, R. B. and St Helen, R. (1971). Mathematical model of the corneal contour. *Br. J. Physiol. Opt.*, **26**, 183–97.

Moore, D. T. (1971). Design of singlets with continuously varying indices of refraction. *J. Opt. Soc. Am.*, **61**, 886–94.

Mutti, D. O., Zadnik, K. and Adams, A. J. (1995). The equivalent refractive index of the crystalline lens in childhood. *Vision Res.*, **35**, 1565–73.

Navarro, R., Santamaría, J. and Bescós, J. (1985). Accommodation-dependent model of the human eye with aspherics. *J. Opt. Soc. Am. A.*, **2**, 1273–81.

Patel, S., Marshall, J. and Fitzke, F. W. (1993). Shape and radius of posterior corneal surface. *Refract. Corn. Surg.*, **9**, 173–81.

Pierscionek, B. K. and Chan, D. Y. C. (1989). Refractive index gradient of human lenses. *Optom. Vis. Sci.*, **66**, 822–9.

Pomerantzeff, O., Fish, H., Govignon, J. and Schepens, C. L. (1971). Wide angle optical model of the human eye. *Ann. Ophthal.*, **3**, 815–19.

Pomerantzeff, O., Fish, H., Govignon, J. and Schepens, C. L. (1972). Wide angle optical model of the eye. *Optica Acta*, **19**, 387–8.

Pomerantzeff, O., Pankratov, M., Wang, G-J. and Dufault, P. (1984). Wide angle optical model of the eye. *Am. J. Optom. Physiol. Opt.*, **61**(3), 166–76.

Prechtel, L. N. and Wesley, N. K. (1970). Corneal topography and its application to contact lenses. *Br. J. Ophthalmol.*, **25**, 117–26.

Raasch, T. and Lakshminarayanan, V. (1989). Optical matrices of lenticular polyincidal schematic eyes. *Ophthal. Physiol. Opt.*, **9**, 61–5.

Rempt, F., Hoogerheide, J. and Hoogenboom, W. P. H. (1971). Peripheral retinoscopy and the skiagram. *Ophthalmologica*, **162**, 1–10.

Sands, P. J. (1970). Third-order aberrations of inhomogenous lenses. *J. Opt. Soc. Am.*, **60**, 1436–43.

Sharma, D. V., Shumar, D. K. and Ghatak, A. K. (1982). Tracing rays through graded index media. *Appl. Opt.*, **21**, 984–7.

Smith, G., Applegate, R. A. and Atchison, D. A. (1998). Assessment of the accuracy of the crossed-cylinder aberroscope technique. *J. Opt. Soc. Am.*, **15**, 2477–87.

Smith, G. and Atchison, D. A. (1983). Construction, specification, and mathematical description of aspheric surfaces. *Am. J. Optom. Physiol. Opt.*, **68**, 125–32.

Smith, G. and Atchison, D. A. (1997a). *The Eye and Visual Optical Instruments*, Chapters 5, 33. Cambridge University Press.

Smith, G. and Atchison, D. A. (1997b). Equivalent power of the crystalline lens of the human eye: comparison of methods of calculation. *J. Opt. Soc. Am. A*, **14**, 2537–46.

Smith, G., Pierscionek, B. K. and Atchison, D. A. (1991). The optical modelling of the human lens. *Ophthal. Physiol. Opt.*, **11**, 359–69.

Stine, G. H. (1934). Tables for accurate retinal localization. *Am. J. Ophthal.*, **17**, 314–24.

Thibos, L. N., Ye, M., Zhang, X. and Bradley, A. (1992). The chromatic eye: a new reduced-eye model of ocular chromatic aberration in humans. *Applied Optics*, **31**, 3594–600.

Thibos, L. N., Ye, M., Zhang, X. and Bradley, A. (1997). Spherical aberration of the reduced schematic eye with elliptical refracting surface. *Optom. Vis. Sci.*, **74**, 548–56.

van Meeteren, A. (1974). Calculations on the optical modulation transfer function of the human eye for white light. *Optica Acta*, **21**, 395–412.

Walsh, G. and Charman, W. N. (1985). Measurement of the axial wavefront aberration of the human eye. *Ophthal. Physiol. Opt.*, **5**, 23–31.

Wang, G., Pomerantzeff, O. and Pankratov, M. M. (1983). Astigmatism of oblique incidence in the human eye. *Vision Res.*, **23**, 1079–85.

Wang, Y-Z. and Thibos, L. N. (1997). Oblique (off-axis) astigmatism of the reduced schematic eye with elliptical refracting surfaces. *Optom. Vis. Sci.*, **74**, 557–62.

Welford, W.T. (1986). *Aberrations of Optical Systems*. Adam Hilger.

17

Chromatic aberrations

Introduction

Like other optical systems, the eye suffers from chromatic aberration as well as from monochromatic aberrations. There are two types of chromatic aberration, **longitudinal** and **transverse**, both of which are manifestations of the dispersion (variation of refractive index with wavelength) of the refracting media of an optical system.

The first two sections of this chapter describe longitudinal and transverse chromatic aberration, and the following two sections discuss their measurement. The effects of these aberrations on visual performance are then discussed, followed by a section on compensation for these effects. Finally, the inclusion of chromatic aberrations in eye modelling is discussed, and this should be considered in conjunction with Chapter 16 on modelling the monochromatic aberrations.

Longitudinal chromatic aberration

Longitudinal chromatic aberration can be explained as follows. Figure 17.1a shows a beam of light from an axial point **O** entering the eye. Because the refractive indices inside the eye vary with wavelength, the path followed by a ray inside the eye depends upon wavelength. As a rule, refractive indices decrease with increase in wavelength, so the eye has lower power as wavelength increases. Regarding the eye as focused on the point **O**

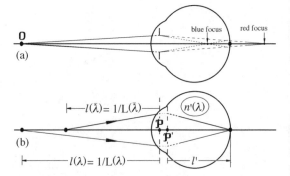

Figure 17.1. Longitudinal chromatic aberration.
a. General effect of longitudinal chromatic aberration.
b. Measuring longitudinal chromatic aberration as a chromatic difference of refraction.

for a yellow wavelength, rays of longer wavelength (e.g. red) are focused behind the retina and shorter wavelength rays (e.g. blue) are focused in front of the retina.

The longitudinal chromatic aberration of the eye can be quantified as the variation in power with wavelength. Thibos *et al.* (1991a) referred to this as **chromatic difference of power**. The aberration can also be quantified as the vergences of the source for which the source is focused at the retina for a range of wavelengths (Figure 17.1b). Thibos *et al.* referred to this as **chromatic difference of refraction**. As for other aberrations of the eye, such as spherical aberration and astigmatism, the second method is how longitudinal chromatic aberration is measured experimentally (see *Measurement of longitudinal chromatic aberration*, this chapter).

A formal definition of chromatic difference of refraction is:

> For any level of ametropia and accommodation, chromatic difference of refraction is the difference between the vergences of the retinal conjugates for a wavelength λ and a reference wavelength $\bar{\lambda}$.

Figure 17.1b shows a general schematic eye and the retinal conjugates for wavelengths λ and $\bar{\lambda}$. These conjugates are at distances $l(\lambda)$ and $l(\bar{\lambda})$ from the eye. Replacing these distances by their corresponding vergences $L(\lambda)$ and $L(\bar{\lambda})$, the chromatic difference of refraction $R_E(\lambda)$ is

$$R_E(\lambda) = L(\lambda) - L(\bar{\lambda}) \tag{17.1}$$

In measurements of chromatic difference of refraction, rather than comparing the results at a wavelength with those of the reference wavelength, it is common to compare measurements between a short and a long wavelength. When doing so, we shall refer to the range of chromatic difference of refraction. It is important to be careful when comparing the ranges obtained in different studies, as these may have used different wavelength ranges.

Longitudinal chromatic aberration has been explained by considering an axial object point, but it should be realized that it is still present as the object moves off-axis.

Transverse chromatic aberration

Transverse chromatic aberration is demonstrated in Figure 17.2a for the case of an eye that is a centred optical system (including pupils), and for an off-axis object point at **Q**. Because of longitudinal chromatic aberration, the different wavelength images of the point are defocused by different amounts relative to the retina. Also, because the power of the eye is less for long wavelengths than for short wavelengths, longer wavelength rays are deviated less than shorter wavelength rays, and meet the retina further from the optical axis.

Transverse chromatic aberration is also demonstrated in Figure 17.2b for the case of an eye that is a centred optical system, except

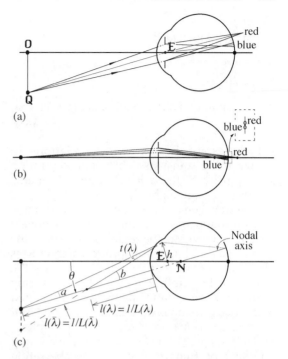

Figure 17.2. Transverse chromatic aberration (greatly exaggerated).
a. Centred pupil and an off-axis object point.
b. Decentred pupil and an on-axis object.
c. Measuring transverse chromatic aberration in object space.

that the pupil is decentred. The object point is on the optical axis. The small pupil in this figure has been decentred so that its position coincides with the top of the pupil in Figure 17.1a.

As happens for longitudinal chromatic aberration, and generally for the monochromatic aberrations, transverse chromatic aberration must be measured outside the eye. This is shown in Figure 17.2c. Two rays, one of wavelength λ and the other of the reference wavelength $\bar{\lambda}$, originate from different positions in object space but pass through the same point in the pupil and intersect at the retina. It can be seen that the transverse chromatic aberration associated with a height h of the rays relative to the nodal ray is given by

$$t(\lambda) = b - a$$

where a and b are the angles subtended by the two rays with the nodal ray in object space.

As

$a \approx hL(\overline{\lambda})$ and $b \approx hL(\lambda)$,

we have

$t(\lambda) \approx h[L(\lambda) - L(\overline{\lambda})]$

Using equation (17.1), it can easily be seen that

$$t(\lambda) \approx hR_E(\lambda) \tag{17.2}$$

which establishes a linear relationship between the transverse chromatic aberration as given by $t(\lambda)$ and longitudinal chromatic aberration as given by $R_E(\lambda)$.

The transverse chromatic aberration that is of most interest is that associated with foveal vision. In this case, the nodal ray becomes the visual axis, and the pupil location of interest is that representative of the light beam – i.e. the centre of the pupil. A method for measuring transverse chromatic aberration associated with foveal vision is described in *Measurement of transverse chromatic aberration*, this chapter.

Thibos *et al.* (1991a) referred to the angular measure of transverse chromatic aberration $t(\lambda)$ as a **chromatic difference of position**.

Transverse chromatic aberration in the eye can be demonstrated by viewing a black–white edge through a small artificial pupil that is decentred. Another way to observe it is to look at a black cross on a pattern consisting of a central red area surrounded by a blue region, as in Figure 17.3a. If the artificial pupil is decentred vertically, the horizontal black line appears deviated as it crosses the boundary between red and blue (Figure 17.3b). A similar effect occurs for the vertical black line when the artificial pupil is decentred horizontally.

Chromatic magnification

As well as an angle, transverse chromatic aberration can be measured as a wavelength-dependent variation in image size of extended objects. Thibos *et al.* (1991a) referred to this as the **chromatic difference of magnification** (*CDM*). In practice, this must be measured in object space.

The chromatic difference of magnification is the transverse chromatic aberration in angular terms $t(\lambda)$, divided by the angular size of the object, that is

$$CDM = t(\lambda)/\theta \tag{17.3}$$

where θ is the angular size of the object subtended at the eye's nodal point. For example, if an object has 10° angular size and the angular transverse chromatic aberration for the edge of the object is 0.1° (0.0017 rad), the chromatic difference of magnification is 1 per cent.

The chromatic difference of magnification can be related directly to the chromatic difference of refraction. In Figure 17.2c

$$\theta \approx h/\mathbf{EN} \tag{17.4}$$

where **EN** is the distance between the entrance pupil at **E** and the front nodal point at **N**, and h is the displacement of the entrance pupil from the visual axis. We can substitute the right-hand side of equation (17.4), together with $h/R_E(\lambda)$ for $t(\lambda)$ from equation (17.2), into equation (17.3) to give

$$CDM = R_E(\lambda)\mathbf{EN} \tag{17.5}$$

Based on a range of chromatic difference of refraction of 2.1 D across the visible spectrum (see next section) and a distance **EN** of 0.004 m (Gullstrand number one eye), the range of *CDM* across the visible spectrum is less than 0.01 (1 per cent). This may rise considerably if artificial pupils are used in visual experiments. Zhang *et al.* (1993) described a method for measuring *CDM*.

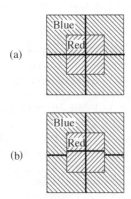

(a)

(b)

Figure 17.3. Demonstration of transverse chromatic aberration.
a. A black cross is placed on a central red area and a blue surround.
b. Appearance of the target when a small pupil is decentred downwards in front of an observer's eye.

Measurement of longitudinal chromatic aberration

Some techniques

Five methods of measuring chromatic difference of refraction are described here.

Best focus method

A target with fine detail, back-illuminated by light of various wavelengths, is moved forwards and backwards in front of an observer until it is judged to be in focus (Figure 17.4a). This can be done using an achromatic Badal lens (e.g. Howarth and Bradley, 1986), which means that the image always subtends the same angle at the eye and that the chromatic difference of refraction is linearly related to the position of the target (see Chapter 8). A clinically related variant of this method is to use trial lenses of different powers in the spectacle plane rather than altering target position (the small chromatic aberration of the lenses should be taken into account).

Laser speckle

When viewing a laser reflected diffusely from a rotating drum, a speckle pattern is seen that generally moves in the same or opposite direction to the drum rotation (see Chapter 8). However, when an eye is focused at the drum, the pattern appears merely to 'boil'. Lasers of different wavelengths are used, and focus is achieved for each wavelength by moving the drum or using auxiliary trial lenses (Gilmartin and Hogan, 1985).

Vernier method

Two narrow test targets of different wavelengths are imaged on the fovea, but light from them is restricted to pass only through a small aperture in front of the eye (Figure 17.4b). The small aperture can be displaced across the pupil perpendicularly to the length of the target. There is one position in the pupil for which the targets are both aligned and appear aligned – this locates the 'foveal achromatic axis', which is usually taken to be the visual axis (see Chapter 4). One of the targets can be displaced perpendicularly to its length. For chosen aperture positions relative to the visual axis, this is done so that the targets appear again to be aligned. If the aperture displacement is h, the target displacement is e, the target distance from the eye is p and the target distance from where the test wavelength ray intersects the axis is x, from similar triangles

$$e/h = x/(x-p) \qquad (17.6)$$

We can replace p by its vergence P where

$$P = 1/p \qquad (17.7)$$

The chromatic difference of refraction $R_E(\lambda)$ is given by

$$R_E(\lambda) = 1/(p-x) - 1/p = x/[(p-x)p] \qquad (17.8)$$

Using the previous two equations (17.7) and (17.8)

$$-R_E(\lambda)/P = x/(x-p) \qquad (17.9)$$

The left-hand side of this equation (17.9) can be substituted for the right-hand side of

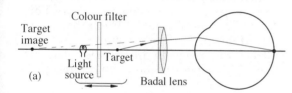

(a)

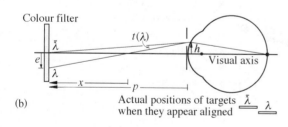

(b)

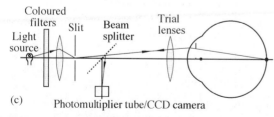

(c)

Figure 17.4. Some techniques for measuring chromatic difference of refraction:
a. Best focus.
b. Vernier alignment.
c. Double-pass technique.

equation (17.6) to obtain

$$-e/h = R_E(\lambda)/P \qquad (17.10)$$

A plot of e as a function of h is only linear in its central region because of the influence of monochromatic aberrations. $R_E(\lambda)$ can be obtained from the slope of this linear section (Thibos *et al.*, 1990). This seems a complicated way to measure the longitudinal chromatic aberration of the eye, but has the advantage that it can be used to determine the transverse chromatic aberration at the same time.

Double pass technique

The image of a narrow illuminated slit is formed on the fundus, which reflects a portion of the light (Figure 17.4c). An aerial image forms outside the eye. Correcting trial lenses can be used to minimize the width of this image for various wavelengths. Charman and Jennings (1976) used this method and found good agreement with their subjective measurements.

Chromo-retinoscopy

Bobier and Sivak (1978, 1980) used retinoscopy and narrow wave-band filters placed in

front of the tested eye to measure the longitudinal aberration in a number of subjects.

Magnitude

Figure 17.5 shows experimental subjective results of chromatic difference of refraction from several studies. These results are for a low level of accommodation stimulus, or under cycloplegia. The data have been adjusted for a common reference wavelength of 589 nm. The figure shows results also for a reduced eye filled with water and a reduced Chromatic eye, which Thibos *et al.* (1992) derived from their experimental data (see *Modelling chromatic aberrations*, this chapter).

There is approximately a 2.1 D range of chromatic difference of refraction between 400 and 700 nm. Although several techniques were used, it is most noticeable that there is little variation between the majority of subjective studies. Only the Gilmartin and Hogan (1985) study, which used the method of laser speckle and obtained results of 1.87 ± 0.26 D between 488 and 633 nm, has results very different from other studies. The intersubject difference in the studies was also small. This small variation is in contrast to the

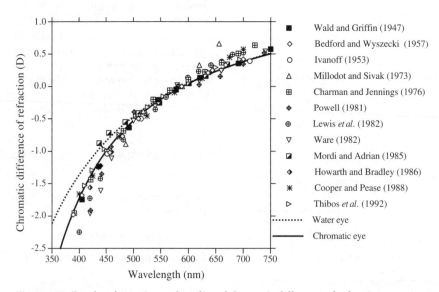

Figure 17.5. Results of experimental studies of chromatic difference of refraction as a function of wavelength. Also shown are the results for an Emsley reduced eye filled with water (Water eye) and the Chromatic eye. Data for Figure 6 of Thibos *et al.* (1992) kindly provided by Larry Thibos, and with permission from The Optical Society of America.

large variation in monochromatic aberrations (see Chapter 15).

The small variation in chromatic aberration is because the main constituent of the ocular media is water, whose dispersion cannot vary between subjects. Despite this, the water eye has insufficient dispersion to fit the experimental results well (Figure 17.5). The Chromatic eye of Thibos *et al.* (1992) provides an excellent fit.

Wavelength in focus

An issue related to longitudinal chromatic aberration is the wavelength at which a white target is in focus at various levels of accommodation. Accommodation response is usually in excess ('lead') for low stimulus levels, while the response is insufficient ('lag') for higher levels of accommodation – for example, Charman and Tucker (1978). Corresponding to this, a long wavelength is usually in focus for low accommodation stimuli and short wavelengths are in focus for higher accommodation stimuli.

Effect of accommodation and refractive error

For optical systems of the same chromatic dispersion, longitudinal chromatic aberration is related linearly to power. Modelling predicts ≈ 2.5 per cent increase in longitudinal chromatic aberration of eyes for each 1 D of accommodation or for each 1 D of refractive error when this is caused by an increase in ocular power (see *Modelling chromatic aberrations*, this chapter).

Jenkins (1963) claimed an early study by Nutting (1914) showed an increase in aberration with accommodation, but the authors believe that Nutting provided insufficient detail to support this claim. Some studies investigating this relationship were flawed in that wavelength-dependent accommodation may have affected measurements (Jenkins, 1963; Millodot and Sivak, 1973; Sivak and Millodot, 1974). Charman and Tucker (1978) found an increase in chromatic aberration of ≈ 0.2 D for a 4 D increase in accommodation for one subject (≈ 3 per cent per dioptre accommodation) between 442 and 633 nm. Wildsoet *et al.* (1993) measured chromatic difference of refraction in right eyes of 34 young subjects consisting of 12 myopes (–3.41 ± 2.62 D), 12 emmetropes (–0.04 ± 0.23 D) and 10 hypermetropes (+2.28 ± 1.43 D), but found no significant differences between groups.

Measurement of transverse chromatic aberration

Compared with longitudinal chromatic aberration, there have been relatively few studies of transverse chromatic aberration associated with foveal vision (Kishto, 1965; Ogboso and Bedell, 1987; Simonet and Campbell, 1990; Thibos *et al.*, 1990; Rynders *et al.*, 1995; Marcos *et al.*, 1999).

Technique

The vernier method used by Thibos *et al.* (1990) can be used as described above (Figure 17.4b). The small aperture displacement h is taken as the distance between the visual axis and the line of sight. The line of sight may be located by some suitable method, such as determining the edges of the pupil by scanning across the pupil with the aperture until the target disappears, and obtaining the mid-point of these limits. The angular transverse chromatic aberration $t(\lambda)$ associated with the line of sight is

$$t(\lambda) = -eP \tag{17.11}$$

Combining equation (17.11) with equation (17.10) gives

$$t(\lambda) \approx hR_{\mathrm{E}}(\lambda) \text{ radians} \tag{17.12}$$

which is the same as equation (17.2).

More sophisticated variations of the vernier method have been used by Simonet and Campbell (1990). Other studies have applied vernier alignment to the whole pupil rather than isolating the line of sight (Hartridge, 1947; Ogboso and Bedell, 1987; Rynders *et al.*, 1995). Such measurements may be influenced by the Stiles–Crawford effect if its peak is decentred from the line-of-sight (Rynders *et al.*, 1995; Marcos *et al.*, 1999).

Table 17.1. Studies of transverse chromatic aberration associated with the fovea. When signs are given, a positive sign indicates that the line of sight is nasal to the optical axis in object space.

Authors	Mean and range (min. arc)	No. subjects	Wavelength range (nm)
Hartridge (1947)	+0.6[a]	1	486–656
Kishto (1965)	+0.3	1	not given
Ogboso and Bedell (1987)	+0.9, +0.6 to +1.2	3	435–572
Thibos *et al.* (1990)	+0.61, –0.36 to +1.67	5	433–622
Simonet and Campbell (1990)	+0.43, –0.20 to +1.28	5	486–656
Rynders *et al.* (1995)	0.8, up to 2.7	85	497–605
Gullstrand No. 1 eye (relaxed)	+1.05[b]		486–656

[a]Hartridge gave his results in 'cone units' (1 cone unit = 0.69 min. arc). He obtained a vertical component also of 0.8 min. arc.
[b]Calculated from Seidel aberration C_T in Appendix 3, using angle α of 5°.

Magnitude

Table 17.1 shows results of experimental studies of foveal transverse chromatic aberration. Although the wavelength range of measurement must be taken into account, it is reasonable to say that the mean results are about half the 1.05 min. arc predicted for schematic eyes (486–656 nm) with centred pupils and the fovea 5° to the optical axis. The probable reasons for this discrepancy are that this angle may be larger than that occurring in many people, and that the pupil is usually decentred nasally and its centre is therefore closer to the visual axis. The main concern with transverse chromatic aberration is for severely decentred natural or artificial pupils. The effect of transverse chromatic aberration on visual performance is discussed in the next section.

Ogboso and Bedell (1987) made experimental measurements of transverse chromatic aberration in the peripheral visual field. The results were very different among their four subjects. Out to 40° object eccentricity, all values were less than 7 min. arc and considerably less than the 11 min. arc predicted from their model eye calculations at 40° eccentricity (wavelength range 435–572 nm).

Effects of chromatic aberrations on vision

Accommodation

Fincham (1951) introduced step changes in accommodative stimulus to his subjects. Most of them made appropriate accommodation responses in white light, but 60 per cent of them were unable to do so in monochromatic light. There is now considerable evidence that the longitudinal chromatic aberration helps the accommodation system respond correctly when there is defocus blur. Accommodation responses to steady and moving targets are more accurate in white or broad wavelength light than in monochromatic light, and doubling the eye's normal chromatic aberration has little effect on accommodative accuracy, whereas correcting or reversing the chromatic aberration leads to poor accommodative response (Kruger and Pola, 1986 and 1987; Kruger *et al.*, 1993, 1995 and 1997; Stone *et al.*, 1993; Aggarwala *et al.*, 1995a and 1995b).

Spatial vision

The effects of chromatic aberration are attenuated by the spectral sensitivity of the eye. For centred pupils, switching from monochromatic light to white light gives a maximum loss to the contrast sensitivity function of only 0.2 log units (Campbell and Gubisch, 1967), and has a negligible effect on visual acuity (Hartridge, 1947; Campbell and Gubisch, 1967). The use of achromatizing lenses makes negligible improvement to visual acuity and contrast sensitivity in white light (Campbell and Gubisch, 1967). Possible reasons include that the potential improvement is small anyway, some of these lenses have transverse chromatic aberration when centred (see the following section), and that additional transverse chromatic aberration is introduced for any of these lenses if they are not carefully centred (Zhang *et al.*, 1991).

Decentring natural or artificial pupils can have devastating effects on foveal spatial vision in white light because large amounts of transverse chromatic aberration are induced. Experimental studies showing up to two-thirds reduction in resolution for ≈ 3 mm displacement of artificial pupils (Green, 1967) or Maxwellian-view instruments (Bradley *et al.*, 1990; Thibos *et al.*, 1991b) are supported theoretically (Thibos *et al.*, 1990).

Some Maxwellian-view projection systems are used clinically to evaluate potential visual acuity in patients with cataract by positioning them so that the light passes through a relatively clear part of the cataractous lens. The experimental and theoretical results just mentioned indicate that those instruments using white light are likely to underestimate potential visual acuity if the light beam enters the pupil well away from its centre.

Theoretically, the transverse chromatic aberration should increase on going further into the peripheral field (Thibos, 1987), with increasingly deleterious effects on image quality. However, the importance of the aberration is likely to be small because of decreasing colour sensitivity and spatial resolution due to neural limitations.

Effects of chromatic aberration on retinal image quality are discussed further in Chapter 18, *Retinal image quality*.

Chromostereopsis

In Chapter 6 (*Binocular vision*) we described stereopsis, in which the two eyes provide the potential for seeing depth in a scene. **Chromostereopsis** is a related binocular phenomenon in which objects at the same distance, but of different colours, are seen in depth. Most commonly, reddish objects appear to be closer than bluish objects. Chromostereopsis is a consequence of transverse chromatic aberration combined with binocular vision.

Figure 17.6a shows the pupil ray paths from red and blue targets at position **O**. The pupil of the eye is decentred temporally relative to the visual axis. The red pupil ray is refracted less than the blue pupil ray, and therefore the red pupil ray intersects the retina to the temporal side of the blue pupil ray. This

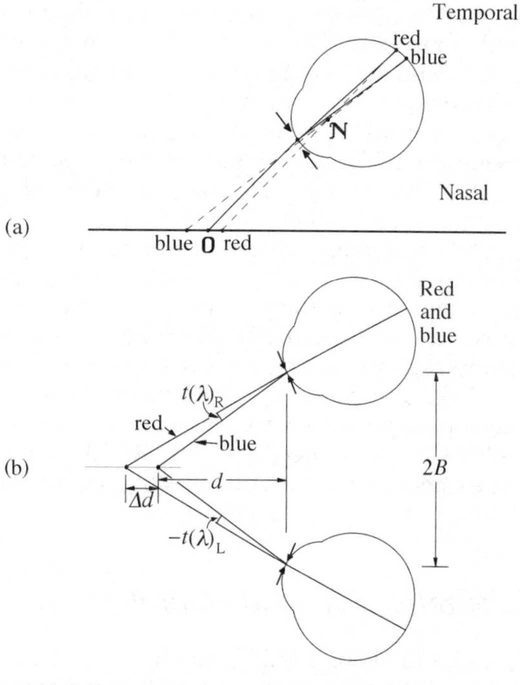

Figure 17.6. Chromostereopsis.
a. An explanation of the source of chromostereopsis.
b. The expected relationship estimating chromo-stereopsis and transverse chromatic aberration induced with small artificial pupils.

retinal disparity is equivalent to the red and blue rays coming from different distances, as shown by the dashed lines in the figure. The retinal disparity leads to an apparent longitudinal displacement when the target is viewed binocularly. The red target appears to be closer than the blue target.

The magnitude of chromostereopsis is predicted by the geometry in Figure 17.6b (Ye *et al.*, 1991). Here, Δd is the amount of chromostereopsis as a distance measurement, $2B$ is the distance between the position of small pupils in front of the two eyes, d is the viewing distance, and $t(\lambda)_R$ and $t(\lambda)_L$ are the right eye and left eye transverse chromatic aberrations. The relationship between these quantities is

$$t(\lambda)_R - t(\lambda)_L = \frac{2B\Delta d}{d^2 + d\Delta d} \tag{17.13}$$

By making measurements of transverse chromatic aberration induced by displace-ment of pinholes from the visual axes

(*Transverse chromatic aberration*, this chapter) and comparing these with measurements of chromostereopsis at these displacements, Ye *et al.* provided experimental support for this equation and for the theory that chromostereopsis with small pupils can be explained by the interocular difference in monocular transverse aberration.

Chromostereopsis often diminishes as pupil size increases, and may even reverse in direction. For natural pupils, this may be attributed at least partly to change in pupil centre as pupil size changes (Chapter 3). Ye *et al.* (1992) attributed the decrease in chromostereopsis, with increase in pupil size, to the Stiles–Crawford effect (see Chapter 13) acting an as anchor to shift the effective centre of pupils closer to the visual axis.

Aberrations of ophthalmic devices

Longitudinal chromatic aberration of correcting ophthalmic lenses is not considered important; spectacle and contact lenses because of their low powers relative to that of the eye, and intraocular lenses because they merely replace the eye's lens. Transverse chromatic aberration is not important in contact or intraocular lenses, because these move with the eye. However, it blurs foveal vision when an eye looks through peripheral

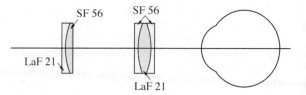

Figure 17.7. Achromatizing lens of Powell (1981).

parts of a spectacle which is made worse when high index, low *V*-value materials are used.

Aberration compensation and correction

Natural compensation mechanism

Chromatic aberration effects are attenuated by the non-uniform spectral sensitivity of the eye (Chapter 11). Thibos *et al.* (1991a) estimated that, when the wavelength with peak sensitivity is in focus, most of the luminance in a white light target is less than 0.25 D out of focus. The yellow macula pigment contributes to the relative luminous efficiency functions, and it's absence in the periphery may remove some of the attenuation.

Table 17.2. Achromatizing lens of Powell (1981). The aperture diameter of both components is 15 mm. Units: millimetres.

glass	n	V	d	r	surface
air	1				
				0.0	1
LaF21	1.788310	47.39	1.0		
				15.5	2
SF56	1.784700	26.08	3.0		
				0.0	3
air	1.0	–	14.5		
				0.0	4
SF56	1.784700	26.08	1.0		
				15.5	5
LaF21	1.788310	47.39	5.0		
				–15.5	6
SF56	1.784700	26.08	1.0		
				0.0	7
air	1.0	–	17.0		
				0.0	8 pupil
air	1.0	–			

Achromatizing correcting lenses

The longitudinal chromatic aberration of the eye can be corrected by a nominally zero power lens, with longitudinal chromatic aberration equal and opposite to that of the eye (van Heel, 1946; Thomson and Wright, 1947; Bedford and Wyszecki, 1957; Fry, 1972; Powell, 1981; Lewis *et al.*, 1982). The Powell (1981) design is given in Table 17.2 and Figure 17.7. It is a modification of the Bedford and Wyszecki triplet design, with a doublet added to reduce the residual longitudinal and transverse chromatic aberration present in the original lens.

These lenses may be assessed by the level of residual power at the reference wavelength, and by the residual chromatic aberration when used with the eye. The Bedford and Wyszecki, Fry, Powell and Lewis *et al.* designs have less than 0.25 D equivalent power at 587.6 nm. The residual variation of power of one lens/eye system is shown in Figure 17.8. The lenses introduce transverse chromatic aberration, with that of the sophisticated

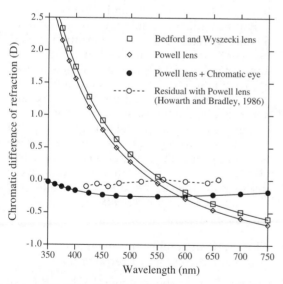

Figure 17.8. The power of the Bedford and Wyszecki (1957) and of the Powell (1981) achromatizing lenses, together with residual chromatic differences of focus for the Powell lens. The latter was obtained by combining the Powell lens with the Chromatic eye of Thibos and from mean experimental results of Howarth and Bradley (1986). The theoretical and experimental residuals differ by 0.1–0.3 D at any wavelength, but neither varies by more than 0.1 D between 400 nm and 700 nm.

Powell lens being much less than those of the other lenses. For a 5° field of view and between wavelengths from 486 to 656 nm, design values are 2.88 min. arc (Powell), 5.23 min. arc (Bedford and Wyszecki), 7.33 min. arc (Fry) and 9.34 min. arc (Lewis *et al.*).

Alignment of such lenses is critical, as otherwise an additional transverse chromatic aberration is induced which is proportional to the decentration. Zhang *et al.* (1991) determined that 0.4 mm of misalignment of an achromatizing lens relative to the eye would cancel any benefit the lens would give to spatial vision.

Modelling chromatic aberrations

Chromatic dispersion

To model the chromatic aberrations of the eye, a knowledge of its dispersive properties is necessary. This can be described by a formula such as

$$n^2(\lambda) = a_1 + a_2\lambda^2 + a_3/\lambda^2 + a_4/\lambda^4 \qquad (17.14a)$$

The advantage of this equation is that it is linear in the co-efficients and therefore, given any data on the relationship between wavelength and index, the *a* co-efficients can easily be found by solving a set of simultaneous linear equations. Other formulas include the Cornu dispersion equation

$$n(\lambda) = n_\infty + K/(\lambda - \lambda_0) \qquad (17.14b)$$

where n_∞, K and λ_0 are constants for a particular medium, and Sellmeier's equation

$$n^2(\lambda) = 1 + \frac{B_1\lambda^2}{\lambda^2 - C_1} + \frac{B_2\lambda^2}{\lambda^2 - C_2} + ... \qquad (17.14c)$$

The dispersion of any optical material is fully described by such equations, provided they are accurate. For some purposes, the dispersion can be reduced to a single number such as the Abbe *V*-value, which is defined as

$$V_d = \frac{n_d - 1}{n_F - n_C} \qquad (17.15)$$

where n_d, n_F and n_C are the refractive indices at the wavelengths 589.3 nm (λ_d), 486.1 nm (λ_F) and 656.3 nm (λ_C), respectively. *V*-values are useful for comparing the amount of dispersion in different optical media and for calculating the Seidel chromatic aberrations.

Bennett and Tucker (1975) used the form of equation (17.14a) to give the refractive index of water as

$$n^2(\lambda) = 1.7642 - 1.38 \times 10^{-8}\lambda^2 + 6.12$$
$$\times 10^{+3}/\lambda^2 + 1.41 \times 10^{+8}/\lambda^4 \qquad (17.16)$$

where the wavelength is in nanometres. Substituting appropriate values obtained from equation (17.16) into equation (17.15) gives $V_d = 55.15$. As shown in Figure 17.6, the dispersion of water is insufficient to account for the longitudinal chromatic aberration of the eye.

Le Grand (1967) presented data designed for his full theoretical eye. He quantified the dispersion of the ocular media using the Cornu dispersion equation (17.14b). His values of n_∞, K and λ_o for each ocular medium and corresponding V-values are given in Table 17.3.

Thibos *et al.* (1992) used their experimental results and the Cornu dispersion equation (17.14b) to describe the refractive index distribution of their Chromatic version of Emsley's reduced eye as

$$n(\lambda) = 1.320535 + \frac{4.685}{(\lambda - 214.102)} \qquad (17.17)$$

where λ has the unit of nanometres. The corresponding V-value is 50.23. The chromatic error of refraction of the Chromatic eye is shown in Figure 17.6.

The high dispersion of the eye has been attributed to a high dispersion of the lens. For example, Sivak and Mandelman (1982) measured V-values of the lens as 29 ± 4 for the periphery and 35 ± 6 for the core. These are much less than the values of Le Grand (1967), given in Table 17.3.

Table 17.3. The values of the parameters in equation (17.15b) for Le Grand's (1967) dispersion of the ocular media.

	n_∞	K	λ_o	V
Cornea	1.3610	7.4147	130.0	56.01
Aqueous	1.3221	7.0096	130.0	53.00
Lens	1.3999	9.2492	130.0	50.01
Vitreous	1.3208	6.9806	130.0	53.00

Schematic eyes

Gaussian properties

There are small, wavelength-dependent changes in the principal and nodal points of schematic eyes. For the Gullstrand number 1 eye, over the wavelength range of 400–700 nm, the front principal point moves just less than 0.0007 mm. Over the same wavelength range, the back principal point moves by 0.013 mm, but this is still small.

Seidel chromatic aberrations

We discussed Seidel monochromatic aberrations in Chapter 16. The Seidel longitudinal (C_L) and transverse (C_T) chromatic aberrations are described by Smith and Atchison (1997). These can be calculated for schematic eyes from constructional and dispersion data, and the values for some schematic eyes are given in Appendix 3. We use the V-value of 50.23 obtained from equations (17.15) and (17.17). Seidel transverse chromatic aberrations, between 486 and 656 nm, are given as percentages of the image sizes at 589 nm. The full schematic, simplified and reduced eyes have similar Seidel chromatic aberrations.

For the Gullstrand number 1 eye at 5° angle, Seidel transverse chromatic aberration is –0.35 per cent, and this can be converted to an angular value of 1.05 min. arc. This is a close approximation to the exact value, and can be used as an estimate of transverse chromatic aberration at the fovea, assuming that the line of sight is 5° to the optical axis and the pupil is centred on the optical axis. This is considerably larger than mean experimental measures (Table 17.1), and reasons for this were discussed earlier in this chapter (*Measurement of transverse chromatic aberration*).

Chromatic difference of power and chromatic difference of refraction

Figure 17.1b shows a general schematic eye and the retinal conjugates for wavelengths λ and $\bar{\lambda}$. We have

$$n'(\lambda)/l' - L(\lambda) = F(\lambda) \text{ and } n'(\bar{\lambda})/l' - L(\bar{\lambda}) = F(\bar{\lambda})$$
$$(17.18a \text{ and } b)$$

For both situations, the distance l' is the distance from the back principal point to the retina and is here assumed to be independent of wavelength. The chromatic difference of refraction $R_E(\lambda)$ is given by equation (17.1), that is

$$R_E(\lambda) = L(\lambda) - L(\overline{\lambda}) \qquad (17.1)$$

The chromatic difference of power $\Delta F(\lambda)$, the difference between the equivalent power $F(\lambda)$ at wavelength λ and the equivalent power $F(\overline{\lambda})$ at the reference wavelength $\overline{\lambda}$, is given by

$$\Delta F(\lambda) = F(\lambda) - F(\overline{\lambda}) \qquad (17.19)$$

Subtracting equation (17.18b) from (17.18a), and after a small amount of manipulation involving equations (17.1) and (17.19), we have

$$R_E(\lambda) = \frac{n'(\lambda) - n'(\overline{\lambda})}{l'} - \Delta F(\lambda) \qquad (17.20)$$

If we replace the length l' using equation (17.18b), equation (17.20) can be written in the form

$$R_E(\lambda) = \frac{[n'(\lambda) - n'(\overline{\lambda})][F(\overline{\lambda}) + L(\lambda)]}{n'(\overline{\lambda})} - \Delta F(\lambda) \qquad (17.21)$$

For an emmetropic eye focused on infinity, $L(\overline{\lambda}) = 0$ and equation (17.21) reduces to

$$R_E(\lambda) = \frac{[n'(\lambda) - n'(\overline{\lambda})]F(\overline{\lambda})}{n'(\overline{\lambda})} - \Delta F(\lambda) \qquad (17.22)$$

This equation shows that there is a difference between the chromatic difference of refraction $R_E(\lambda)$ and the chromatic difference of power $\Delta F(\lambda)$, apart from a change in sign.

Using appropriate chromatic dispersions of the media, paraxial schematic eyes are excellent at estimating the chromatic difference of refraction of real eyes. As an example, Atchison *et al.* (1993) used the Gullstrand number 1 eye with its refractive indices, but scaled the variations in refractive index so that the chromatic dispersion was the same as for equation (17.18). This gave a range of chromatic difference of refraction of 1.94 D between 400 and 700 nm. This is probably a slight underestimation of chromatic difference of focus in most eyes.

Atchison *et al.* (1993) determined the effect of refractive error on change in range of chromatic difference of refraction for schematic eyes, modified to have axial ametropia and refractive ametropia. The latter was

modelled by altering corneal curvature. For the Gullstrand number 1 eye, changes occurring were 0.012 D (0.56 per cent) per dioptre of axial ametropia and 0.047 D (2.4 per cent) per dioptre of refractive ametropia. Similar results were obtained for reduced eyes. The accommodated version of the Gullstrand eye gave a range of chromatic difference of refraction 0.55 D greater than the relaxed, emmetropia eye, which corresponds to 0.050 D (2.6 per cent) increase per dioptre of accommodation.

Chromatic difference of refraction of reduced schematic eyes

If the corneal radius of curvature of the reduced eye is r, the equivalent power $F(\lambda)$ as a function of wavelength is simply

$$F(\lambda) = [n'(\lambda) - 1]/r \qquad (17.23)$$

where $n'(\lambda)$ is given by equations such as equation (17.17). The radius can be given in terms of the reference power $F(\overline{\lambda})$ as

$$r = [n'(\overline{\lambda}) - 1]/F(\overline{\lambda}) \qquad (17.24)$$

The equivalent power of the eye $F(\lambda)$ as a function of wavelength is then

$$F(\lambda) = \frac{[n'(\lambda) - 1]F(\overline{\lambda})}{[n'(\overline{\lambda}) - 1]} \qquad (17.25)$$

and the chromatic difference of power $\Delta F(\lambda)$ is

$$\Delta F(\lambda) = \frac{F(\overline{\lambda})[n'(\lambda) - n'(\overline{\lambda})]}{n'(\overline{\lambda}) - 1} \qquad (17.26)$$

Equation (17.26) can be rearranged to give

$$F(\overline{\lambda}) = \frac{\Delta F(\lambda)[n'(\overline{\lambda}) - 1]}{n'(\lambda) - n'(\overline{\lambda})} \qquad (17.27)$$

Substituting the right-hand side of this equation (17.27) for $F(\overline{\lambda})$ into equation (17.21) gives

$$R_E(\lambda) = \frac{[n'(\lambda) - n'(\overline{\lambda})]L(\overline{\lambda}) - \Delta F(\lambda)}{n'(\overline{\lambda})} \qquad (17.28)$$

For an emmetropic eye focused on infinity, $L(\overline{\lambda}) = 0$ and equation (17.28) reduces to

$$R_E(\lambda) = -\Delta F(\lambda)/n'(\overline{\lambda}) \qquad (17.29)$$

Using a value of 1.333 for $n'(\overline{\lambda})$ shows that the chromatic difference of refraction is three-quarters of the chromatic difference of power.

Chromatic and Indiana reduced eyes of Thibos *et al.* (1992, 1997)

Some of the details of these reduced eyes were provided in Chapter 16. The refractive index distribution is given by equation (17.17), and the chromatic difference of refraction (see Figure 17.6) is given in dioptres by

$$R_E(\lambda) = 1.68524 - \frac{633.46}{(\lambda - 214.102)} \qquad (17.30)$$

where the reference wavelength is 589 nm and the wavelength λ is in nanometres. To obtain good predictions of transverse chromatic aberration of their eyes according to equations (17.2) and (17.5), Thibos *et al.* placed the stop 1.91 mm inside the eye so that the distance **EN** of 3.98 mm between the entrance pupil and the nodal point was similar to that of more sophisticated schematic eyes.

To allow for variations in transverse chromatic aberration, the pupils of the chromatic eye do not need to be on the optical axis. Thibos *et al.* (1992) included a number of additional axes: line of sight, visual axis and achromatic axis (see Chapter 4). The cornea has an asphericity Q of –0.56 to correct spherical aberration at the reference wavelength of 589 nm.

The Indiana eye varies from the chromatic eye in that the optical axis, visual axis and line of sight are now coincident and the cornea has a variable asphericity (Thibos *et al.*, 1997).

Summary of main symbols

$t(\lambda)$ (angular) transverse chromatic aberration

CDM   chromatic difference of magnification

EN   distance between entrance pupil at **E** and front nodal point at **N**

λ wavelength, usually expressed in nanometres

$\bar{\lambda}$ reference wavelength at which the reference power $F(\bar{\lambda})$ of the eye is defined

$F(\lambda)$ equivalent power of a schematic eye as a function of wavelength

$\Delta F(\lambda)$ chromatic difference of power; the difference in equivalent power between that at the wavelength λ and that at the reference wavelength $\bar{\lambda}$

$R_E(\lambda)$ chromatic difference of refraction

References

Aggarwala, K. R., Kruger, E. S., Mathews, S. and Kruger, P. B. (1995a). Spectral bandwidth and ocular accommodation. *J. Opt. Soc. Am. A.*, **12**, 450–55.

Aggarwala, K. R., Nowbotsing, S. and Kruger, P. B. (1995b). Accommodation to monochromatic and white-light targets. *Invest. Ophthal. Vis. Sci.*, **36**, 2695–705.

Atchison, D. A., Smith, G. and Waterworth, M. D. (1993). Theoretical effect of refractive error and accommodation on longitudinal chromatic aberration of the human eye. *Optom. Vis. Sci.*, **70**, 716–22.

Bedford, R. E. and Wyszecki, G. (1957). Axial chromatic aberration of the human eye. *J. Opt. Soc. Am.*, **47**, 564–5.

Bennett, A. G. and Tucker, J. (1975). Correspondence: chromatic aberration of the eye between 200 and 2000 nm. *Br. J. Physiol. Opt.*, **30**, 132–5.

Bobier, C. W. and Sivak, J. G. (1978). Chromoretinoscopy. *Vision Res.*, **18**, 247–50.

Bobier, C. W. and Sivak, J. G. (1980). Chromoretinoscopy and its instrumentation. *Am. J. Optom. Physiol. Opt.*, **57**, 106–8.

Bradley, A., Thibos, L. N. and Still, D. L. (1990). Visual acuity measured with clinical Maxwellian-view systems: effects of beam entry location. *Optom. Vis. Sci.*, **67**, 811–17.

Campbell, F. W. and Gubisch, R. W. (1967). The effect of chromatic aberration on visual acuity. *J. Physiol. (Lond.)*, **192**, 345–58.

Charman, W. N. and Jennings, J. A. M. (1976). Objective measurements of the longitudinal chromatic aberration of the human eye. *Vision. Res.*, **16**, 999–1005.

Charman, W. N. and Tucker, J. (1978). Accommodation and color. *J. Opt. Soc. Am.*, **68**, 459–71.

Cooper, D. P. and Pease, P. L. (1988). Longitudinal chromatic aberration of the human eye and wavelength in focus. *Am. J. Optom. Physiol. Opt.*, **65**, 99–107.

Fincham, E. F. (1951). The accommodation reflex and its stimulus. *Br. J. Ophthalmol.*, **35**, 381–93.

Fry, G. A. (1972). Visibility of color contrast borders. *Am. J. Optom. Arch. Am. Acad. Optom.*, **49**, 401–6.

Gilmartin, B. and Hogan, R. E. (1985). The magnitude of longitudinal chromatic aberration of the human eye between 458 and 633 nm. *Vision Res.*, **25**, 1747–55.

Green, D. G. (1967). Visual resolution when light enters the eye through different parts of the pupil. *J. Physiol. (Lond.)*, **192**, 345–58.

Hartridge, H. (1947). The visual perception of fine detail. *Phil. Trans. R. Soc. B.*, **232**, 519–671.

Howarth, P. A. and Bradley, A. (1986). The longitudinal chromatic aberration of the human eye, and its correction. *Vision Res.*, **26**, 361–6.

Ivanoff, A. (1953). Les aberrations de l'oeil. Leur role dans l'accommodation. *Éditions de la Revue d'Optique Théorique et Instrumentale*, Paris.

Jenkins, T. C. A. (1963). Aberrations of the eye and their effects on vision – Part II. *Br. J. Physiol. Optics*, **20**, 161–201.

Kishto, B. N. (1965). The colour stereoscopic effect. *Vision Res.*, **5**, 313–29.

Kruger, P. B., Aggarwala, K. R., Bean, S. and Mathews, S. (1997). Accommodation to stationary and moving targets. *Optom. Vis. Sci.*, **74**, 505–10.

Kruger, P. B., Mathews, S., Aggarwala, K. R. and Sanchez, N. (1993). Chromatic aberration and ocular focus: Fincham revisited. *Vision Res.*, **33**, 1397–1411.

Kruger, P. B., Nowbotsing, S., Aggarwala, K. R. and Mathews, S. (1995). Small amounts of chromatic aberration influence dynamic accommodation. *Optom. Vis. Sci.*, **72**, 656–69.

Kruger, P. B. and Pola, J. (1986). Stimuli for accommodation: Blur, chromatic aberration and size. *Vision Res.*, **26**, 957–71.

Kruger, P. B. and Pola, J. (1987). Dioptric and non-dioptric stimuli for accommodation: target size alone and with blur and chromatic aberration. *Vision Res.*, **27**, 555–67.

Le Grand, Y. (1967). *Form and Space Vision*. Revised edition (translated by M. Millodot and G. Heath). Indiana University Press.

Lewis, A. L., Katz, M. and Oehrlein, C. (1982). A modified achromatizing lens. *Am. J. Optom. Physiol. Opt.*, **59**, 909–11.

Marcos, S., Burns, S. A., Moreno-Barriuso, E. and Navarro, R. (1999). A new approach to the study of ocular chromatic aberrations. *Vision Res.*, **39**, 4309–23.

Millodot, M. and Sivak, J. G. (1973). Influence of accommodation on the chromatic aberration of the eye. *Br. J. Physiol. Opt.*, **28**, 169–74.

Mordi, J. A. and Adrian, W. K. (1985). Influence of age on chromatic aberration of the human eye. *Amer. J. Optom. Physiol. Opt.*, **62**, 864–9.

Nutting, P. G. (1914). The axial chromatic aberration of the eye. *Proc. R. Soc. Lond. (Biol.)*, **90**A, 440–42.

Ogboso, Y. U. and Bedell, H. E. (1987). Magnitude of lateral chromatic aberration across the retina of the human eye. *J. Opt. Soc. Am. A.*, **4**, 1666–72.

Powell, I. (1981). Lenses for correcting chromatic aberration of the eye. *Appl. Opt.*, **20**, 4152–5.

Rynders, M., Lidkea, B., Chisholm, W. and Thibos, L. N. (1995). Statistical distribution of foveal tranverse chromatic aberration, pupil centration, and angle ψ in a population of young adult eyes. *J. Opt. Soc. Am. A.*, **12**, 2348–57.

Simonet, P. and Campbell, M. C. W. (1990). The optical transverse chromatic aberration on the fovea of the human eye. *Vision Res.*, **30**, 187–206.

Sivak, J. G. and Mandelman, T. (1982). Chromatic dispersion of the ocular media. *Vision Res.*, **22**, 997–1003.

Sivak, J. G. and Millodot, M. (1974). Axial chromatic aberration of eye with achromatizing lens. *J. Opt. Soc. Am.*, **64**, 1724–5.

Smith, G. and Atchison, D. A. (1997). Aberration theory. In *The Eye and Visual Optical Instruments*. Cambridge University Press pp. 601–46.

Stone, D., Mathews, S. and Kruger, P. B. (1993). Accommodation and chromatic aberration: effect of spatial frequency. *Ophthal. Physiol. Opt.*, **13**, 244–52.

Thibos, L. N. (1987). Calculation of the influence of lateral chromatic aberration on image quality across the visual field. *J. Opt. Soc. Am. A.*, **4**, 1673–80.

Thibos, L. N. (1990). Optical limitations of the Maxwellian view interferometer. *Applied Optics*, **29**, 1411–19.

Thibos, L. N., Bradley, A., Still, D. L. *et al.* (1990). Theory and measurement of ocular chromatic aberration. *Vision Res.*, **30**, 33–49.

Thibos, L. N., Bradley, A. and Zhang, X. (1991a). Effect of ocular chromatic aberration on monocular visual performance. *Optom. Vis. Sci.*, **68**, 599–607.

Thibos, L. N., Bradley, A. and Still, D. L. (1991b). Interferometric measurement of visual acuity and the effect of ocular chromatic aberration. *Applied Opt.*, **30**, 2079–87.

Thibos, L. N., Ye, M., Zhang, X. and Bradley, A. (1992). The chromatic eye: a new reduced-eye model of ocular chromatic aberration in humans. *Applied Optics*, **31**, 3594–600.

Thibos, L. N., Ye, M., Zhang, X. and Bradley, A. (1997). Spherical aberration of the reduced schematic eye with elliptical refracting surface. *Optom. Vis. Sci.*, **74**, 548–56.

Thomson, L. C. and Wright, W. D. (1947). The colour sensitivity of the retina within the central fovea of man. *J. Physiol. (Lond.)*, **105**, 316–31.

van Heel, A. C. S. (1946). Correcting the spherical and chromatic aberrations of the eye. *J. Opt. Soc. Am.*, **36**, 237–9.

Wald, G. and Griffin, D. R. (1947). The change in refractive power of the human eye in dim and bright light. *J. Opt. Soc. Am.*, **37**, 321–36.

Ware, C. (1982). Human axial chromatic aberration found not to decline with age. *Graefe's Arch. Clin. Exp. Ophthal.*, **218**, 39–41.

Wildsoet, C. F., Atchison, D. A., Collins, M. J. (1993). Longitudinal chromatic aberration as a function of refractive error. *Clin. Exp. Optom.*, **76**, 119–22.

Ye, M., Bradley, A., Thibos, L. N. and Zhang, X. (1991). Interocular differences in transverse chromatic aberration determine chromostereopsis for small pupils. *Vision Res.*, **31**, 1787–96.

Ye, M., Bradley, A., Thibos, L. N. and Zhang, X. (1992). The effect of pupil size on chromostereopsis and chromatic diplopia; interaction between the Stiles–Crawford effect and chromatic aberrations. *Vision Res.*, **32**, 2121–8.

Zhang, X., Bradley, A. and Thibos, L. N. (1991). Achromatizing the human eye: the problem of chromatic parallax. *J. Opt. Soc. Am. A*, **8**, 686–91.

Zhang, X., Bradley, A. and Thibos, L. N. (1993). Experimental determination of the chromatic difference of magnification of the human eye and the location of the anterior nodal point. *J. Opt. Soc. Am.*, **10**, 213–20.

18

Retinal image quality

Introduction

The quality of the visual system depends upon a combination of optical and neural factors, with subjective measures depending also upon psychological factors.

The optical factors that determine the retinal image quality and affect visual system quality are refractive errors, ocular aberrations, diffraction and scatter. The levels of the first three depend upon wavelength and pupil size, and can be easily quantified. Scatter is complex, and depends upon the level and nature of the turbidity of the ocular media, in particular the size and spatial distribution of the scattering centres.

The neural factors affecting visual system quality include sizes and spacing of retinal cells, the degree of spatial summation at the various levels of processing from the retina to the visual cortex, and higher level processing.

The relative influences of optical and neural factors upon visual system quality vary with retinal position and the criterion used for assessing quality. In the foveal region, the in-focus retinal image quality appears well matched to the neural network's resolution at optimum pupil sizes of 2–3 mm (Campbell and Green, 1965; Campbell and Gubisch, 1966), but resolution in the peripheral visual field is limited much more by neural factors than by optical factors. For example, Green (1970) found that 'bypassing' the optics did not improve the resolution of sinusoidal gratings beyond about 5° degrees from the fovea. By comparison, the quality of the optics has a large influence on detection in the periphery (Wang *et al.*, 1997).

Direct measurement of retinal image quality is not possible because of the inaccessibility of the retina. The retinal image quality can be estimated from aberrations. The aerial image of the retinal image can be analysed; techniques using this approach are referred to as **double-pass** techniques, and also as ophthalmoscopic techniques. Another possibility is psychophysical measurement of visual performance in which two similar methods are used, one of which bypasses the optics of the eye; comparison of the results from the two methods yields the retinal image quality.

The retinal light distribution is not the same as the perceived light distribution, partly because of the Stiles–Crawford effect, which describes the luminous efficiency $L_e(r)$ of rays entering the eye through different heights r in the pupil (Chapter 13). The Stiles–Crawford effect is a retinal phenomenon, but for some purposes it can be considered as a pupil apodization; that is, as a filter of transmittance $L_e(r)$ placed over the pupil (Westheimer, 1959). As such, it is often included in calculations of retinal image quality.

In this chapter we examine retinal image quality criteria that are common in the analysis of general optical systems. These are the **point** and **line spread functions** and the **optical transfer function**. Equations for calculating the point spread function and the optical transfer function from the aberrations of an optical system are given in Appendix 4. Relationships between image quality criteria and measurements are shown in Figure 18.1. The chapter is completed with an evaluation of the retinal image quality of the eye.

The point and line spread functions

The point spread function is the illuminance or luminance distribution in the image of a point source of light, while the line spread function is the distribution in the image of a line (of zero width) source of light. The abbreviations PSF and LSF are often used for the point spread function and line spread function, respectively.

The form of the PSF depends upon diffraction, defocus, aberrations and scattered light. In the absence of defocus, aberrations and scatter, the PSF is called the **diffraction-limited PSF**. Defocus, aberrations and scattered light broaden the PSF. The form of the PSF also depends upon the shape and diameter of the aperture stop. In the following

discussion, it is assumed that the pupil is circular.

The diffraction-limited PSF (monochromatic light)

For a circular aperture or pupil, the diffraction-limited PSF is a radially symmetric function. For a monochromatic source, the relative light level $L(\zeta)$ at a distance ζ from the centre of the PSF is given by the equation

$$L(\zeta) = [2J_1(\zeta)]^2 / \zeta^2 \qquad (18.1)$$

where $J_1(\zeta)$ is a Bessel function. Tabulated values of $J_1(\zeta)$ can be found in books such as Abramowitz and Stegun (1965), and it is well approximated by polynomials such as that given in Table 18.1.

In object space with the object at infinity,

$$\zeta = 2\pi\theta\bar{\rho}/\lambda = \pi\theta D/\lambda \qquad (18.2)$$

where

$$\theta = \text{angular distance (radian)} = \frac{\zeta\lambda}{2\pi\bar{\rho}} = \frac{\zeta\lambda}{\pi D}$$

$$(18.2a)$$

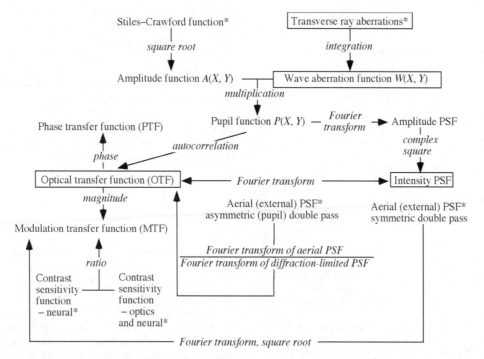

Figure 18.1. Relationships between image quality criteria. Main image quality criteria are in boxes, operations are in italics, and quantities obtained by measurement are marked by *.

Table 18.1. Polynomial approximation to the Bessel function $J_1(\zeta)$, from Abramowitz and Stegun (1965).

If $(\zeta < 3)$ or $(\zeta = 3)$, then
$$y = \zeta/3$$
$$x = 0.5 - 0.56249985y^2 + 0.21093573y^4 - 0.03954289y^6 + 0.00443319y^8 - 0.00031761y^{10} + 0.00001109y^{12}$$
$$J_1 = zx$$
Otherwise
$$y = 3/\zeta$$
$$g = +0.79788456 + 0.00000156y + 0.01659667y^2 + 0.00017105y^3 - 0.00249511y^4 + 0.00113653y^5 - 0.00020033y^6$$
$$w = z - 2.35619449 + 0.12499612y + 0.0000565y^2 - 0.00637879y^3 + 0.00074348y^4 + 0.00079824y^5 - 0.00029166y^6$$
$$J_1 = g\cos(w)/\sqrt{\zeta}$$

and $\bar{p}$ is the radius of the entrance pupil of eye, D is the diameter of the entrance pupil ($=2\bar{p}$), and λ is the wavelength in a vacuum. If we wish to convert the angular distance θ in object space to a distance on the retina, we can use the conversion equation

retinal distance = θF (18.3)

where F is the equivalent power of the eye.

This diffraction-limited PSF is plotted in Figure 18.2. The figure shows that the light distribution consists of a central peak and central disc of light, known as the **Airy disc**. This is surrounded by a number of rings of light of ever-decreasing light level.

The outer limit of the Airy disc occurs when the above function (that is, the light level) first goes to zero, which occurs at

$\zeta = 3.8317$ (18.4)

From equation (18.2), the corresponding value of θ at which this zero occurs is given by the equation

$\theta = 1.22\, \lambda/D$ rad   (18.5)

This is the angular radius of the Airy disc. Considering only the effect of diffraction, equation (18.5) shows that the PSF decreases in width as the aperture stop diameter increases in size.

The diffraction-limited PSF can be observed by looking at a bright monochromatic point source against a dark background through a small artificial pupil. To be able to resolve the Airy disc and the surrounding rings, the disc must be several times larger than the smallest resolvable detail, which is often taken as 1 min. arc. Assuming that the disc is 4 min. arc in diameter, equation (18.5) predicts that the pupil diameter should be about 1.2 mm diameter at a wavelength of 550 nm.

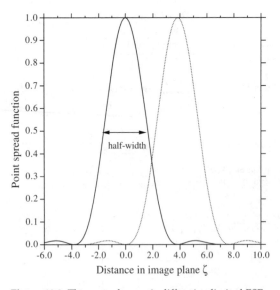

Figure 18.2. The monochromatic diffraction limited PSFs for two light sources. The sources are separated so that the first zero of one source falls on the peak value of the other source (Rayleigh criterion). The half-width is also shown.

The aberrated PSF

For pupil diameters greater than about 2 mm, or in polychromatic light, aberrations cannot be neglected, and the point spread function is not accurately described by the above diffraction-limited equation. The effect of any aberration is to spread light out more than predicted by diffraction. Therefore, the aberrated PSF is broader and the peak is lowered, relative to the diffraction-limited case.

The PSF and its use in quantifying image quality

The PSF of the eye is affected by defocus, aberrations and scatter, and is usually formed by polychromatic light. Thus it is not generally well described by the diffraction-limited PSF. Furthermore, because of asymmetries in the function, it is difficult often to compare the PSF under different conditions. Comparisons are much easier if the PSF can be reduced to a single number that specifies the image quality on some meaningful scale. Three of these are the **Rayleigh criterion**, **half-width** and the **Strehl intensity ratio**.

The Rayleigh criterion (diffraction-limited and monochromatic sources)

The Rayleigh resolution criterion applies only to monochromic point sources and states that, for a diffraction-limited system, two point sources can just be resolved if the peak of one of the PSFs lies on the first minimum of the other. For two sources of the same wavelength, the situation is shown in Figure 18.2. Since the radius of the first dark ring of the diffraction-limited PSF is given by equation (18.5), it follows that this is the minimum angular resolution according to the Rayleigh criterion.

The half-width

Once the influence of aberrations, scatter and polychromatic light are included, the Airy disc ceases to exist because the PSF has, in general, no well-defined zeros. The width of the PSF is then often taken as the half-width, which is the width at half the peak height. If the diffraction-limited PSF is analyzed, we find that the half-width $\Delta\zeta$ is

$$\Delta\zeta = 3.2327 \tag{18.6}$$

which is less than the diameter of the Airy disc (equation (18.4)). With this value, the diffraction-limited angular half-width $\Delta\theta$ is given by the equation

$$\Delta\theta = \frac{1.029\lambda}{D} \text{ rad or } = \frac{3537\lambda}{D} \text{ min. arc} \tag{18.7}$$

The half-width of the diffraction-limited PSF is shown in Figure 18.2. If aberrations are introduced, the half-width increases.

When astigmatism and coma are present, the half-width should be considered in two mutually perpendicular directions, where the width is minimum and maximum. These can be reduced to a single number by taking the arithmetic or geometric mean of the two widths.

The Strehl intensity ratio

The Strehl intensity ratio is a measure of the effect of aberrations on reducing the maximum or peak value of the PSF. It is defined as follows:

$$E = \frac{\text{maximum light level value of aberrated PSF}}{\text{maximum light level value of unaberrated PSF}} \tag{18.8}$$

The Strehl intensity ratio has an advantage over the half-width by always being a single number, even if the PSF is not rotationally symmetric.

Since the effect of aberrations is to spread out the PSF and decrease the maximum peak height, the Strehl intensity ratio is always less than or equal to one. The greater the aberrations, the lower the value of the Strehl intensity ratio and the poorer the image quality. A criterion for a good, near to diffraction-limited system is that the Strehl intensity ratio has a value of ≥ 0.8.

The PSF and LSF of eyes

The light distribution of a point source at the retina cannot be measured directly, but the light passing back out of the eye (the aerial or external image) is measurable. Because the light has passed twice through the eye's optical system, this method is known as a double-pass method. The light is doubly aberrated, and the aerial PSF is wider than the retinal PSF. It has long been thought that the retinal PSF is given by the inverse Fourier transform (FT^{-1}) of the square root of the Fourier transform (FT) of the aerial PSF, which is expressed mathematically as

$$\text{PSF} = FT^{-1}\sqrt{[FT(\text{aerial PSF})]} \tag{18.9a}$$

This is not correct, because the aerial image loses the information of asymmetric aberrations, such as coma, which results in loss of phase information (Artal *et al.*, 1995a). This does not affect the determination of the modulation transfer function, but it does affect the phase transfer function so that earlier determinations of this are incorrect (e.g. Artal *et al.*, 1988). To overcome this problem, Artal and co-workers used different diameters of the aperture stops for light entering and leaving the eye, one of which was small enough to be considered diffraction limited (e.g. 1 mm diameter). They called this a 'one-and-a-half pass' method (Artal *et al.*, 1995b; Navarro and Losada, 1995) and an 'asymmetric (pupil) double-pass method'. Using this method, the retinal PSF with the larger aperture stop is obtained by dividing the Fourier transform of the aerial PSF by the Fourier transform of the diffraction-limited PSF, and then obtaining the inverse Fourier transform of this result. This is expressed mathematically as

$$\text{PSF} = FT^{-1}[FT(\text{aerial PSF})/ \\ FT(\text{diffraction-limited PSF})] \qquad (18.9b)$$

Early measurements of the eye's LSF were made by Flamant (1955), Krauskopf (1962, 1964), and Westheimer and Campbell (1962). Estimates of the modulation transfer function (see next section) were made by taking the square root of a one-dimensional Fourier transform of the aerial LSF. LSF measurements preceded measurements of the PSF by about 30 years (Santamaría *et al.*, 1987) because of the problem of low light levels. With the development of lasers and more sensitive detectors, it is now possible to measure PSFs in monochromatic light, and detectors are sensitive enough for accurate recording within a few minutes of arc of the centre of the PSF. This is the region influenced by diffraction, aberrations and small angle scatter. Diffraction and aberrations have almost no influence on image quality at angles larger than a few minutes of arc, and light beyond this distance is due to scatter alone. Technical issues involved in the measurement of the PSF are described by Artal *et al.* (1993), Navarro *et al.* (1993) and Williams *et al.* (1994, 1996).

Sophisticated techniques are being devel-

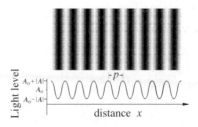

Figure 18.3. A one-dimensional pattern with a sinusoidally varying light level.

oped to derive the aberrations of the eye from the PSF (Iglesias *et al.*, 1998a and b).

The optical transfer function

Figure 18.3 shows a one-dimensional grating pattern with a light level that varies sinusoidally. The variation of this light level with distance x can be described by the equation

$$\text{Light level } (x) = A_o + A \sin(2\pi x/p + \delta) \qquad (18.10)$$

where A is the amplitude of the variation and its value may be negative, δ is a phase factor, and p is the period of this pattern whose reciprocal is the spatial frequency σ, that is

$$\sigma = 1/p \qquad (18.10a)$$

In object space, the period is in units of angle (e.g. radians, degrees, minutes of arc), and thus the units of spatial frequency are cycles/units of angle (e.g. c/rad, c/deg, and c/min. arc).

If this pattern is imaged by an optical system, and providing the aberrations do not change too rapidly over the field of the sinusoidal pattern, the image is also sinusoidal but now has amplitude A', phase factor δ' and period p', and can be represented by the equation

$$\text{Light level } (x') = A_o' + A' \sin(2\pi x'/p' + \delta') \qquad (18.11)$$

The **modulation transfer function** is defined as the amplitude A' of the image divided by the amplitude A of the object, and it is a function of spatial frequency. In one dimension, we denote the modulation transfer function by the symbol $G(\sigma)$ and so

$$G(\sigma) = A'/A \qquad (18.12)$$

Because this will depend upon light attenuation in the system, the modulation transfer function is normalized so that $G(0) = 1$.

Different aberrations have different effects on the image. Spherical aberration and defocus cause a decrease in the amplitude, but coma causes both a decrease in the amplitude and a transverse shift from the Gaussian (or aberration-free) image position. Astigmatism is a defocus that varies with azimuth (meridian) in the pupil, and field curvature is a defocus that is independent of this azimuth. Distortion causes a transverse shift only. Those aberrations that produce a transverse shift produce an effective phase shift in the image – i.e. δ and δ' have different values. The phase shift across a range of spatial frequencies is the **phase transfer function**.

The **optical transfer function** (OTF) is a complex quantity that includes both the modulation transfer function (MTF) and the phase transfer function (PTF). In some situations, for example on-axis in a rotationally symmetric optical system, there is no change in phase with spatial frequency. In these situations the OTF is identical to the MTF, and we can use the terms interchangeably.

The MTF is closely associated with the **contrast threshold function**, which is the visual threshold contrast of sinusoidal patterns as a function of spatial frequency. This function depends upon neural factors as well as optical effects. The reciprocal of the contrast threshold function is called the **contrast sensitivity function** (CSF).

The diffraction-limited OTF with no Stiles–Crawford effect

Using the theory presented in Appendix 4, one can easily show that the monochromatic diffraction-limited optical transfer function, without any Stiles–Crawford effect, is given by the equation

$$G(\sigma) = [\Gamma - \sin(\Gamma)]/\pi \qquad (18.13)$$

where

$$\Gamma = 2\cos^{-1}[\sigma\lambda/(2\bar{\rho})] \qquad (18.13a)$$

It is common practice to express the diffraction-limited OTF in terms of a 'reduced spatial frequency' s, which is defined in terms of the actual spatial frequency σ, by the equation

$$s = \sigma\lambda/\bar{\rho} \qquad (18.14)$$

Equation (18.13) can still be used, but with $G(\sigma)$ replaced by $G(s)$ to calculate the OTF in terms of s, and the equation of Γ becomes

$$\Gamma = 2\cos^{-1}(s/2) \qquad (18.14a)$$

This is an example in which there is no phase shift with spatial frequency, and the MTF and the OTF are the same.

The function $G(s)$ giving the diffraction-limited modulation transfer function is plotted in Figure 18.4, and it follows from this figure that the upper limit of s is 2.0, which corresponds to the resolution limit of the optical system. The corresponding actual spatial frequency or resolution limit σ_{max} is thus

$$\sigma_{max} = 2\bar{\rho}/\lambda \text{ or } = D/\lambda \text{ c/rad} \qquad (18.15)$$

and this equation can be used to predict the theoretical OTF resolution limit of the eye for any pupil size and wavelength.

Determination of the OTF

The OTF can be determined in three ways (Figure 18.1).

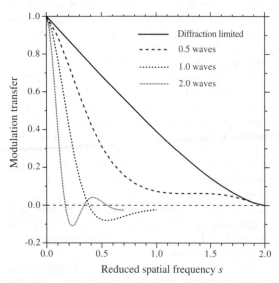

Figure 18.4. Examples of the defocused modulation transfer function for three values of $_0W_{2,0}$ in wavelength units.

Determining the OTF from the measured wave aberrations

The OTF can be calculated theoretically from the aberrations, and the mathematical basis of this is described briefly in Appendix 4.

Determining the OTF from the aerial PSF

(See, for example, Artal *et al.*, 1995a.)

The OTF is the Fourier transform of the PSF. However, as described in the previous section, with a single aperture stop for both ingoing and outgoing light, phase information is lost. The full retinal OTF cannot be determined, but the MTF is the square root of the Fourier transform of the aerial PSF. Using the asymmetric double-pass method in which either the ingoing or outgoing light beam is diffraction limited, the OTF is the ratio of the Fourier transforms of the aerial and diffraction-limited PSFs.

Determining the OTF from psychophysical comparison

(See, for example, Arnulf and Dupuy, 1960; Campbell and Green, 1965; Bour, 1980; Williams *et al.*, 1994.)

The CSF is measured for sinusoids viewed naturally (e.g. created on a video screen), and by using an interferometer with Maxwellian view which bypasses the optics and projects sinusoidal fringes directly on the retina. The first function includes both the optics and neural factors, and the second function involves only the neural factors.

For the second function, two mutually coherent point sources are produced near the nodal points, and the two resulting beams overlap on the retina to produce a series of parallel fringes with angular separation $\gamma = \lambda/a$, where λ is the source wavelength and a is the source separation in air (Le Grand, 1935 (translated Charman and Simonet, 1997); Smith and Atchison, 1997). Assuming the two sources have equal intensity, the fringes have a contrast of 1. The fringe contrast is reduced by adding light from an incoherent source of the same wavelength.

Denoting the CSF determined with both optics and neural factors as CSF_{o+n} and the CSF determined with only the neural factors as CSF_n, the modulation transfer function is simply the ratio of these two functions; that is

$$MTF = CSF_{o+n}/CSF_n \qquad (18.16)$$

CSF_{o+n} must be measured for each pupil size of interest. Campbell and Green's (1965) CSF results for one subject are shown in Figure 18.5a, with the derived MTFs for a range of pupil sizes appearing in Figure 18.5b.

OTF in the presence of defocus

To examine the optical transfer function with some defocus, we must add a $W_{2,0}$ term to the wave aberration function (Appendix 2), and this is related to the defocus expressed as a power ΔF by equation (A2.5). This is another example where the MTF and OTF are identical.

Results are shown in Figure 18.4 for different levels of defocus. For higher levels of defocus, the MTF eventually becomes negative, and then has an oscillatory nature with a decreasing amplitude. When the MTF is negative, the image pattern has reversed contrast compared with that of the object. This means that the brighter parts of the object become the darker parts of the image, and the darker parts of the object become the brighter parts of the image. The spatial frequency at which the modulation transfer function first goes to zero is the resolution limit. Any resolution of higher frequency patterns is called **spurious resolution**.

Spurious resolution can be seen with the Siemen's star pattern in Figure 18.6 when this is defocused severely by using lenses or by viewing from a close distance within the accommodation limit. Some regions in the pattern show contrast reversal. If eyes were rotationally symmetric, the regions of contrast reversal would form concentric annuli. However, because real eyes are asymmetric, particular the aberrations, these annuli have irregularities. The presence of the asymmetries means that the phase transfer function is not zero.

The geometrical optical approximation for defocus

The phenomenon of spurious resolution can be investigated by a much simpler but

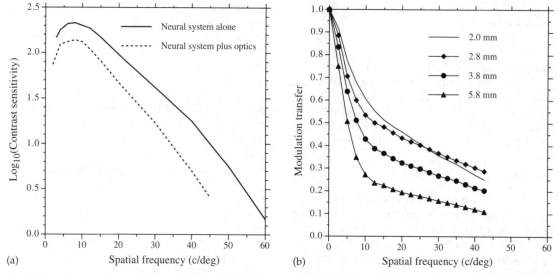

(a) Spatial frequency (c/deg)   (b) Spatial frequency (c/deg)

Figure 18.5.
a. Results of Campbell and Green (1965) showing the contrast threshold functions for the whole eye; that is, the combined neural and optical systems, and the neural system alone. For the former the subject viewed sinusoidal gratings on a television monitor with a green phosphor through a 2 mm artificial pupil, while for the latter the fringes were generated by interferometry using monochromatic light (wavelength 633 nm).
b. Modulation transfer functions from a range of pupil sizes derived from the ratio of the two types of curves shown in Figure 18.5a.

approximate process if it is assumed that the defocus is large. In this case, the PSF is a uniformly illuminated disc. In Chapter 9, we showed that the angular diameter Φ of the defocus blur disc was related to the level of

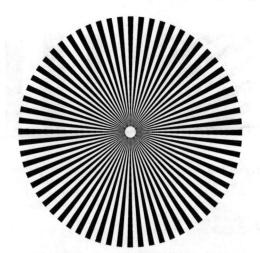

Figure 18.6. The Siemen's star, which can be used for observing spurious resolution.

refractive error ΔL and pupil diameter D, by equation (9.17), that is

$$\Phi = \Delta L \, D \tag{18.17}$$

In the simple aberration and diffraction-free defocused system, the PSF is the defocus blur disc of diameter Φ. The OTF is the Fourier transform of this PSF. For a circular uniform function with a diameter Φ, the OTF $G(\sigma)$ is given by the equation

$$G(\sigma) = \frac{J_1(\pi\Phi\sigma)}{\pi\Phi\sigma} \tag{18.18}$$

where J_1 is the same Bessel function as in equation (18.1). For distance viewing, i.e. Φ is in radians, the spatial frequency σ is in cycles/radian. The first zero of this equation occurs at

$$\pi\Phi\sigma = 3.83$$

and thus

$$\sigma = \frac{3.83}{\pi\Phi} = \frac{1.22}{\Phi} \tag{18.19}$$

Replacing the blur disc diameter Φ by the right-hand side expression from equation

(18.17), we have

$$\sigma = \frac{1.22}{\Delta LD} \text{ c/rad} \qquad (18.20)$$

This value of σ is the resolution limit.

As an example, let us calculate the resolution limit of an eye with a pupil diameter of 4 mm and 1 D of defocus. In equation (18.20), we put $\Delta L = 1$ D and $D = 0.004$ m, and thus the resulting resolution limit is

$$\sigma = 305 \text{ c/rad} = 5.32 \text{ c/deg}$$

Figure 18.7 shows the expected region of spurious resolution in an aberration-free eye according to physical and geometric optics predictions (Smith, 1982). Geometric optics approximations become more accurate for higher levels of defocus and lower spatial frequencies.

Retinal image quality

To appreciate the limits that the optics of the eye place on vision, we also need some understanding of the limits provided by the retina. To be able to resolve the detail provided by a pattern of light imaged upon the retina, the adjacent 'receptor units' must be sufficiently close together to correctly interpret the pattern. In Figure 18.8, oblique square wave light patterns imaged on a square array of receptor units are shown. In Figure 18.8a, the pattern repeats every four units in the vertical meridian. Another way of putting this is that the receptor units are a quarter of a cycle apart. The visual system interprets the spatial frequency and orientation of the pattern correctly (the term **veridically** is sometimes used). In Figure 18.8b, the pattern repeats every two units in the vertical direction. For every two receptor units in the vertical direction struck by adjacent light bars, there is a receptor unit between them which is struck by a dark bar (and *vice versa*). The visual system is just able to resolve the pattern; that is, vision is again veridical. In Figure 18.8c, the sinusoidal pattern is yet finer, repeating every receptor

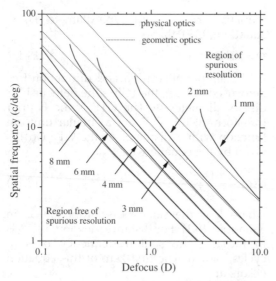

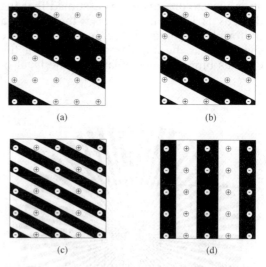

Figure 18.7. Physical and geometrical optical predictions of the boundaries of spurious resolution for an aberration-free system and for different pupil diameters as marked (mm). Spurious resolution occurs above the boundaries. The physical optical predictions are given by the curves. The geometrical optics approximations given by the straight lines are increasingly accurate as pupil size increases, defocus increases, and spatial frequency decreases. Wavelength is 550 nm (based on Smith, 1982).

Figure 18.8. Oblique square wave patterns are imaged on a square array of receptor units. The receptor units are excited by the bright bars and inhibited by dark bars.
a. The pattern repeats itself every four units in the vertical direction.
b. The pattern repeats itself every two units in the vertical direction.
c. The pattern repeats itself every unit in the vertical direction.
d. An aliased perception of the pattern in (c).

unit in the vertical meridian, and now the sampling rate of the receptor units is inadequate to correctly interpret the pattern. The visual system 'undersamples' the pattern, which may be perceived to have a much lower spatial frequency and a different orientation such as that in Figure 18.8d. This incorrect interpretation of the pattern is referred to as **aliasing**. Another way of considering this is that the visual system cannot distinguish between the light patterns shown in Figures 18.8c and d.

Figure 18.8b shows the finest light pattern that can be correctly resolved by the retina. Its spatial frequency is called the **Nyquist limit** (*NL*), and is given by

$$NL = 1/(2c_s) \tag{18.21a}$$

where c_s is the centre-to-centre spacing of the receptor units.

The 'receptor unit' that correlates best with resolution is the spacing between ganglion cells (Thibos *et al.*, 1987). At the fovea there is a one to one correspondence between cones and ganglion cells, so the cone spacing can be used to determine resolution limits. Because of the tight hexagonal packing of cones, the previous equation needs to be modified to

$$NL = 1/(\sqrt{3}c_s) \tag{18.21b}$$

Williams (1985) calculated the Nyquist limit to be 56 c/deg in object space (or subtense at back nodal point), by assuming that the closest spacing of human foveal cones is 3 μm and that 0.29 mm on the retina corresponds to 1°. The resolution limit drops quickly away from the fovea because of the rapid decrease in ganglion cell density (Curcio and Allen, 1990).

There are two major types of spatial tasks that are performed by the visual system. Resolution has already been referred to; the other type is detection. Perimetry is an example of a detection task in which a patient must detect that a spot of light is present; details such as the shape of the spot are usually unimportant. Although in Figure 18.8c the pattern is not seen veridically, it is still seen, provided that the contrast is sufficiently high. It is likely that the highest spatial frequency that can be detected by the retina is limited by the size of photoreceptors (Still, 1989). Visual acuity involves resolution, as a patient must be able to resolve detail of a target. It can be argued that visual acuity is more than a resolution task, as identifying the arrangement of resolved elements is important for identification of a letter.

The relative importance of optical and neural limitations to visual performance can be determined by using the CSF both as a resolution task and as a detection task. In the detection task, the subject is asked which of two presentations contains a grating. In the resolution task, the subject is asked to determine the orientation of a sinusoidal grating; for example, whether it is horizontal or vertical. For normal presentation of the gratings on a monitor, when the two CSFs are essentially the same, the optics act as a filter to provide the main limitation to both detection and resolution (see central curves in Figure 18.9). However, if the detection CSF is superior to the resolution CSF, then resolution, although not necessarily detection, is limited by the sampling rate of the receptor elements (see peripheral curves in Figure 18.9).

This issue was discussed in detail by Thibos and Bradley (1993), who recommended using

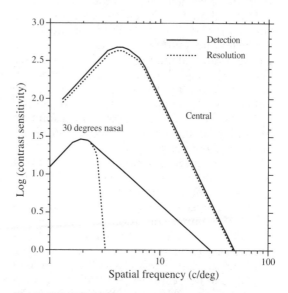

Figure 18.9. Normal contrast sensitivity functions for resolution and detection tasks for the centre and periphery (30° nasal in object space) of the visual field. The region between the two peripheral vision curves indicates the spatial frequencies for which aliasing occurs. Representation is based on results of Thibos *et al.* (1996) in which measurements in the periphery were done after careful refraction.

the distinction between resolution and detection to design clinical tests to determine at which stage (detection, resolution or identification) an abnormal visual system is breaking down.

Central vision

Despite being carried out in the mid-1960s, the classic work of Campbell and colleagues is still considered to provide good data on the quality of the optics of the eye. Figure 18.5b shows the psychophysically determined modulation transfer functions of Campbell and Green (1965) for one subject. Optical performance is near diffraction-limited for 2 mm diameter pupils. As pupil size increases, aberrations cause performance to decrease relative to diffraction-limited performance, with optimum quality occurring for 2.0–2.8 mm pupil diameters. The maximum spatial frequency at which resolution of the pattern is possible is approximately 60 c/deg. Using an improved technique with reduced spatial noise masking effects, which can affect the CSF measured by bypassing the optics, Williams (1985) showed that the neural ability is better than that given by Campbell and Green beyond 40 c/deg. This indicates that the retinal image quality beyond 40 c/deg is worse than calculated by Campbell and Green. Although both the optics and neural factors contribute to the normal CSF, the optics are the major limitation to central vision because both detection and resolution CSFs give similar results – that is, there is no aliasing (Thibos *et al.*, 1996).

The aberration methods of determining image quality might be expected to over-estimate image quality because media scattering effects are ignored. The psycho-physical comparison method has several considerations. Again, the scattering effects may be ignored, assuming that they affect the two CSFs equally. There is also the problem of making the two contrast sensitivity measure-ments equivalent for subjects to perform. The ophthalmoscopic techniques involve assump-tions, including that the retina acts as a diffuse reflector and that scatter is similar for both directions of light. They may be affected by a retinal effect similar to the Stiles–Crawford function (Artal, 1989). They also involve

imaging manipulations to remove influences of forward- and back-scattered light.

Williams *et al.* (1994) found that the double-pass method produced slightly lower MTFs than the psychophysical method in red light (633 nm) for three subjects with 3 mm diameter pupils. They attributed the differ-ence to light scattered back from the choroid, because repeating the PSF measurements in green light (543 nm), which reduces the choroidal contribution to the fundus reflect-ance, gave results which were consistent with the psychometric results. Their MTFs were much lower than studies using the aberro-scope technique to determine MTFs (Figure 18.10), and were lower than a subsequent investigation by Liang and Williams (1997) using the wave-front sensor technique.

There is considerable variation in retinal image quality between different eyes, as shown in Figure 18.10 for 3 mm diameter pupils (Walsh and Charman, 1985).

Although much of our emphasis is on the modulation transfer function, the phase transfer function is an aspect of image quality that should not be neglected. Phase transfer

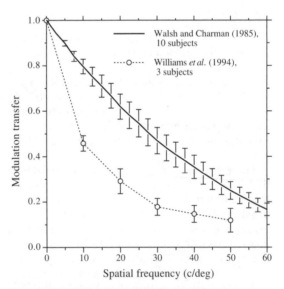

Figure 18.10. Comparison of MTFs obtained for 3 mm diameter pupils from the psychophysical comparison method (Williams *et al.*, 1994) and the aberroscope technique (Walsh and Charman, 1985). Results show means and standard deviations. Vertical grating orientation. For the Walsh and Charman study, the MTFs were determined from the 10 subjects' aberration co-efficients.

functions of eyes are very different from zero, corresponding to the presence of coma-like aberrations (Walsh and Charman, 1985; Charman and Walsh, 1985). This is very important in recognition of complex objects, which do not look like the originals because of different phases at different spatial frequencies.

Liang *et al.* (1997) used adaptive optics in conjunction with the wave-front sensor technique to correct the aberrations of four subjects. They were able substantially to correct the aberrations of the eyes, obtaining near diffraction-limited performance with 6 mm diameter pupils. Contrast sensitivity and resolution limits were improved markedly with the adaptive optics, and retinal cones could be seen easily with a fundus camera through the adaptive optics. An interesting phenomenon they noticed illustrates their success in correcting the eye's optics. A steadily fixated red laser light appeared to fluctuate in colour between red and green – this was due to fixational eye movements shifting the retinal location between long and medium wavelength cones.

Defocus

The most important optical defect affecting retinal image quality is defocus. Fluctuations in the modulation transfer function (e.g. Figure 18.4) produced by defocus can be expected to be accompanied by fluctuations in the CSF. Few studies dealing with defocus have shown dips (or notches) in the CSF, probably because of limitations in technique such as sampling rate and quality of equipment. Apkarian *et al.* (1987) and Bour and Apkarian (1996) showed notches in the CSF in the presence of astigmatism. Woods *et al.* (1996) and Atchison *et al.* (1998b) were able to show up to four notches in the CSF (Figure 18.11) which generally coincided well with predictions from MTFs. Even in less well-controlled experiments, which are much closer to the usual clinical situation, it is still possible to show these fluctuations in the CSF (Woods *et al.*, in press). Even small levels of defocus (0.5 D) can produce quite marked losses, demonstrating that it is important carefully to correct even small refractive errors to prevent incorrect attribution of losses to retinal/neural pathological causes.

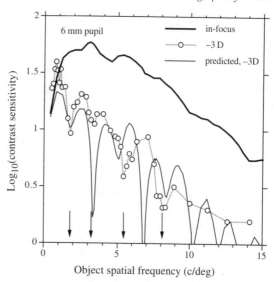

Figure 18.11. Measured monochromatic CSFs for one subject for in-focus condition (0 D) and defocus condition (–3 D). Also shown is the predicted monochromatic CSF for the defocus condition. This was obtained by multiplying the CSF for the in-focus condition by the ratio of MTFs for the defocused and in-focus conditions. The MTFs were themselves obtained from aberration measurements. The arrows indicate spatial frequencies corresponding to four 'notches' in the CSF; these correspond well with those predicted from theory. Unpublished data of the study of Atchison *et al.* (1998b).

Polychromatic light

On the basis of theoretical considerations, van Meeteren (1974) considered that chromatic aberration is the major optical limitation to in-focus retinal image quality. Thibos *et al.* (1991) showed theoretically that, with 2.5 mm centred pupils, the longitudinal chromatic aberration would have similar effects in white light to 0.2 D defocus in monochromatic light (Figure 18.12). They obtained a maximum contrast sensitivity loss of 0.2 log unit and a visual acuity loss of ~ 10 per cent (< 0.05 log unit) relative to those in monochromatic light, similar to the experimental findings of Campbell and Gubisch (1967).

As mentioned in Chapter 17 (*Effects of chromatic aberrations on vision*), decentration of natural or artificial pupils in white light can have devastating effects on retinal image quality. Large levels of transverse chromatic aberration produce wavelength-dependent spatial phase shifts of the image of a

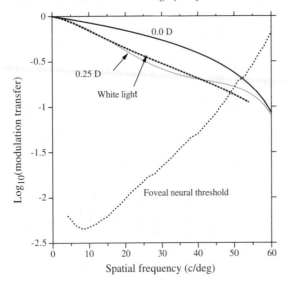

Figure 18.12. Comparison of in-focus white-light MTF with defocused monochromatic MTFs for the Chromatic eye, which is free of monochromatic aberrations (pupil diameter 2.5 mm, white light provided by a P4 phosphor, reference wavelength 589 nm). Also shown is the neural contrast threshold of one subject from Campbell and Green (1965). Intersection of the MTF curves with the neural contrast threshold predicts the cut-off spatial frequency. Based on Figure 4 of Thibos *et al.* (1991), with data kindly provided by Larry Thibos and with permission from The American Academy of Optometry.

sinusoidal target, leading to loss of image contrast. This has its greatest effects for target orientation at right angles to the decentration direction, with up to three times loss of resolution for 3 mm displacements of small artificial pupils (Figure 18.13)(Green, 1967; Thibos *et al.*, 1991).

The Stiles–Crawford effect

The Stiles–Crawford effect has often been implicated by vision researchers to explain the difference between expected and actual findings – for example, the failure of depth-of-field to decrease with increase in pupil size as quickly as expected (Campbell, 1957; Tucker and Charman, 1975; Charman and Whitefoot, 1977; Legge *et al.*, 1987). However, the results of theoretical investigations using the apodiz-ation model suggest that the Stiles–Crawford effect is not important for spatial resolution for in-focus imagery, even in the presence of considerable aberrations (Metcalf, 1965;

Krakau, 1974; van Meeteren, 1974; Carroll, 1980). Even in the presence of defocus, the influence of the Stiles–Crawford function should be small (e.g. van Meeteren, 1974; Atchison *et al.*, 1998a) (Figure 18.14). The Stiles–Crawford effect is expected to influence optimal refraction in the presence of aberrations, but the magnitude is likely to be small – for example, approximately 0.2 D at 10 c/deg in Figure 18.14.

Pupil decentration

Decentration of the eye's pupil induces additional optical aberrations, such as trans-verse chromatic aberration and coma, which decrease spatial visual performance (Green, 1967; van Meeteren and Dunnewold, 1983; Artal *et al.*, 1996). The Stiles–Crawford effect may be of assistance to spatial vision by reducing the influence of the aberrations of the parts of the pupil furthest from the peak of the Stiles–Crawford effect; Bradley and

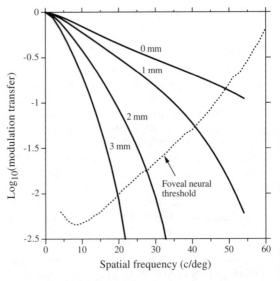

Figure 18.13. White-light MTFs for the Chromatic eye, which is free of monochromatic aberrations, for various displacements of a 2.5 mm diameter pupil perpendicular to the grating orientation (white light provided by a P4 phosphor, reference wavelength 589 nm). Also shown is the neural contrast threshold of one subject from Campbell and Green (1965). Intersection of the MTF curves with the neural contrast threshold predicts the cut-off spatial frequency. Based on Figure 9 of Thibos *et al.* (1991), with data kindly provided by Larry Thibos and with permission from The American Academy of Optometry.

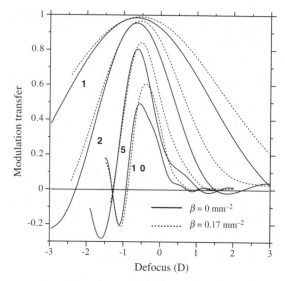

Figure 18.14. Modulation transfer as a function of defocus at various object spatial frequencies (cycles/degree) when there is +1.0 D of primary spherical aberration at the edge of a 6 mm diameter pupil in 605 nm wavelength light. Results are shown with and without Stiles–Crawford apodization of β = 0.17, which is near the 97.5 per cent upper limit (Applegate and Lakshminarayanan, 1993). The Stiles–Crawford effect has only a small influence on image quality, which is greater when the defocus and spherical aberration are in the same direction than when they are opposed. Data from Figure 6 of Atchison *et al.* (1998a), with permission from The Optical Society of America.

Thibos (1995) refer to this as an anchoring role. A number of studies have shown that subjective transverse chromatic aberration declines as pupil size increases; for example, Ye *et al.* (1992). This effect reduces as luminance is reduced, thus indicating that it is a retinal effect and due to the Stiles–Crawford effect.

Peripheral vision

The optics associated with the peripheral retina are poor, mainly because of focusing errors in the form of oblique astigmatism and field curvature (see Chapter 15). Retinal image quality declines steadily with object angle (Jennings and Charman 1978, 1981; Navarro *et al.*, 1993 and 1998). However, as shown in Figure 18.15, when the periphery is carefully refracted, the image quality

improves considerably (Jennings and Charman, 1978 and 1981; Still, 1989; Williams *et al.*, 1996). Navarro *et al.* (1998) found that the root-mean-squared wave aberration increases by a factor of only two from the central visual field out to 40° in the periphery when astigmatism and field curvature/defocus are corrected (6.7 mm diameter pupil). The importance of the peripheral optics has often been discounted because improving them has given little improvement in resolution (see, for example, Green, 1970). However, marked improvement in detection occurs (Williams *et al.*, 1996; Wang *et al.*, 1997).

Curve fitting of modulation transfer function results

Jennings and Charman (1997) listed a number of mathematical fits that have been proposed for experimentally determined modulation transfer functions, both for the centre and periphery of the visual field. As an example, Jennings and Charman (1974) examined

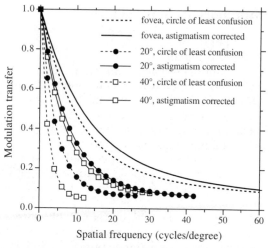

Figure 18.15. Fits of computed MTFs, averaged over two subjects, for different horizontal object angles, from the results of Williams *et al.* (1996). MTFs were determined from PSFs. The circle of least confusion plots are orientation-averaged MTFs obtained without correcting oblique astigmatism at a refractive state corresponding to the circle of least confusion. The astigmatism-corrected plots are effectively those obtained when defocus and oblique astigmatism are corrected. The off-axis correction gives considerable improvement in image quality. Pupil diameter 3 mm, wavelength 543 nm.

fitting central modulation transfer functions of the eye by the function

$$\text{MTF}(\sigma) = \exp[-(\sigma/\sigma_c)^n] \qquad (18.22a)$$

where σ is the spatial frequency, σ_c is a spatial frequency scaling constant at each pupil size, and n is a shape factor constant. Their fits are accurate only for lower spatial frequencies. At higher frequencies, errors arise because actual modulation transfer functions have a finite resolution limit and the above function does not. Later, Jennings and Charman (1997) found that this approximation was useful for the peripheral field, with n remaining relatively constant at about 0.9 out to 40° eccentricity and σ_c declining steeply over this range. Navarro *et al.* (1993) and, later, Williams *et al.* (1996) used the fit

$$\text{MTF}(\sigma) = (1 - C)\exp(-A\sigma) + C\exp(-B\sigma) \qquad (18.22b)$$

where σ is again the spatial frequency in cycles/degrees and A, B and C are constants for a particular object angle for a range of object angles. The results of these are shown in Figure 18.15.

Summary of main symbols

PSF point spread function
LSF line spread function
CSF contrast sensitivity function
MTF modulation transfer function
OTF optical transfer function
PTF phase transfer function
$G(\sigma)$ optical transfer function
σ spatial frequency (c/radian)
s corresponding modified spatial frequency, called 'reduced spatial frequency', related to σ by equation (18.14)
Φ angular diameter of defocus blur disc
$\bar{\rho}$ radius of entrance pupil
D diameter of entrance pupil

References

Abramowitz, M. and Stegun, I. A. (1965). *Handbook of Mathematical Functions with Formulas, Graphs and Mathematical Tables*, p. 370. US Government Print Office.

Apkarian, P., Tijssen, R., Spekreijse, H. and Regan, D. (1987). Origin of notches in CSF: Optical or neural? *Invest. Ophthal. Visual. Sci.*, **28**, 607–12.

Applegate, R. A. and Lakshminarayanan, V. (1993). Parametric representation of Stiles–Crawford functions: normal variation of peak location and directionality. *J. Opt. Soc. Am. A.*, **10**, 1611–23.

Arnulf, A. and Dupuy, O. (1960). La transmission des contrastes par le système optique de l'œil et les seuils des contrastes rétiniens. *C. R. Acad. Sci. Paris*, **250**, 2757–9.

Artal, P. (1989). Incorporation of directional effects of the retina into computations of optical transfer functions of human eyes. *J. Opt. Soc. Am. A.*, **6**, 1941–4.

Artal, P., Santamaría, J. and Bescós, J. (1988). Phase-transfer function of the human eye and its influence on point-spread function and wave aberration. *J. Opt. Soc. Am. A.*, **5**, 1791–5.

Artal, P., Ferro, M., Miranda, I. and Navarro, R. (1993). Effects of aging in retinal image quality. *J. Opt. Soc. Am. A.*, **10**, 1656–62.

Artal, P., Marcos, S., Navarro, R. and Williams, D. R. (1995a). Odd aberrations and double-pass measurements of retinal image quality. *J. Opt. Soc. Am. A.*, **12**, 195–201.

Artal, P., Iglesias, I. and López-Gil, N. (1995b). Double-pass measurements of the retinal-image quality with unequal entrance and exit pupil sizes and the reversibility of the eye's optical system. *J. Opt. Soc. Am. A.*, **12**, 2358–66.

Artal, P., Marcos, S., Iglesias, I. and Green, D. G. (1996). Optical modulation transfer and contrast sensitivity with decentered small pupils in the human eye. *Vision Res.*, **36**, 3575–86.

Atchison, D. A., Smith, G. and Joblin, A. (1998a). Influence of Stiles–Crawford apodization on spatial visual performance. *J. Opt. Soc. Am. A.*, **15**, 2545–51.

Atchison, D. A., Woods, R. L. and Bradley, A. (1998b). Predicting the effects of optical defocus on human contrast sensitivity. *J. Opt. Soc. Am. A.*, **15**, 2536–44.

Bour, L. J. (1980). MTF of the defocused optical quality of the human eye for incoherent monochromatic light. *J. Opt. Soc. Am.*, **70**, 321–8.

Bour, L. J. and Apkarian, P. (1996). Selective broad-band spatial frequency loss in contrast sensitivity functions. *Invest. Ophthal. Vis. Sci.*, **37**, 2475–84.

Bradley, A. and Thibos, L. N. (1995). Modelling off-axis vision – I: The optical effects of decentring visual targets or the eye's entrance pupil. In *Vision Models for Target Detection and Recognition*, pp. 313–37. World Scientific Press.

Campbell, F. W. (1957). The depth of field of the human eye. *Optica Acta*, **4**, 157–66.

Campbell, F. W. and Green, D. G. (1965). Optical and retinal factors affecting visual resolution. *J. Physiol. (Lond.)*, **181**, 576–93.

Campbell, F. W. and Gubisch, R. W. (1966). Optical quality of the human eye. *J. Physiol. (Lond.)*, **186**, 558–78.

Campbell, F. W. and Gubisch, R. W. (1967). The effect of

chromatic aberration on visual acuity. *J. Physiol. (Lond.)*, **192**, 345–58.

Carroll, J. P. (1980). Apodization model of the Stiles–Crawford effect. *J. Opt. Soc. Am.*, **70**, 1155–6.

Charman, W. N. and Simonet, P. (1997). Yves Le Grand and the assessment of retinal acuity using interference fringes. *Ophthal. Physiol. Opt.*, **17**, 164–8.

Charman, W. N. and Walsh, G. (1985). The optical transfer function of the eye and perception of spatial phase. *Vision Res.*, **25**, 619–23.

Charman, W. N. and Whitefoot, H. (1977). Pupil diameter and the depth-of-focus of the human eye for Snellen letters. *Optica Acta*, **24**, 1211–16.

Curcio, C. A. and Allen, K. A. (1990). Topography of ganglion cells in human retina. *J. Comp. Neurology*, **300**, 5–25.

Flamant, F. (1955). Étude de la répartition de lumière dans l'image rétienne d'une fente. *Rev. Opt. Théor. Instrum.*, **34**, 433–59.

Green, D. G. (1967). Visual resolution when light enters the eye through different parts of the pupil. *J. Physiol. (Lond.)*, **192**, 345–58.

Green, D. G. (1970). Regional variations in the visual acuity for interference fringes on the retina. *J. Physiol.(Lond.)*, **207**, 351–6.

Iglesias, I., López-Gil, N. and Artal, P. (1998a). Reconstruction of the point-spread function of the human eye from two double-pass retinal images by phase retrieval algorithms. *J. Opt. Soc. Am. A.*, **15**, 326–39.

Iglesias, I., Berrio, E. and Artal, P. (1998b). Estimates of the ocular wave aberration from pairs of double pass retinal images. *J. Opt. Soc. Am. A.*, **15**, 2466–76.

Jennings, J. A. M. and Charman, W. N. (1974). Analytic approximation of the off-axis modulation transfer function of the eye. *Br. J. Physiol. Opt.*, **29**, 64–72.

Jennings, J. A. M. and Charman, W. N. (1978). Optical image quality in the peripheral retina. *Am. J. Optom. Physiol. Opt.*, **55**, 582–90.

Jennings, J. A. M. and Charman, W. N. (1981). Off-axis image quality in the human eye. *Vision Res.*, **21**, 445–55.

Jennings, J. A. M. and Charman, W. N. (1997). Analytic approximation of the off-axis modulation transfer function of the eye. *Vision Res.*, **37**, 697–704.

Krakau, C. E. T. (1974). On the Stiles–Crawford phenomenon and resolution power. *Acta Ophthalmol.*, **52**, 581–3.

Krauskopf, J. (1962). Light distribution in human retinal images. *J. Opt. Soc. Am.*, **52**, 1046–50.

Krauskopf, J. (1964). Further measurements of human retinal images. *J. Opt. Soc. Am.*, **54**, 715–16.

Legge, G. E., Mullen, K. T., Woo, G. C. and Campbell, F. W. (1987). Tolerance to visual defocus. *J. Opt. Soc. Am. A.*, **4**, 851–63.

Le Grand, Y. (1935). Sur la mesure de l'acuité visuelle au moyen de franges d'interférence. *C. R. Acad. Sci. Paris*, **200**, 490–91 (translated by W. N. Charman and P. Simonet, 1997).

Liang, J. and Williams, D. R. (1997). Aberrations and retinal image quality of the normal human eye. *J. Opt. Soc. Am. A.*, **14**, 2873–83.

Liang, J., Williams, D. R. and Miller, D. T. (1997). Supernormal vision and high-resolution retinal imaging through adaptive optics. *J. Opt. Soc. Am. A.*, **14**, 2884–92.

Metcalf, H. (1965). Stiles–Crawford apodization. *J. Opt. Soc. Am.*, **55**, 72–4.

Navarro, R. and Losada, M. A. (1995). Phase transfer and point-spread function of the human eye determined by a new asymmetric double-pass method. *J. Opt. Soc. Am. A.*, **12**, 2385–92.

Navarro, R., Artal, P. and Williams, D. R. (1993). Modulation transfer of the human eye as a function of retinal eccentricity. *J. Opt. Soc. Am. A.*, **10**, 201–12.

Navarro, R., Moreno, E. and Dorronsoro, C. (1998). Monochromatic aberrations and point-spread functions of the human eye across the visual field. *J. Opt. Soc. Am. A.*, **15**, 2522–9.

Santamaría, J., Artal, P. and Bescós, J. (1987). Determination of the point-spread function of the human eyes using a hybrid optical-digital method. *J. Opt. Soc. Am. A.*, **4**, 1109–14.

Smith, G. (1982). Ocular defocus, spurious resolution and contrast reversal. *Ophthal. Physiol. Opt.*, **2**, 5–23.

Smith, G. and Atchison, D. A. (1997). *The Eye and Visual Optical Instruments*, pp. 517–24. Cambridge University Press.

Still, D. L. (1989). Optical limits to contrast sensitivity in human peripheral vision. Unpublished PhD thesis, University of Indiana.

Thibos, L. N. and Bradley, A. (1993). New methods of discriminating neural and optical losses of vision. *Optom. Vis. Sci.*, **70**, 279–87.

Thibos, L. N., Bradley, A. and Zhang, X. (1991). Effect of ocular chromatic aberration on monocular visual performance. *Optom. Vis. Sci.*, **68**, 599–607.

Thibos, L. N., Cheney, F. E. and Walsh, D. (1987). Retinal limits to the detection and resolution of gratings. *J. Opt. Soc. Am. A.*, **A4**, 1524–9.

Thibos, L. N., Still, D. L. and Bradley, A. (1996). Characterization of spatial aliasing and contrast sensitivity in peripheral vision. *Vision Res.*, **36**, 249–58.

Tucker, J. and Charman, W. N. (1975). The depth-of-focus of the eye for Snellen letters. *Am. J. Optom. Physiol. Opt.*, **52**, 3–21.

van Meeteren, A. (1974). Calculations on the optical modulation transfer function of the human eye for white light. *Optica Acta*, **21**, 395–412.

van Meeteren, A. and Dunnewold, C. J. W. (1983). Image quality of the human eye for eccentric entrance pupils. *Vision Res.*, **23**, 573–9.

Walsh, G. and Charman, W. N. (1985). Measurement of the axial wavefront aberration of the human eye. *Ophthal. Physiol. Opt.*, **5**, 23–31.

Wang, Y.-Z., Thibos, L. N. and Bradley, A. (1997). Effects of refractive error on detection acuity and resolution acuity in peripheral vision. *Invest. Ophthalmol. Vis. Sci.*, **38**, 2134–43.

Westheimer, G. (1959). Retinal light distribution for circular apertures in Maxwellian view. *J. Opt. Soc. Am.*, **49**, 41–4.

Westheimer, G. and Campbell, F. W. (1962). Light distribution in the image formed by the living human eye. *J. Opt. Soc. Am.*, **52**, 1040–45.

Williams, D. R. (1985). Visibility of interference fringes near the resolution limit. *J. Opt. Soc. Am. A.*, **2**, 1087–93.

Williams, D. R., Artal, P., Navarro, R. *et al.* (1996). Off-axis optical quality and retinal sampling in the human eye. *Vision Res.*, **36**, 1103–14.

Williams, D. R., Brainard, D. H., McMahon, M. J. and Navarro, R. (1994). Double pass and interferometric measures of the optical quality of the eye. *J. Opt. Soc. Am. A.*, **11**, 3123–35.

Woods, R. L., Bradley, A. and Atchison, D. A. (1996). Consequences of the monocular diplopia for the contrast sensitivity function. *Vision Res.*, **36**, 3587–96.

Woods, R. L., Strang, N. C. and Atchison, D. A. (in press). Measuring contrast sensitivity with inappropriate optical correction. *Ophth. Physiol. Opt.*

Ye, M., Bradley, A., Thibos, L. N. and Zhang, X. (1992). The effect of pupil size on chromostereopsis and chromatic diplopia: interaction between the Stiles–Crawford effect and chromatic aberrations. *Vision Res.*, **32**, 2121–8.

Section 5:

Miscellaneous

19

Depth-of-field

Introduction

In any optical system, the ultimate precision in focusing is set by the ability to detect errors in focus. The range of distances over which the system's detector cannot detect any change in focus is called the depth-of-field, and this range may be specified by a movement of the object plane or by the corresponding movement of the image plane. Because these two distances are usually different, some textbooks differentiate between depth-of-field, a movement of the object plane, and depth-of-focus, a movement of the image plane. In vision science, depth-of-field is usually expressed as a change in vergence, which has the same value in both object and image space. Distinctions may still have to be made between object and image space quantities in some circumstances, such as when using visual optical instruments. However, in this chapter there is no need to distinguish between object and image situations.

The definition adopted here for depth-of-field is the vergence range of focusing error ΔL, which does not result in objectionable deterioration in retinal image quality. This is sometimes referred to as the **total** depth-of-field. This can be determined according to a number of criteria (*Experimental results*, this chapter). Some studies mentioned in this chapter used half the total depth-of-field and expressed values as $\pm\Delta L$ (e.g. Campbell, 1957). When referring to such studies in this chapter,

their numbers have been doubled. This is satisfactory where depth-of-field is measured in just one direction from a focus position, or where simple theory is used in which the depth-of-field is symmetrical about the position of focus.

The depth-of-field sets the precision to which refractive state, including the amplitude of accommodation, can be measured by subjective methods. It also determines the distance range for which a target can be seen clearly when using visual optical instruments, such as simple magnifiers, microscopes and telescopes. For example, the depth-of-field of a simple magnifier or microscope of magnification M can be given as a total distance Δl_{m} in object space. This distance is related to the depth-of-field of the eye ΔL by the approximate equation (Smith and Atchison, 1997)

$$\Delta l_{m} = \Delta L / (16M^2) \tag{19.1a}$$

As another example, the depth-of-field of a two-lens afocal telescope of magnification M can be given as a total vergence in object space ΔL_{t}, and this is related to the depth-of-field of the eye ΔL by

$$\Delta L_{t} = \Delta L / M^2 \tag{19.1b}$$

Increasing the depth-of-field is advantageous in some circumstances. For example, the age-related reduction in amplitude of accommodation can be ameliorated by increasing depth-of-field. One way to do this is to introduce additional aberrations. This approach has been used with contact lenses for presbyopes but, unfortunately, this reduces peak visual performance (Bradley *et al.*, 1993; Plakitsi and Charman, 1995).

Depth-of-field depends upon several factors, including the following:

1. Optical properties of the eye
     pupil diameter (interacts with the other optical properties)
     accommodation level
     monochromatic and chromatic aberrations
     diffraction.
2. Retinal and visual processing properties
     photoreceptor size and ganglion cell density
     visual acuity and contrast thresholds
     disease in ocular pathway.
3. Target properties
     luminance
     spatial detail
     contrast
     spectral profile, e.g. colour.

Depth-of-field in the eye can be explained at a simple level using the defocus blur disc model of defocused systems (Chapter 9) and the size of the detector elements in the image plane. In an aberration and diffraction-free system, the image of a defocused point is a defocus blur disc. If this disc is smaller than a detector element, the system will not be able to detect defocus. Defocus will be detectable only once the defocus blur disc overlaps at least two detectors. Because this model neglects aberrations, diffraction and how the visual system processes retinal images (e.g. interactions between adjacent receptors), it is a crude model and cannot be expected to predict accurately the depth-of-field of the eye.

In the following sections we look at experimentally determined values, and consider models, such as the above defocus blur disc model, that can be used to predict depth-of-field.

Experimental results

There are several criteria for measuring depth-of-field according to a focusing error range that do not cause an 'objectionable deterioration in retinal image quality'. Six of these are considered here. Because these criteria

may depend upon different optical, neural and psychological factors, it is not always meaningful to try to compare depth-of-field results based on different criteria. The common feature of experimental results according to most criteria is that depth-of-field decreases as pupil size increases, at least out to 5–6 mm pupil diameters.

Criterion 1: the range of focusing errors for which no perceptible blur of a target is noticeable

This criterion is relevant to subjective refraction and determining the amplitude of accommodation. The vergence of the target is varied, and the extremes at which the target first appears to be blurred are measured. The

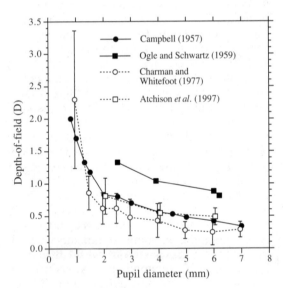

Figure 19.1. Depth-of-field as a function of pupil size. Details of studies are as follows:

Campbell (1957): threshold blur, retinal illuminance constant (corresponding to 318 cd/m² at 1 mm pupil diameter), one subject.

Ogle and Schwartz (1959): 50 per cent probability limits of correctly resolving checkerboard with equivalent letter size 6/7.5, subject JTS.

Charman and Whitefoot (1977): limits of depth-of-field give 95 per cent correct identification of the direction of movement of laser speckle, mean of six subjects, error bars indicate ±1 standard deviation of subjects.

Atchison *et al.* (1997): threshold blur, 6/7.5 letter E, mean of five subjects, error bars indicate ±1 standard deviation of subjects.

details of presentation can vary. The target can be moved backwards and forwards to locate the range within which it appears to be in focus (Campbell, 1957; Atchison *et al.*, 1997). Two targets may be presented, either in succession or simultaneously side-by-side, one in focus and the other with various levels of defocus, and the subject is asked to decide which is not in focus (Jacobs *et al.*, 1989).

Studies using this criterion show that the depth-of-field decreases with increase in pupil diameter (Campbell, 1957; Atchison *et al.*, 1997) (Figure 19.1), increasing target luminance and correction of longitudinal chromatic aberration of the eye (Campbell, 1957). As an example of the dependence on pupil size, in Campbell's study the depth-of-field decreases from 1.7 D to 0.3 D between the pupil diameters of 1 mm and 7 mm (Figure 19.1). Depth-of-field is smallest for target sizes near the visual acuity limit, and increases slowly with increase in target size (Jacobs *et al.*, 1989; Atchison *et al.*, 1997) (Figure 19.2). Jacobs and colleagues (1989) measured the threshold of just detectable change in defocus of an already defocused target and found that the threshold was slightly less than the depth-of-field.

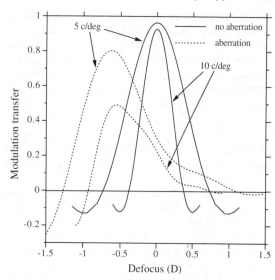

Figure 19.3. Theoretical modulation transfer as a function of defocus at 5 and 10 c/deg when there is 0D or +1.0 D of primary spherical aberration at the edge of a 6 mm diameter pupil in 605 nm wavelength light. Results are shown without Stiles–Crawford apodization. Data of Figures 5 and 6 of Atchison *et al.* (1998), with permission from The Optical Society of America.

Criterion 2: the range of focusing errors for which the visual acuity or contrast sensitivity does not decrease below a particular level or by more than a certain amount

This criterion has two aspects, which can be explained with reference to Figure 19.3. This figure shows theoretical 'through-focus' modulation transfer as a function of two levels of spherical aberration for spatial frequencies of 5 and 10 c/deg. Considering just the 10 c/deg plots and adopting an absolute level of depth-of-field as that for which modulation transfer values are greater than 0.5, the no-aberration condition has a depth-of-field of 0.4 D. However, the aberration condition has a depth-of-focus of 0 D because its modulation transfer is always less than 0.5. If the modulation transfer requirement is lowered to 0.3, the aberration condition has greater depth-of-field (0.7 D) than does the no-aberration condition (0.5 D).

If we adopt either a relative loss in modulation transfer or a particular proportional loss in modulation transfer, relative to the

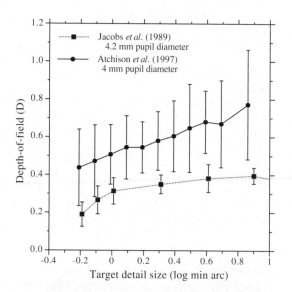

Figure 19.2. Depth-of-field as a function of target size. Jacobs *et al.* (1989) measured the depth-of-field in only one direction from the optimum focus, and their results have been doubled so that they are comparable with those of Atchison *et al.* (1997).

peak value, the no-aberration condition always has smaller depth-of-field than the aberration condition (considering only the defocus region within which the modulation transfers first fall to zero). This is because the rate of loss with modulation transfer away from the peak value is always slower for the former than for the latter condition. This aspect of criterion 2 has been used in some studies comparing the depths-of-field for different bifocal contact lenses, e.g. Plakitsi and Charman (1995).

A couple of studies are now mentioned which use the first aspect of criterion 2. Ogle and Schwartz (1959) determined the defocus providing 50 per cent and 99 per cent probability levels for correct recognition of checkerboard patterns of various sizes. As expected, depth-of-field was larger for the 50 per cent level. The depth-of-field decreased with increase in pupil size (Figure 19.1) and with decrease in target size. Tucker and Charman (1975) found similar results with letter targets.

Tucker and Charman (1986) estimated depth-of-field using the visibility of sinusoidal modulated (80 per cent) luminance targets as the criterion. As spatial frequency increased, the depth-of-field decreased. For example, at a 10 cd/m^2 luminance level, the depth-of-field was zero for 30 c/deg, 1 D at 20 c/deg, and 5 D for 10 c/deg. Increasing target luminance from 0.001 to 10 cd/m^2 increased depth-of-field. Tucker and Charman found little difference in depth-of-field between 3 mm and 7 mm pupil diameters.

Criterion 3: the range of focusing errors for which changes in contrast are not detected for a target in longitudinal sinusoidal motion

The subject views a target through a Badal optical system. The target is usually periodic – i.e. the luminance profile is generally that of a sine wave or square wave. As measured as an image vergence at the eye, the target is moved forwards and backwards in sinusoidal motion. The peak-to-peak amplitude of the movement is varied until the subject can detect apparent variation in the target's contrast (for non-periodic targets some other

criterion can be used, such as the appearance of blur or changes in target shape).

Similar to the results of Jacobs *et al.* (1989) with criterion 1, the depth-of-field is a minimum when the centre of the range is slightly off-set to one side of the optimal focus (Campbell and Westheimer, 1958; Walsh and Charman, 1988). Typically, the depth-of-field at optimal focus is 0.6 D, while the minimum depth-of-field is approximately 0.2 D (Walsh and Charman, 1988). The effect of increasing pupil size is to decrease the difference between the optimum focus and the centre of the range at which the minimum depth-of-field occurs. Walsh and Charman investigated a range of variables, including target colour, luminance and temporal frequency.

Criterion 4: the range of focusing errors for which a laser speckle pattern appears to be stationary

The laser speckle method for measuring refractive errors was described in Chapter 8. Briefly, a subject views a speckle pattern produced by a laser beam reflected diffusely from a moving surface such as a rotating drum. The speckle pattern appears to move at increasing velocity as the refractive error relative to the surface increases. This technique can be adapted to depth-of-field measurement by determining the focus range over which the subject cannot reliably distinguish the pattern's direction of movement.

Results with this technique show that pupil size has a strong effect on depth-of-field (Ronchi and Fontana, 1975; Charman and Whitefoot, 1977). Charman and Whitefoot (1977) found that depth-of-field decreased with increase in pupil size up to about 5 mm diameter; their values are slightly smaller than Campbell (1957) using criterion 1 for nearly all pupil sizes (Figure 19.1).

Criterion 5: the range of focusing errors for which the accommodation response does not change

Accommodation response can occur for target movements as small as 0.1 D (Ludlum *et al.*,

1968), even if this produces no perceptible blur (Kotulak and Schor, 1986).

Criterion 6: the range of focusing errors which degrades retinal image quality below a particular level or by more than a certain amount

The retinal image quality referred to here may be measured by the point spread function, line spread function or modulation transfer function, or by their derivations, such as half-width of the point spread function (see Chapter 18). The modulation transfer function is closely related to the contrast sensitivity function mentioned with criterion 2, and we used the modulation transfer function to explain two aspects of criterion 2.

Using the double-pass point spread function technique, Artal *et al.* (1995) determined through-focus modulation transfer at 2.6 c/deg in patients with monofocal and multifocal intraocular lenses. Marcos *et al.* (1999) used the criterion of a quantity, similar to the peak of the double-pass intensity point spread function, decreasing to 80 per cent of its value at optimum focus. They found that rather than decreasing, the average depth-of-field for three subjects increased slightly (although non-significantly) for increase in pupil diameter from 4 mm to 6 mm.

Modelling depth-of-field

Various models will be discussed here that can be used in understanding the factors that affect depth-of-field, by examining the optics of defocused images using two image quality criteria at various levels of complexity.

Criterion 1: The range of focusing errors for which no perceptible blur of a target is noticeable

The threshold of blur can be modelled by examining the image of a defocused point source of light and making assumptions about the threshold of defocus. We will begin by considering the simplest of models, assuming

that the system is aberration- and diffraction-free and, therefore, a point is imaged as a point. When this point is defocused, its image is a uniformly illuminated blur disc as already referred to in the previous section.

In Chapter 9, equation (9.17), the angular diameter Φ of the defocus blur disc was given as

$$\Phi = D \, \Delta L \qquad (19.2)$$

where D is pupil diameter and ΔL is refractive error. Using (total) depth-of-field to replace the refractive error, this equation becomes

$$\Phi = D \, \Delta L / 2 \qquad (19.2a)$$

We will now assume that the depth-of-field is set by the range over which this defocus blur disc is smaller than a certain threshold diameter. If this diameter is Φ_{th}, the depth-of-field is

$$\Delta L = 2\Phi_{th}/D \qquad (19.3)$$

This equation predicts that the depth-of-field is inversely proportional to the pupil diameter.

The smallest meaningful estimate of Φ_{th} is obtained using the diameter of a foveal cone, which is approximately 0.003 mm (Polyak, 1941). At the back nodal point, a distance of 0.003 mm subtends an angular diameter of

$$\approx 0.003/17 \approx 0.000176 \text{ rad } (\approx 0.61 \text{ min. arc})$$

where 17 mm is the approximate distance from the back nodal point to the retina. Substituting this value for Φ_{th} in equation (19.3) gives the threshold of defocus as

$$\Delta L = 0.000352/D \qquad (19.3a)$$

If we use a pupil diameter of 3 mm, i.e. $D = 0.003$ m, this equation gives a depth-of-field of 0.116 D, which is much less than the experimental values given in the preceding section. Therefore, there are serious flaws in this model.

Effect of diffraction and aberrations

Because of diffraction and aberrations, the focused image of a point is not a point but a patch of light – the point spread function as discussed in Chapter 18. The size of this patch depends upon the pupil diameter, since both diffraction and aberrations depend upon the size of the pupil.

In the presence of diffraction and aberrations, the point spread function is much more complex than a uniform disc (see Chapter 18), and this complexity presents problems in measuring its diameter. In such cases, the diameter or width is often represented by its half-width, which is the width at which the light level drops to half the central or maximum value. In-focus point spread functions have half-widths of about 2–3 minutes of arc.

We will now adopt the defocus, which would produce a blur disc equal to the half width of the in-focus point spread function, for our blur detection model. Any defocus with a blur disc less than this size can be expected to have little chance of being detected. Taking the threshold of blur disc size Φ_{th} as 2 min. arc (i.e. 0.000582 rad), we put $\Phi_{th} = 0.000582$ in equation (19.3) to obtain

$$\Delta L = 0.00116/D \qquad (19.3b)$$

For a pupil diameter of 3 mm this equation gives a depth-of-field value of 0.38 D, which is much closer to experimental values (Figure 19.1).

Influence of diffraction alone at small pupil diameters

At small pupil diameters, e.g. 2 mm, the threshold value Φ_{th} is governed by diffraction and not by aberrations. Diffraction theory predicts that the width of the point spread function is proportional to wavelength and inversely proportional to pupil diameter (equation (18.5)). Thus, on assuming that Φ_{th} follows the same trend, equation (19.3) becomes

$$\Delta L \propto \lambda/D^2 \qquad (19.4)$$

This equation predicts that, for small pupil sizes, the depth-of-field is inversely proportional to the square of pupil diameter.

Influence of aberrations alone at large pupil diameters

As pupil diameter increases, the effects of diffraction become less and the influence of aberrations increases. For larger pupil diameters, the point spread function can be regarded as being affected by aberrations alone.

As aberrations usually increase with pupil diameter, the size of the focused point spread function is expected to increase with pupil diameter, and the threshold diameter Φ_{th} of the defocus blur disc is expected to increase. In the presence of primary spherical aberration, the transverse aberration at the edge of the pupil is proportional to the cube of the pupil diameter. Therefore, we could expect that Φ_{th} would show some higher order dependence on pupil diameter. For large pupil sizes, from equation (19.3), it is expected that depth-of-field increases with increase in pupil diameter. However, from the results of Figure 19.1, this does not happen out to at least 5–6 mm in diameter. This may be because the aberrations of the eye are too low to have a large effect, or because the aberrations are too irregular. The Stiles–Crawford effect (Chapter 13) may play a small role here by reducing the effect of aberrations and defocus at larger pupil sizes.

More complex objects

We have so far examined the effect of defocus only on the image of a point object. This is not realistic, since few scenes are composed of point sources. On the other hand, edges are very common, and we will consider a sharp luminous edge of high contrast. Using the defocus blur disc model, a luminance profile slope forms at the edge, and the width of this edge is equal to the width of the corresponding defocus blur disc. The threshold for defocus will depend in some complex manner on the width of the image edge and on the image's contrast.

Now suppose that the edge is the edge of a bar of a finite width (e.g. in a letter). The defocus now has two phases. In the first phase (low levels of defocus), only the edge of the image is affected. The second phase begins once the defocus reaches the level when the two sloping edges (on either side of the bar) of the image meet in the centre. Once this occurs, the contrast of the bar is reduced. The narrower the bar, the sooner this second phase occurs. Depending upon how the visual system detects defocus, it may be more sensitive to this reduction in image contrast than on the profile of the image's edge.

These considerations suggest that depth-of-field depends on target size. Atchison *et al.*

CRITERION

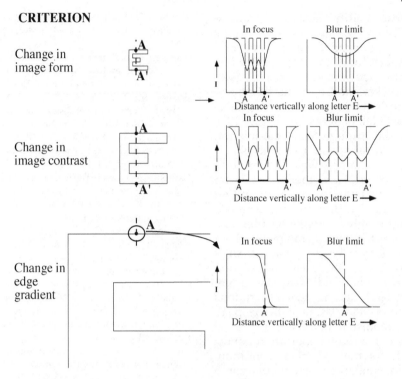

Figure 19.4. A model of a person's determination of what is perceptible blur of a letter. For a small letter (top), the low spatial frequency information in the letter is used; for an intermediate-sized letter (middle), the contrast between light and dark bars in the image is used; for a large letter (bottom), the luminance slope at the image's edges is used.

(1997) developed a model to describe how the visual system might change its criterion of what is perceptible blur, according to the size of letter targets (Figure 19.4). According to this model, for very small letter sizes (e.g. < 0.0 log min. arc of target detail), the perception of blur is based on low spatial frequency information in the letters. This low spatial frequency information affects mainly the overall contrast of the retinal image of the letter against its background. As letter size increases, the fundamental spatial frequency of the pattern moves into the spatial frequency range at which modulation transfer is very sensitive to defocus, and thus the contrast between dark and light bars of an image is important. For even larger letter sizes (e.g. > 1.0 log min. arc of target detail), the spatial frequency of the fundamental is so low that its modulation transfer is relatively unaffected by defocus. However, higher order harmonics in the letter will be at spatial frequencies whose modulation transfer is affected by defocus. These are important to the detection of edges, so the perception of blur may be now based on edge sharpness rather than bar contrast.

Criterion 6: the range of focusing errors which degrades retinal image quality below a particular level or by more than a certain amount

The point spread function, line spread function and the modulation transfer function were discussed in Chapter 18. Using the modulation transfer function image quality criterion, we can investigate the effect of small levels of defocus on the contrast of sinusoidal patterns as a function of spatial frequency. This is a much more advanced approach than the simple defocus blur disc model, since it can readily take into account aberrations (including chromatic), diffraction and the Stiles–Crawford effect. Furthermore, with a knowledge of the retinal contrast sensitivity function we can readily calculate the threshold of visibility of sinusoidal patterns (criterion 2) as a function of defocus and spatial frequency, and the results can be compared with experimental measures (see, for example, Tucker and Charman, 1986).

As an example, we consider the depth-of-field for sinusoidal patterns in Figure 19.3, where theoretical through-focus modulation transfer is shown for spatial frequencies of 5 and 10 c/deg (this example was introduced in the previous section). Here, there is either no aberration or 1 D primary spherical aberration at the edge of a 6 mm diameter pupil in 605 nm wavelength light. If we consider the depth-of-focus as the defocus range for which the modulation transfer is greater than a certain proportion of the peak modulation transfer for a set of conditions, the figure shows the general finding that aberrations increase depth-of-field. Using half the peak value as this proportion, depths-of-field at 10 c/deg are 0.4 D for the no-aberration condition and 0.8 D for the aberration condition, respectively. A similar pattern occurs for 5 c/deg to that for 10 c/deg. The Stiles–Crawford effect increases these ranges slightly for most spatial frequencies (Figure 19.4). We note, however, that using experimentally-determined wave aberrations and a criterion based on the point spread function, Marcos *et al.* (1999) calculated that the Stiles–Crawford function decreased depth-of-field at 6 mm by 3 per cent and 7 per cent in two subjects.

Summary of main symbols

D pupil diameter
ΔL (Total) depth-of-field
Φ angular diameter of defocus blur disc
Φ_{th} detection threshold value of Φ

References

Artal, P., Marcos, S., Navarro, R. *et al.* (1995). Through-focus image quality of eyes implanted with monofocal and multifocal intraocular lenses. *Opt. Eng.*, **34**, 772–8.

Atchison, D. A., Charman, W. N. and Woods, R. L. (1997). Subjective depth-of-focus of the eye. *Optom. Vis. Sci.*, **74**, 511–20.

Atchison, D. A., Smith, G. and Joblin, A. (1998). Influence of Stiles–Crawford apodization on spatial visual performance. *J. Opt. Soc. Am. A*, **15**, 2545–51.

Bradley, A., Rahman, H. A., Soni, P. S. and Zhang, X. (1993). Effects of target distance and pupil size on letter contrast sensitivity with simultaneous vision bifocal contact lenses. *Optom. Vis. Sci.*, **70**, 476–81.

Campbell, F. W. (1957). The depth of field of the human eye. *Optica Acta*, **4**, 157–64.

Campbell, F. W. and Westheimer, G. (1958). Sensitivity of the eye to differences in focus. *J. Physiol.*, **143**, 18.

Charman, W. N. and Whitefoot, H. (1977). Pupil diameter and the depth-of-field of the human eye as measured by laser speckle. *Optica Acta*, **24**, 1211–16.

Jacobs, R. J., Smith, G. and Chan, C. D. C. (1989). Effect of defocus on blur thresholds and on thresholds of perceived change in blur: comparison of source and observer methods. *Optom. Vis. Sci.*, **66**, 545–53.

Kotulak, J. C. and Schor, C. M. (1986). The accommodative response to subthreshold blur and to perceptual fading during the Troxler phenomenon. *Perception*, **15**, 7–15.

Ludlum, W. M., Wittenberg, S., Giglio, E. J. and Rosenberg, R. (1968). Accommodative responses to small changes in dioptric stimulus. *Am. J. Optom. Arch. Am. Acad. Optom.*, **45**, 483–506.

Marcos S., Moreno, E. and Navarro, R. (1999). The depth-of-field of the human eye with polychromatic light from objective and subjective measurements. *Vision Res.*, **39**, 2039–49.

Ogle, K. N. and Schwartz, T. J. (1959). Depth of focus of the human eye. *J. Opt. Soc. Am.*, **49**, 273–80.

Plakitsi, A. and Charman, W. N. (1995). Comparison of the depths of focus with the naked eye and with three types of presbyopic contact lens correction. *J. Br. Cont. Lens Assoc.*, **18**, 119–25.

Polyak, S. L. (1941). *The Retina*. University of Chicago Press.

Ronchi, L. and Fontana, A. (1975). Laser speckles and the depth-of-field of the human eye. *Optica Acta*, **22**, 243–6.

Smith, G. and Atchison, D. A. (1997). *The Eye and Visual Optical Instruments*, pp. 703–4. Cambridge University Press.

Tucker, J. and Charman, W. N. (1975). The depth-of-focus of the human eye for Snellen letters. *Am. J. Optom. Physiol. Opt.*, **52**, 3–21.

Tucker, J. and Charman, W. N. (1986). Depth of focus and accommodation for sinusoidal gratings as a function of luminance. *Am. J. Optom. Physiol. Opt.*, **63**, 58–70.

Walsh, G. and Charman, W. N. (1988). Visual sensitivity to temporal change in focus and its relevance to the accommodation response. *Vision Res.*, **28**, 1207–21.

20

The aging eye

Introduction

Age-related optical changes in the eye were mentioned briefly in earlier chapters, but here we will give a fuller account, with emphasis on changes occurring in the adult eye. Many of these changes produce progressive reduction in visual performance. A number of changes in the optical properties may be regarded as pathological, e.g. cataract, but these will not be considered here. Neural properties also change with age, but these are beyond the scope of this book. For those particularly interested in the subject of the aging eye, we recommend two books by Weale (1982 and 1992).

Cornea

With increasing age, there is decreased spacing between collagen fibrils of the stroma, some fibre degeneration, and increases in the cross-sectional area of collagen fibres (Kanai and Kaufman, 1973; Malik et al., 1992). Descemet's membrane increases in thickness with age (Cogan and Kuwabara, 1971). Possibly the most important age-related change is endothelial degeneration. The size of endothelial cells becomes more variable (**polymegathism**), because some cells either increase in size or fuse (Daus and Völcker, 1987). Eventually endothelial function may be impaired, and then aqueous humour may

seep into the cornea, disrupting the structural order and increasing light scatter (Pierscionek, 1996).

Corneal thickness

There is no clear trend of thickness changes with increasing age. Findings include no change (Kruse Hansen, 1971; Olsen, 1982; Siu and Herse, 1993), increase (Koretz et al., 1989), and slow decrease (Alsbirk, 1978; Olsen and Ehlers, 1984).

Corneal shape

In young eyes the curvature of the anterior surface is usually greater in the vertical meridian than that in the horizontal meridian, but this tends to reverse with increase in age (Phillips, 1952; Lyle, 1971; Anstice, 1971; Baldwin and Mills, 1981; Kame et al., 1993; Goh and Lam, 1994; Lam et al., 1994). Kiely et al. (1984) and Hayashi et al. (1995) found that the cornea becomes more curved with age, but more so in the horizontal meridian than in the vertical meridian.

The aberrations due to the cornea seem to increase with age, and this is due to the coma-like aberration contribution rather than spherical aberration-like contribution (Oshika et al., 1999).

Transmittance

Most studies of corneal transmittance have found that there is no significant variation with age (Boettner and Wolter, 1962; Beems and van Best, 1990; van den Berg and Tan, 1994). However, Boettner and Wolter found a decrease in the direct (non-scattered) light with increased age.

Lens

The most dramatic age-related optical changes in the eye occur in the lens. Its shape, size and mass alter markedly, its ability to vary its shape (i.e. accommodation) diminishes, and its light transmission reduces considerably, particularly at short wavelengths.

Lenticular transmittance, scatter and fluorescence

The transmittances of both ultraviolet and visible wavelengths decrease with increase in age, with the lens becoming more yellow, particularly in the nucleus (Said and Weale, 1959; Boettner and Wolter, 1962; Mellerio, 1971 and 1987; Pokorny et al., 1987; Sample et al., 1988). There is an increase in both forward and backward scattered light with age, particularly after the age of 40 years (Bena-Sira et al., 1980; IJspeert et al., 1990; Fujisawa and Sasaki, 1995). There is increased fluorescence with increase in age (Hockwin et al., 1984).

Thickness

The lens increases in volume and mass throughout life, with most of this being due to increase in axial thickness of the cortex (Brown, 1973a; Niesel, 1982; Cook et al., 1994). Koretz et al. (1989) found an increase in axial thickness of 13 μm per year. The anterior chamber depth decreases throughout life approximately at the same rate as the lens axial thickness increases (Koretz et al., 1989). Brown (1973a) and Weekers et al. (1973), but not Koretz et al. (1989), found a small decrease in vitreous chamber depth with increase in age.

Shape

Brown (1974) found a linear reduction in the central anterior lens radius of curvature of emmetropic, unaccommodated eyes with increase in age. This changed from 16.0 mm at 8 years to 8.3 mm at 82 years of age. Changes in radius of the posterior surface with increase in age were less marked, decreasing from approximately 8.6 mm at 8 years to 7.5 mm at 82 years. Cook et al. (1991) obtained similar results.

As age increases, the maximum possible changes in lens shape decline (Koretz et al., 1997), reflecting the decrease in amplitude of accommodation with age.

Magnetic resonance imaging shows no change in unaccommodated lens diameter, but increase in accommodated lens diameter, with age (Strenk et al., 1999).

Refractive index distribution

Models for the refractive index distribution of the lens were discussed in Chapters 2 and 16. Based on the increasing thickness and surface curvatures of the lens with age, it would be expected that eyes should become more myopic. However, the general shift is in the other direction, with Saunders (1986a) finding a mean hypermetropic shift of 2 D between the ages of 30 and 60 years (Figure 20.1). This is the 'lens paradox', and it is not known why this occurs. Grosvenor (1987) proposed that there is a decline in axial length during adult life, but another possibility is a change in the refractive index distribution of the lens. This could be by a reduced magnitude of refractive index variation across the lens as proposed by Koretz and Handelman (1988), or by a change in the refractive index pattern with increasing age (Pierscionek, 1990). The latter was modelled by Smith et al. (1992), with the gradient index profile becoming flatter near the middle of the lens and then increasing in steepness towards the edge (see *Schematic eyes*, this chapter), and there is some clinical support for this (Hemenger et al., 1995).

The zones in the lens seen with the slit-lamp, which become more obvious and greater in number with increasing age, are of considerable interest. Although several reasons for their appearance have been

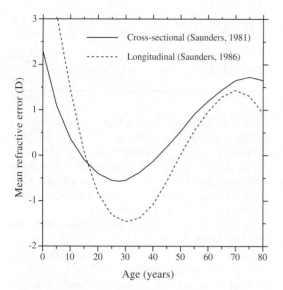

Figure 20.1. Change in mean refractive error with age. Cross-sectional data of Saunders (1981) and longitudinal data of Saunders (1986a). 'Cross-sectional' means that data are collected from each subject once, while 'longitudinal' means that each subject is followed over a period of time.

suggested, including refractive index discontinuities, the nature and origin of these is not yet known (Pierscionek and Weale, 1995).

Refractive errors and axial length

Refractive errors are relatively stable between the ages of 20 and 40 years (Grosvenor, 1991), after which there is a shift in the hypermetropic direction (Saunders, 1986a) (Figure 20.1). After the approximate age of 70 years, there is some shift of the mean refractive error in the myopic direction associated with the development of nuclear cataract (Brown and Hill, 1987). The distribution of refractive errors of a young adult population is steeper than a normal distribution (**leptokurtosis**). The distribution of refractive errors becomes more normal with increasing age, with increases in the proportions of both myopes and hypermetropes (Grosvenor, 1991).

Age-related changes in the corneal shape, discussed earlier in this chapter, are reflected in the astigmatism of the eye (e.g. Hirsch, 1959; Anstice, 1971; Saunders, 1981 and 1986b; Fledelius, 1984). Most measurable astigmatism is with-the-rule up to 40 years of age, after which the prevalence of against-the-rule astigmatism increases (Goss, 1998).

Grosvenor (1987) re-analyzed Sorsby and co-workers' (1957, 1962) data, and found that the mean axial length of emmetropic eyes decreased after the age of approximately 20 years, with a difference of 0.6 mm between a 20–29 years age group and a 50+ age group. He cited other studies with similar results. However, Koretz *et al.* (1989) did not find significant change in the axial length of emmetropes with age. Also, Ooi and Grosvenor (1995) did not find a significant difference between the axial lengths of young and old adult groups, in which the two groups were matched on the basis of sex and refractive error.

Accommodation and presbyopia

Accommodation is the ability of the eye to change its power to bring objects of interest at different distances into focus. As such, it makes an essential contribution to visual performance. Our understanding of its mechanism is based on Helmholtz's (1909) theory. In the unaccommodated form, with the focus of the eye at its far point, the zonules connecting the lens and ciliary body pull on the lens and flatten it. When changing focus from far to near vision, the ciliary muscle contracts, thus reducing the tension on the zonules. Because of the elastic properties of the capsule of the lens, the lens takes on a more rounded shape. Thus, both the lens and the eye increase in refractive power.

When the eye accommodates, the anterior surface moves forward and takes on a more hyperboloid form (Brown, 1973b). Axial thickness changes are confined to the nucleus (Brown, 1973b; Koretz *et al.*, 1997). The equatorial diameter of the overall lens and the nucleus are reduced (Brown, 1973b). Most of the curvature change occurs at the front surface, with Brown (1973b) obtaining changes in anterior and posterior radii of curvature of 12.8 mm to 7.7 mm and 7.1 mm to 6.5 mm, respectively, in the eye of a 19-year-old subject upon accommodation of 6 D. As age increases, the maximum possible change in lens movement declines (Koretz *et al.*, 1997).

Uncertainty still exists about the exact interaction between the zonules and the ciliary body (Atchison, 1995).

Presbyopia

The range or amplitude of accommodation reaches a peak early in life, then gradually declines. The decline in accommodation becomes a problem for most people in their forties, when they can no longer see clearly to perform near tasks. This condition is called presbyopia. The age at which this occurs for any particular person depends on the refractive error, nature of close work and, probably, on genetic and environmental factors. Accommodation is completely lost in the fifties, well before most other physiological functions are appreciably affected. However, as discussed below, most clinically related studies do not show this complete loss.

There have been many studies of the reduction in the amplitude of accommodation with age. Figure 20.2 shows the data of Ungerer (1986). The authors chose these results because they are for a large number of people (1285) who were not part of a clinical population. They were predominantly civil servants, mainly Anglo-Celtic, in the coastal Australian city of Melbourne (latitude 38°S).

Ungerer fitted an exponential function for the expected mean between the ages of 20 and 60 years of

$$amplitude \text{ (dioptres)} = \exp[1.93 + 0.0401 \, age - 0.00119 \, (age)^2]$$

(20.1)

This equation predicts mean amplitudes of accommodation of 9.5 D at 20 years, 3.7 D at 45 years, 2.6 D at 50 years and 1.0 D at 60 years. Using a 3.75 D amplitude of accommodation limit as the criterion for presbyopia, she found that only 2 per cent of those over 50 years were not presbyopic.

Studies such as Ungerer's overestimate the amplitude of accommodation due to depth-of-field effects. Figure 20.3 shows Hamasaki and co-workers' (1956) results for subjects between the ages of 42 and 60 years, using a stigmatoscopic method and the conventional clinical push-up method. Linear fits are shown also for Sun and co-workers' (1988) results for subjects between the ages of 13 and 46 years using the stigmatoscopic method and the push-up method. The stigmatoscopic method, designed to eliminate depth-of-field effects, reduced the estimate of amplitude by approximately 2 D across the range of ages. Studies such as those carried out by Hamasaki *et al.* and Sun *et al.* also indicate that accom-

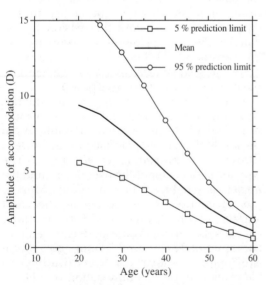

Figure 20.2. Amplitude of accommodation with age. Results of Ungerer (1986).

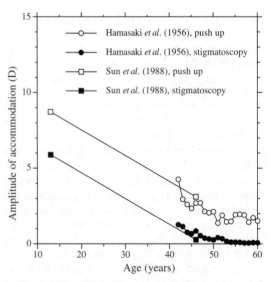

Figure 20.3. Amplitude of accommodation with age. Results of Hamasaki *et al.* (1956) and Sun and co-workers' (1988) data fit.

modation does not occur beyond the early 50s.

Cross-sectional studies mask the age-related decline in amplitude of individual subjects. They show a non-linear trend in the mean amplitude with age, but with the rate of decline decreasing as presbyopia is approached (Figure 20.2). Two small-scale longitudinal studies (Hofstetter, 1965; Ramsdale and Charman, 1989) found that individual subjects have a linear decrease of accommodation with age. The non-linear trend in cross-sectional studies is probably due to artefacts introduced by the averaging process (Charman, 1989). At any age beyond that at which some individuals no longer accommodate, the distribution of amplitudes is truncated, because these individuals cannot contribute negative values to it.

The rate of amplitude decline varies considerably, and may be affected by several factors. The rate of progression of presbyopia is faster the closer people live to the equator, and faster for people living at low altitudes than at higher altitudes. These findings indicate that ambient temperature may affect the progression of presbyopia (Miranda, 1979; Weale, 1981).

Presbyopia theories

Current theories of the development of presbyopia can be categorized as follows (Atchison, 1995):

1. Lenticular theories
   a. Mechanical changes in lens and capsule
      i. Hess-Gullstrand theory
      ii. Fincham theory
   b. Geometric theory.
2. Extra-lenticular theories
   a. Changes in ciliary muscle – Duane theory
   b. Changes in elastic components of zonule and/or ciliary body.

The development of presbyopia is generally regarded as originating in the 'plant' of the accommodative system, either within the lens and its capsule or within their support structures. Because the optical parameters of the eye are involved in several of these theories, they are discussed briefly below. For a more extensive coverage and full reference details, see Atchison (1995).

Lenticular theories

Mechanical changes in lens and capsule

The lens is purported to become more rigid with age and to be increasingly resistant to the elastic forces of the capsule upon it. Ronald Fisher's *in vitro* measurements of the mechanics of the various parts of the accommodative 'plant' provide evidence for this group of theories: the ciliary muscle does not lose its power with age; the lens behaves as a simple elastic body, which requires more energy to deform it with increasing age; and the capsule's elasticity declines so that it is less able to provide this deforming energy.

Hess–Gullstrand theory

The amount of muscle contraction required for a given change in accommodation is purported to remain constant throughout life (Hess, 1904 (cited by Alpern, 1962); Gullstrand, 1909). This theory predicts that an increasing proportion of ciliary muscle contraction will be 'latent', i.e. it does not affect accommodative status. This theory is distinct from all other theories of presbyopia, which predict that the maximum possible amount of ciliary muscle contraction is required to produce maximum accommodation at any age.

The Hess–Gullstrand theory would be supported by evidence that the ciliary muscle increases its contraction at accommodation stimulus levels beyond those which produce the maximal accommodation response, but this evidence is limited. Some studies have found electrical changes in the region of the equator of the eyeball for stimuli beyond those producing the maximal response, but whether this indicates ciliary muscle activity has been disputed.

The Hess–Gullstrand theory predicts that zonule slackness should be more apparent in older subjects trying to accommodate beyond the amplitude limit, but the reverse has been noted in monkeys without irises. Similarly, the predicted increased zonule slackness upon accommodation in older subjects should allow the lens to be more influenced by gravity for older rather than younger subjects, and again the reverse seems to occur.

Fincham theory

According to the mechanical change theories,

the lens becomes more resistant to change in shape with age. Fincham (1937) believed that greater pressure from the capsule, necessary with increase in age to achieve a given level of accommodation, can only be achieved by further releasing the zonular tension on the capsule. This means that the changes responsible for the decline in accommodation reside in the lens and capsule, but ciliary muscle contraction required for a given change in accommodation increases throughout life.

This theory is supported by studies of the effect of age and drugs on the accommodation–convergence synkinesis. For example, the response AC/A ratio (amount of convergence induced by 1 D change in accommodation response) increases with age, as predicted if increasing innervation to the ciliary muscle is required to produce a unit change in accommodation response as age increase. By contrast, the Hess–Gullstrand theory predicts that this ratio should be unaffected by age. The evidence supporting the Fincham theory, at the expense of the Hess–Gullstrand theory, also supports the following theories.

Geometric theory

This attributes the decline in amplitude with age mainly to increased size and curvature of the lens (see *Lens*, this chapter). Koretz and Handelmann (1986 and 1988) suggested that the increasing curvature and the likely change in orientation of the zonules due to shifting zonule insertions means that zonules apply tension less radially to the capsule's surface. This means that, upon ciliary muscle contraction, the zonule relaxation may have smaller effects on the lens shape.

Schachar (1992) developed a variation of the geometric theory. He rejected the Helmholtzian explanation for accommodation, believing instead that the ciliary body moves away from the lens upon increased accommodation, so that zonular tension increases and the lens becomes spindle-shaped. Increasing lens diameter with age will restrict the ability of the zonules to provide this tension. Schachar has published a number of experimental and theoretical papers claiming to support his theory. The experiments of Fisher (1977) and Glaser and Campbell (1998), which showed that stretch-ing human lenses decreases the power rather than increasing it, would seem to provide overwhelming evidence against Schachar's theory.

Extra-lenticular theories

These theories attribute accommodation amplitude decline either to weakening of the ciliary muscle or to loss of elasticity of zonules or ciliary body components. Workers using the rhesus monkey as an animal model for human accommodation found that electrically stimulating the mid-brain region that influences accommodation produced axial thickening of the lens, narrowing of the ciliary ring, and zonule slackening at high amplitudes. As the monkeys' age increased, these findings were less noticeable. Lenticular theories do not predict the decline in the narrowing of the ciliary ring.

Changes in ciliary muscle – Duane theory

Duane (1922 and 1925) believed that the ciliary muscle weakens with increased age. However, Fisher (1977) found that the strength of muscle contraction should decline only slightly before 45–50 years of age, and anatomical studies of the ciliary muscle and surrounding tissue suggest that its possible movement should not decrease markedly with increase in age.

Changes in elastic components of zonules and/or ciliary body

Bito and Miranda (1989) claimed that presbyopia is a loss of the ability to relax accommodation, rather than loss of the ability to increase accommodation, which is opposite to the usual way in which presbyopia is considered. This occurs through deterioration of elastic components in the ciliary body and choroid. As age increases, the lens takes up a more curved shape under its elastic forces, even when ciliary muscle contraction does not occur, because the elastic antagonists of the ciliary muscle in the ciliary body and choroid are not doing their work. The theory ignores changes in lens and capsule elasticity.

Some anatomical studies have found age-related changes in the attachments to the ciliary muscle. As discussed earlier in this chapter, the lens certainly does become more curved with increasing age.

Summary

Presbyopia possibly has more than one cause – for example, changes in capsule and lenticular elasticity combined with changes in lens geometry. There is considerable evidence against the Hess–Gullstrand theory, and it is unlikely that changes in ciliary muscle contractility contribute significantly to presbyopia. A lenticular origin of presbyopia according to the Fincham theory seems most likely, with recent experiments indicating that it is possible to restore a measure of accommodation by an intraocular lens, which can be moved or adjusted in shape within the lens capsule under the influence of the ciliary body (Koprowski, 1995; Cumming and Kamman, 1996). Glasser and Campbell (1998) have confirmed Fisher's (1977) finding that, with increasing age, the ability to change *in vitro* lens power by stretching will decrease at a rate which is similar to the decrease in amplitude of accommodation. Although the forces acting on the *in vitro* lenses are not necessarily the same as those occurring in the eye, this evidence tends to discount the need for an extralenticular role in presbyopia.

Pupil diameter

Pupil size decreases with increased age (Birren *et al.*, 1950; Kumnick, 1954; Kadlecova *et al.*, 1958; Leinhos, 1959; Said and Sawires, 1972; Winn *et al.*, 1994) (Figure 20.4). This is referred to as **senile miosis**. In addition, the speed and extent of pupillary reactions decrease with increase in age (e.g. Kumnick, 1954). The maximum pupil size in dark-adapted eyes is reached in the teenage years, after which it declines (Kadlecova *et al.*, 1958; Said and Sawires, 1972). For example, Kadlecova *et al.* (1958) found maximum diameters ranging from about 7.5 mm at 10 years of age to about 5 mm at 80 years of age. As age increases, the variation in pupil diameter with change in luminance decreases (Figure 20.4).

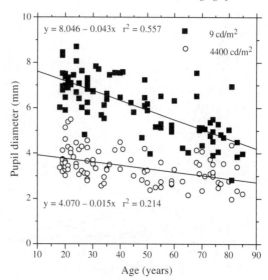

Figure 20.4. Effect of age on pupil size. Ninety-one subjects viewed a 10° field monocularly in Maxwellian view with relaxed accommodation. Results, including regression equations, are shown for luminance levels of 9 cd/m^2 and 4400 cd/m^2. Data from Figures 2a and 2e of Winn *et al.* (1994), kindly provided by Barry Winn and with permission from the Association for Research in Vision and Ophthalmology.

Aberrations and retinal image quality

Jenkins (1963) used retinoscopy to investigate the direction of spherical aberration of 133 subjects between the ages of 2 and 60 years. He found that negative spherical aberration predominated before the age of 6 years, but after this age, a dramatic shift occurred to positive spherical aberration. He claimed that, after about 35 years of age, there was a considerable increase in positive spherical aberration. In support of increasing positive spherical aberration with increase in age, Chateau *et al.* (1998) found that optimum contrast sensitivity (at 12 c/deg) was produced with contact lenses which increased in negative asphericity as age increased.

Artal *et al.* (1993) and Guirao *et al.* (1999) determined modulation transfer functions (MTFs) from point spread functions for subjects in different age groups and found much poorer retinal image quality for the oldest group at any particular pupil size (Figure 20.5). Having corrected their results for scatter, Artal *et al.* attributed the

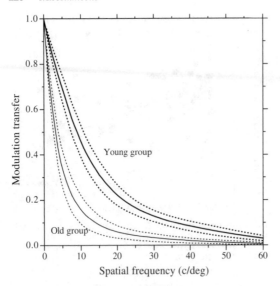

Figure 20.5. Modulation transfer functions (averaged in all meridians) for a young subject group (20–30 years of age) and for an old subject group (60–70 years of age) using 543 nm laser light and a 4 mm pupil. The dashed lines indicate 1 standard deviation from the mean. Data of Guirao *et al.* (1999) kindly provided by Pablo Artal and with permission from the Association for Research in Vision and Ophthalmology.

age-related decline to increase in aberrations. Using the aberroscope technique, Calver *et al.* (1999) found MTFs to be lower in an old (68 ± 5 years) than in a young age group (24 ± 3 years) at any particular pupil size, but senile miosis caused the older eyes to have the lower aberration levels at natural pupil sizes.

Some studies have found a decrease in longitudinal chromatic aberration with age (Millodot and Sivak, 1973; Millodot, 1976; Mordi and Adrian, 1985), but a majority of studies have found no change (Lau *et al.*, 1955; Ware, 1982; Pease and Cooper, 1986; Howarth *et al.*, 1988; Morrell *et al.*, 1991).

Photometry

Retinal illumination decreases with age due to two factors. One is the reduction of pupil diameter with age, particularly at low light levels. The other factor is the decrease in ocular transmittance with age (Chapter 12).

The data of Winn *et al.* (1994), shown in Figure 20.4, can be used to predict the effect of changing pupil size. At 9 cd/m² background luminance, the pupil diameter decreased approximately linearly with age from 20 years to 60 years by about 25 per cent. This corresponds to a light loss at the retina of more than 43 per cent at low light levels.

The decrease in ocular transmittance with age is due mainly to the lens, particularly for the shorter wavelengths (Figure 20.6). Said and Weale (1959) found that the lens transmittance decreases by about 25 per cent between the ages of 20 and 60 years (558 nm) (Figure 20.6).

Combining the pupil size and ocular transmittance changes with age given above indicates a reduction in light level reaching the retina, between the ages of 20 and 60 years, of approximately 60 per cent at lower light levels. This is similar to an earlier determination by Weale (1961).

Effect of light loss on visual performance

Spatial visual performance decreases with increase in age (Blackwell and Blackwell,

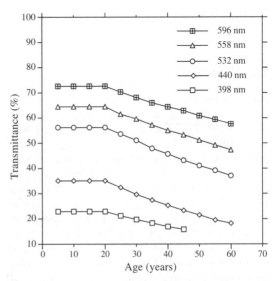

Figure 20.6. Variation in lens transmittance with age at different wavelengths. Data of Said and Weale (1959), after conversion from densities to transmittances. The technique was based on the relative brightnesses of the third and fourth Purkinje images.

1971; Richards, 1977; Owsley *et al.*, 1983; Elliot, 1987; Elliot *et al.*, 1993 and 1995; Haegerstrom-Portnoy *et al.*, 1999). This has both optical and neural causes (Elliot, 1987; Sloane *et al.*, 1988). The loss in performance is much more marked at low than at higher luminances (Weston, 1948; Guth, 1957; Blackwell and Blackwell, 1971; Richards, 1977; Sloane *et al.*, 1987), so that transmittance decreases at lower light levels can be compensated to a large extent by increasing the light level. An example of this is given by Guth (1957), concerning visibility of words. The greater loss in transmittance at the shorter wavelengths affects colour perception, reducing the ability to discriminate shades of greens and blues (Knoblauch *et al.*, 1987).

The decrease in transmittance has two contributions; absorption and backward scatter. Unlike these, increasing the light level cannot compensate for the forward scatter. Forward scatter produces a veiling glare over the retina, which reduces the contrast of the retinal image. Low-contrast objects may become invisible. This becomes worse at low ambient light levels when bright lights are in the field of view, e.g. on dark streets with streetlamps.

With increase in age, there is an increase in the amount of forward light scatter from the lens, so that K increases in the equivalent veiling luminance equation (13.15)

$$L_v(\theta) = KE/\theta^n \tag{20.2}$$

although the angular dependency remains similar (Fisher and Christie, 1965; IJspeert *et al.*, 1990). For example, Christie and Fisher found that K increased linearly with age, but that n was essentially independent of age. K increased by a factor of 1.9 to 3.3 in their experiments between the ages of 20 and 70 years.

Stiles–Crawford effect

Two longitudinal studies have shown that the β co-efficient (equation (13.29)) is relatively unaffected by age for healthy eyes (Rynders *et al.*, 1995; DeLint *et al.*, 1997).

Schematic eyes

The structures of paraxial and finite schematic eyes were discussed in Chapters 5 and 16, respectively, and the dimensions of many of these eyes are listed in Appendix 3. We found in the preceding section that many dimensions of the eye depend upon age, but designers of most schematic eyes gave no indication that a particular age was modelled. An exception is the finite eye of Liou and Brennan (1997), which contains ocular parameters for an eye near the age of 45 years. Also, Blaker (1991), Smith *et al.* (1992) and Smith and Pierscionek (1998) designed model eyes adapted for age. Rabbetts (1998) presented an 'elderly' version of the Bennett and Rabbetts' simplified eye. Any selection of parameters is complicated by other factors, such as sex and race. As examples, female eyes are shorter and hence have higher powers than male eyes (Koretz *et al.*, 1989), and there are many racial variations including pupil size (Said and Sawires, 1972) and refractive error distributions. A very sophisticated schematic eye would be adaptable for these effects.

We include a brief description of an age-dependent, relaxed, emmetropic, paraxial schematic eye based on Smith *et al.* (1992). Age-dependent parameters are shown in Table 20.1 for 20-, 40- and 60-year-old eyes. The eye has an equivalent power of 60 D at the age of 20 years.

Table 20.1. Age-dependent parameters in age-dependent schematic eye.

	Age (years)		
	20	40	60
Anterior chamber depth (mm)	3.38	3.12	2.86
Lens anterior radius of curvature (mm)	14.735	12.655	10.575
Lens posterior radius of curvature (mm)	–8.419	–8.119	–7.819
Lens thickness (mm)	3.72	3.98	4.24
Refractive index of lens	1.4506	1.4398	1.4280

Radii

Cornea

Some decrease in radius occurs with age, as discussed earlier in this chapter, but this is small, and the Gullstrand number one schematic eye values of 7.7 mm and 6.8 mm are used for the anterior and posterior surfaces, respectively.

Lens

The lens radii are taken from Brown's (1974) study:

$$R_1 \text{ (mm)} = 16.815 - 0.104 \times age \text{ (years)} \quad (20.3a)$$

$$R_2 \text{ (mm)} = -8.719 + 0.015 \times age \text{ (years)} \quad (20.3b)$$

Distances/thicknesses

Cornea

Because of the contradictory results of studies regarding this parameter, we have kept this constant at the Gullstrand number one schematic eye value of 0.5 mm.

Anterior chamber

This is represented by the equation

$$\begin{aligned} anterior\ chamber \\ depth \text{ (mm)} = 3.64 - 0.013 \times age \end{aligned} \quad (20.4)$$

Lens

The lens thickness is represented by the equation

$$lens\ thickness \text{ (mm)} = 3.46 + 0.013 \times age \quad (20.5)$$

Vitreous chamber

This has been kept constant at 16.6 mm to keep the axial length at 24.2 mm for all ages.

Refractive index

Cornea, aqueous and vitreous

In the absence of any data indicating age-related change, we have retained those of the Gullstrand number one schematic eye. These are 1.376 for the cornea and 1.336 for the aqueous and vitreous.

Lens

We use an age-dependent uniform index. From the data given for radii and distances, the eye will remain emmetropic if

$$\begin{aligned} refractive\ index\ of\ lens = \\ 1.4608 - 0.000488 \times age - 0.00000097 \times (age)^2 \end{aligned} \quad (20.6)$$

This is a high refractive index compared with other schematic eyes, indicating that some of the other parameters in the model may not be very accurate.

References

Alpern, M. (1962). Accommodation in muscular mechanisms. *The Eye*, 2nd edn (H. Davson, ed.), vol 3, pp. 191–229. Academic Press.

Alsbirk, P. H. (1978). Corneal thickness. I. Age variation, sex difference and oculometric correlations. *Acta Ophthal.*, **56**, 95–104.

Anstice, J. (1971). Astigmatism – its components and their changes with age. *Am. J. Optom. Arch. Am. Acad. Optom.*, **48**, 1001–6.

Artal, P., Ferro, M., Miranda, I. and Navarro, R. (1993). Effect of aging in retinal image quality. *J. Opt. Soc. Am. A.*, **10**, 1656–62.

Atchison, D. A. (1995). Review of accommodation and presbyopia. *Ophthal. Physiol. Opt.*, **15**, 255–72.

Baldwin, W. R. and Mills, D. (1981). A longitudinal study of corneal astigmatism and total astigmatism. *Am. J. Opt. Physiol. Opt.*, **58**, 206–11.

Beems, E. M. and van Best, J. A. (1990). Light transmission of the cornea in whole human eyes. *Exp. Eye Res.*, **50**, 393–5.

Bena-Sira, I., Weinberger, D., Bodenheimer, J. and Yassur, Y. (1980). Clinical method for measurement of light back-scattering from the *in vivo* human lens. *Invest. Ophthal. Vis. Sci.*, **19**, 435–7.

Birren, J. E., Casperson, R. C. and Botwinick, J. (1950). Age changes in pupil size. *J. Gerontol.*, **5**, 216–221.

Bito, L. Z. and Miranda, O. C. (1989). Accommodation and presbyopia. In *Ophthalmology Annual* (R. D. Reinecke, ed.), pp. 103–28. Raven Press.

Blackwell, O. M. and Blackwell, H. R. (1971). Visual performance data for 156 normal observers of different ages. *J. Illum. Eng. Soc.*, **1**, 3–13.

Blaker, J. W. (1991). A comprehensive model of the aging, accommodative adult eye. In *Technical Digest on Ophthalmic and Visual Optics*, vol. 2, pp. 28–31. Optical Society of America.

Boettner, E. A. and Wolter, J. R. (1962). Transmission of the ocular media. *Invest. Ophthal.*, **1**, 776–83.

Brown, N. (1973a). Lens changes with age and cataract; slit-image photography. In *The Human Lens in relation to Cataract*, pp. 65–78. Elsevier, CIBA Symposium Foundation.

Brown, N. (1973b). The change in shape and internal form of the lens of the eye on accommodation. *Exp. Eye Res.*, **15**, 441–59.

Brown, N. (1974). The change in lens curvature with age. *Exp. Eye Res.*, **19**, 175–83.

Brown, N. A. P. and Hill, A. R. (1987). Cataract: the relation between myopia and cataract morphology. *Br. J. Ophthal.*, **71**, 405–14.

Calver, R. I., Cox, M. J. and Elliot, D. B. (1999). Effect of aging on the monochromatic aberrations of the human eye. *J. Opt. Soc. Am. A.*, **16**, 2069–78.

Charman, W. N. (1989). The path to presbyopia: straight or crooked? *Ophthal. Physiol. Opt.*, **9**, 424–30.

Chateau, N., Blanchard, A. and Baude, D. (1998). Influence of myopia and aging on the optimal spherical aberration of soft contact lenses. *J. Opt. Soc. Am. A*, **15**, 2589–96.

Cogan, D. G. and Kuwabara, T. (1971). Growth and regenerative potential of Descemet's membrane. *Trans. Ophthal. Soc. U.K.*, **91**, 875–94.

Cook, C. A., Koretz, J. F. and Kaufman, P. L. (1991). Age-dependent and accommodation dependent increases in sharpness of human crystalline lens curvatures. *Invest. Ophthal. Vis. Sci.*, **32**, 358.

Cook, C. A., Koretz, J. F., Pfahnl, A. *et al.* (1994). Aging of the human crystalline lens and anterior segment. *Vision Res.*, **34**, 2945–54.

Cumming, J. S. and Kamman, J. (1996). Experience with an accommodating IOL. *J. Cat. Refract. Surg.*, **22**, 1001.

Daus, W. and Völcker, H. E. (1987). Entstehung der Zell-Polymorphie im menschlichen Hornhautendothel. *Klin. Mbl. Augenheilk.*, **191**, 216–21.

DeLint, P. J., Vos, J. J., Berendschot, T. T. J. M. and van Norren, D. (1997). On the Stiles–Crawford effect with age. *Invest. Ophthal. Vis. Sci.*, **38**, 1271–4.

Duane, A. (1922). Studies in monocular and binocular accommodation with their clinical applications. *Am. J. Ophthal.*, **5**, 865–77.

Duane, A. (1925). Are the current theories of accommodation correct? *Am. J. Ophthal.*, **8**, 196–202.

Elliot, D. B. (1987). Contrast sensitivity decline with ageing: a neural or optical phenomenon? *Ophthal. Physiol. Opt.*, **7**, 415–19.

Elliot, D. B., Yang, K. C. H. and Whitaker, D. (1995). Visual acuity changes throughout adulthood in normal, healthy eyes: seeing beyond 6/6. *Optom. Vis. Sci.*, **72**, 186–91.

Elliott, D. B., Yang, K. C. H., Dumbleton, K. and Cullen, A. P. (1993). Ultraviolet-induced lenticular fluorescence: intraocular straylight affecting visual function. *Vision Res.*, **33**, 1827–33.

Fincham, E. F. (1937). The mechanism of accommodation. *Br. J. Ophthal. Suppl.*, **8**, 5–80.

Fisher, A. J. and Christie, A. W. (1965). A note on disability glare. *Vision Res.*, **5**, 565–71.

Fisher, R. F. (1977). The force of contraction of the human ciliary muscle during accommodation. *J. Physiol. (Lond.)*, **270**, 51–74.

Fledelius, H. C. (1984). Prevalences of astigmatism and anisometropia in adult Danes. *Acta Ophthalmol.*, **62**, 391–400.

Fujisawa, K. and Sasaki, K. (1995). Changes in light scattering intensity of the transparent lenses of subjects selected from population-based surveys depending on age: analysis through Scheimpflug images. *Ophthal. Res.*, **27**, 89–101.

Glasser, A. and Campbell, M. C. W. (1998). Presbyopia and the optical changes in the human crystalline lens with age. *Vision Res.*, **38**, 209–29.

Goh, W. S. H. and Lam, C. S. Y. (1994). Changes in refractive trends and optical components of Hong Kong Chinese aged 19–39 years. *Ophthal. Physiol. Opt.*, **14**, 378–82.

Goss, D. A. (1998). Development of the ametropias. Chapter 3. In *Borish's Clinical Refraction*. (W. J. Benjamin, ed.), pp. 47–76. W. B. Saunders.

Grosvenor, T. (1987). Reduction in axial length with age: an emmetropizing mechanism for the adult eye? *Am. J. Optom. Physiol. Opt.*, **64**, 657–63.

Grosvenor, T. (1991). Changes in spherical refraction during the adult years. In *Refractive Anomalies. Research and Clinical Applications* (T. Grosvenor and M. C. Flom, eds), pp. 131–45. Butterworth-Heinemann.

Guirao, A., González, C., Redondo, M., Geraghty, E., Norrby, S. and Artal, P. (1999). Average optical performance of the human eye as a function of age in a normal population. *Invest. Ophthal. Vis. Sci.*, **40**, 203–13.

Gullstrand, A. (1909). Appendix I: Optical imagery. In *Helmholtz's Handbuch der Physiologischen Optik*, vol. 1, 3rd edn (English translation edited by J. P. Southall, Optical Society of America, 1924).

Guth, S. K. (1957). Effects of age on visibility. *Am. J. Optom. Arch. Am. Acad. Optom.*, **34**, 463–77.

Haegerstrom-Portnoy, G., Schneck, M. and Brabyn, J. A. (1999). Seeing into old age: Vision function beyond acuity. *Optom. Vis. Sci.*, **76**, 141–58.

Hamasaki, D., Ong, J. and Marg, E. (1956). The amplitude of accommodation in presbyopia. *Am. J. Optom. Arch. Am. Acad. Optom.*, **33**, 3–14.

Hayashi, K., Hayashi, H. and Hayashi, F. (1995). Topographic analysis of the changes in corneal shape due to aging. *Cornea*, **14**, 527–32.

Helmholtz, H. von (1909). *Handbuch der Physiologischen Optik*, vol. 1, 3rd edn (English translation edited by J. P. Southall, Optical Society of America, 1924).

Hemenger, R. P., Garner, L. F. and Ooi, C. S. (1995). Change with age of the refractive index gradient of the human ocular lens. *Invest. Ophthal. Vis. Sci.*, **36**, 703–7.

Hess, C. (1904). Arbeiten aus dem Gebiete der Accommodationslehre. *Graefe's Arch. Klin. Exp. Ophthal.*, **52**, 143–74 (cited by M. Alpern, 1962).

Hirsch, M. J. (1959). Changes in astigmatism after the age

of forty. *Am. J. Optom. Arch. Am. Acad. Optom.*, **36**, 395–405.

Hockwin, O., Lerman, S. and Ohrloff, C. (1984). Investigations on lens transparency and its disturbances by microdensitometric analyses of Scheimpflug photographs. *Curr. Eye Res.*, **3**, 15–22.

Hofstetter, H. W. (1965). A longitudinal study of amplitude changes in presbyopia. *Am. J. Optom. Arch. Am. Acad. Optom.*, **42**, 3–8.

Howarth, P. A., Zhang, X., Bradley, A. *et al.* (1988). Does the chromatic aberration of the eye vary with age? *J. Opt. Soc. Am. A.*, **5**, 2087–92.

IJspeert, J. K., de Waard, P. W. T., van den Berg, T. J. T. P. and de Jong, P. T. V. M. (1990). The intraocular straylight function in 129 healthy volunteers; dependence on angle, age and pigmentation. *Vision Res.*, **30**, 699–707.

Jenkins, T. C. A. (1963). Aberrations of the eye and their effects on vision: part 1. *Br. J. Physiol. Opt.*, **20**, 59–91.

Kadlecova, V., Peleska, M. and Vasko, A. (1958). Dependence on age of the diameter of the pupil in the dark. *Nature*, **182**, 1520–21.

Kame, R. T., Jue, T. S. and Shigekuni, D. M. (1993). A longitudinal study of corneal astigmatism changes in Asian eyes. *J. Am. Optom. Assoc.*, **64**, 215–19.

Kanai, A. and Kaufman, H. E. (1973). Electron microscopic studies of corneal stroma: aging changes of collagen fibres. *Ann. Ophthal.*, **5**, 285–92.

Kiely, P. M., Smith, G. and Carney, L. G. (1984). Meridional variations of corneal shape. *Am. J. Optom. Physiol. Optics*, **61**, 619–25.

Knoblauch, K., Saunders, F., Kusuda, M. *et al.* (1987). Age and illuminance effects in the Farnsworth-Munsell 100-hue test. *Appl. Opt.*, **26**, 1441–8.

Koprowski, G. (1995). Primate study shows future directions for accommodative IOL. *Ocular Surgery News*, international edn, March issue, p. 9.

Koretz, J. F. and Handelman, G. H. (1986). Modeling age-related accommodative loss in the human eye. *Math. Modelling*, **7**, 1003–14.

Koretz, J. F. and Handelman, G. H. (1988). How the human eye focuses. *Sci. Am.*, **256** (7), 64–71.

Koretz, J. F., Cook, C. A. and Kaufman, P. L. (1997). Accommodation and presbyopia in the human eye. Changes in the anterior segment and crystalline lens with focus. *Invest. Ophthal. Vis. Sci.*, **38**, 569–78.

Koretz, J. F., Kaufman, P. L., Neider, M. W. and Goeckner, P. A. (1989). Accommodation and presbyopia in the human eye – aging of the anterior segment. *Vision Res.*, **29**, 1685–92.

Kruse Hansen, F. (1971). A clinical study of the normal human central corneal thickness. *Acta Ophthal.*, **49**, 82–9.

Kumnick, L. S. (1954). Pupillary psychosensory restitution and aging. *J. Opt. Soc. Am.*, **44**, 735–41.

Lam, C. S. Y., Goh, W. S. H., Tang, Y. K. *et al.* (1994). Changes in refractive trends and optical components of Hong Kong Chinese aged over 40 years. *Ophthal. Physiol. Opt.*, **14**, 383–8.

Lau, E., Mütze, K. and Weber, G. (1955). Die chromatische Aberration des menschlichen Auges. *Graefe's Arch. Klin. Exp. Ophthal.*, **157**, 39–41.

Leinhos, R. (1959). Die Altersabhängigheit des Augenpupillendurchmessers. *Optik*, **16**, 669–71.

Liou, H.-L. and Brennan, N. A. (1997). Anatomically accurate, finite model eye for optical modeling. *J. Opt. Soc. Am. A.*, **14**, 1684–95.

Lyle, W. M. (1971). Changes in corneal astigmatism with age. *Am. J. Optom. Arch. Am. Acad. Optom.*, **48**, 467–78.

Malik, N. S., Moss, S. J., Ahmed, N. *et al.* (1992). Ageing of the human corneal stroma: structural and biochemical changes. *Biochim. Biophys. Acta*, **1138**, 222–8.

Mellerio, J. (1971). Light absorption and scatter in the human lens. *Vision Res.*, **11**, 129–41.

Mellerio, J. (1987). Yellowing of the human lens: nuclear and cortical contributions. *Vision Res.*, **27**, 1581–7.

Millodot, M. (1976). The influence of age on the chromatic aberration of the eye. *Graefe's Arch. Klin. Exp. Ophthal.*, **198**, 235–43.

Millodot, M. and Sivak, J. G. (1973). Influence of accommodation on the chromatic aberration of the eye. *Brit. J. Physiol. Opt.*, **28**, 169–74.

Miranda, M. N. (1979). The geographic factor in the onset of presbyopia. *Trans. Am. Ophthal. Soc.*, **7**, 603–21.

Mordi, J. A. and Adrian, W. K. (1985). Influence of age on the chromatic aberration of the human eye. *Am. J. Optom. Physiol. Opt.*, **62**, 864–9.

Morrell, A., Whitefoot, H. D. and Charman, W. N. (1991). Ocular chromatic aberration and age. *Ophthal. Physiol. Opt.*, **11**, 385–90.

Niesel, P. (1982). Visible changes of the lens with age. *Trans. Ophthal. Soc. UK*, **102**, 327–30.

Ooi, C. S. and Grosvenor, T. (1995). Mechanisms of emmetropization in the aging eye. *Optom. Vis. Sci.*, **72**, 60–6.

Olsen, T. (1982). Light scattering from the human cornea. *Invest. Ophthal. Vis. Sci.*, **23**, 81–6.

Olsen, T. and Ehlers, N. (1984). The thickness of the human cornea as determined by a specular method. *Acta Ophthal.*, **62**, 859–71.

Oshika, T., Klyce, S. D., Applegate, R. A. and Howland, H. C. (1999). Changes in corneal wavefront aberrations with aging. *Invest. Ophthal. Vis. Sci.*, **40**, 1351–5.

Owsley, C., Sekuler, R. and Siemsen, D. (1983). Contrast sensitivity throughout adulthood. *Vision Res.*, **23**, 689–99.

Pease, P. L. and Cooper, D. P. (1986). Longitudinal chromatic aberration and age. *Am. J. Optom. Physiol. Opt.*, **63**, 106P.

Phillips, R. A. (1952). Changes in corneal astigmatism. *Am. J. Optom. Arch. Am. Acad. Optom.*, **29**, 379–80.

Pierscionek, B. K. (1990). Presbyopia – effect of refractive index. *Clin. Exp. Optom.*, **73**, 23–30.

Pierscionek, B. K. (1996). Aging changes in the optical elements of the eye. *J. Biomed. Optics*, **1**, 147–56.

Pierscionek, B. K. and Weale, R. A. (1995). The optics of the eye lens and lenticular senescence. *Doc. Ophthal.*, **89**, 321–35.

Pokorny, J., Smith,V. C. and Lutze, M. (1987). Aging of the human lens. *Applied Optics*, **26**, 1437–40.

Rabbetts, R. B. (1998). *Bennett and Rabbetts' Clinical Visual Optics*, 3rd edn, pp. 209–13. Butterworth-Heinemann.

Ramsdale, C. and Charman, W. N. (1989). A longitudinal study of the changes in the static accommodation response. *Ophthal. Physiol. Opt.*, **9**, 255–63.

Richards, O. W. (1977). Effects of luminance and contrast on visual acuity, ages 16 to 90 years. *Am. J. Optom. Physiol. Opt.*, **54**, 178–84.

Rynders, M., Grosvenor, T. and Enoch, J. M. (1995). Stability of the Stiles–Crawford function in a unilateral amblyopic subject over a 38-year period: a case study. *Optom. Vis. Sci.*, **72**, 177–85.

Said, F. S. and Sawires, W. S. (1972). Age dependence of changes in pupil diameter in the dark. *Optica Acta*, **19**, 359–61.

Said, F. S. and Weale, R. A. (1959). The variation with age of the spectral transmissivity of the living human crystalline lens. *Gerontologia*, **3**, 213–31.

Sample, P. A., Esterson, F. D., Weinreb, R. N. and Boynton, R. M. (1988). The aging lens: *in vivo* assessment of light absorption in 84 human eyes. *Invest. Ophthal. Vis. Sci.*, **29**, 1306–11.

Saunders, H. (1981). Age-dependence of human refractive errors. *Ophthal. Physiol. Opt.*, **1**, 159–74.

Saunders, H. (1986a). A longitudinal study of the age dependence of human ocular refraction. 1. Age-dependent changes in the equivalent sphere. *Ophthal. Physiol. Opt.*, **6**, 39–46.

Saunders, H. (1986b). Changes in the orientation of the axis of astigmatism associated with age. *Ophthal. Physiol. Opt.*, **6**, 343–4.

Schachar, R. A. (1992). Cause and treatment of presbyopia with a method for increasing the amplitude of accommodation. *Ann. Ophthal.*, **24**, 445–52.

Siu, A. and Herse, P. (1993). The effect of age on human corneal thickness. Statistical implications of power analysis. *Acta Ophthal.*, **71**, 51–6.

Sloane, M.E., Owsley, C. and Alvarez, S. L. (1988). Aging, senile miosis and spatial contrast sensitivity at low luminance. *Vision Res.*, **28**, 1235–46.

Smith, G., Atchison, D. A. and Pierscionek, B. K. (1992). Modeling the power of the aging human eye. *J. Opt. Soc. Am. A*, **9**, 2111–17.

Smith, G. and Pierscionek, B. K. (1998). The optical structure of the lens and its contribution to the refractive status of the eye. *Ophthal. Physiol. Opt.*, **18**, 21–9.

Sorsby, A., Sheridan, M. and Leary, G. A. (1962). *Refraction and its Components in Twins*. HMSO.

Sorsby, A., Benjamin, J. B., Davey, M., Sheridan, M. and Tanner, J. M. (1957). *Emmetropia and its Aberrations*. HMSO.

Strenk, S. A., Semmlow, J. L., Strenk, L. M. *et al.* (1999). Age-related changes in human ciliary muscle and lens: a magnetic resonance imaging study. *Invest. Ophthalmol. Vis. Sci.*, **40**, 1162–9.

Sun, F., Stark, L., Nguyen, A. *et al.* (1988). Changes in accommodation with age: static and dynamic. *Am. J. Optom. Physiol. Opt.*, **65**, 492–8.

Ungerer, J. (1986). The optometric management of presbyopic airline pilots. Unpublished MSc Optom thesis, University of Melbourne.

van den Berg ,T. J. T. P. and Tan, K. E. W. P. (1994). Light transmittance of the human cornea from 320 to 700 nm for different ages. *Vision Res.*, **34**, 1453–6.

Ware, C. (1982). Human axial chromatic aberration found not to decline with age. *Graefe's Arch. Klin. Exp. Ophthalmol.*, **218**, 39–41.

Weale, R. A. (1961). Retinal illumination and age. *Trans Illum. Eng. Soc.*, **26**, 95–100.

Weale, R. A. (1981). Human ocular ageing and ambient temperature. *Br. J. Ophthalmol.*, **65**, 869–70.

Weale, R. A. (1982). *A Biography of the Eye*. H. K. Lewis and Co.

Weale, R. A. (1992). *The Senescence of Vision*. Oxford University Press.

Weekers, R., Delmarcelle, Y., Luyckx-Bacus, J. and Collignon, J. (1973). Morphological changes of the lens with age and cataract. In *The Human Lens in relation to Cataract*, pp. 25–40. Elsevier, CIBA Symposium Foundation.

Weston, H. C. (1949). On age and illumination in relation to visual performance. *Trans. Illum. Eng. Soc.*, **14**, 281–7.

Winn, B., Whitaker, D., Elliot, D. B. and Phillips, N. J. (1994). Factors affecting light-adapted pupil size in normal human subjects. *Invest. Ophthal. Vis. Sci.*, **35**, 1132–7.

Appendices

A1

Paraxial optics

Introduction

The study of the image formation by optical systems can be reduced to the imagery of selected points in the object space or field. The study of the image formation of an object point can be reduced to tracing a number of rays from this point, through the system, and examining their paths in image space. Such a situation is shown in Figure A1.1, which shows an object point **Q** and a set of three image-forming rays. Ideally, these rays should be concurrent at some point – say **Q'** – in the image space, as shown in the figure. However, they are not usually concurrent, and this is due to what are known as **aberrations**. The greater the spread of the rays in the image plane, the greater the aberrations. Usually the aberrations increase as the light beam widens and the object point **Q** moves further away from the optical axis. If rays are traced very close to the axis, aberrations are reduced the ray-trace equations can be simplified by making some simple approximations called paraxial approximations.

In this book, exact or actual rays are referred to as **finite** rays, and rays traced using the paraxial approximations as **paraxial** rays.

Finite ray tracing

The tracing of a finite ray through an optical system involves a number of steps:

1. Choosing an origin or starting point and a direction for the ray, such as the point **O** and angle u, shown in Figure A1.2 (sometimes the starting point may be off-axis).
2. Locating the point of intersection **B** of the ray with the surface, using trigonometry, algebra and a knowledge of the surface position and shape.
3. Determining the angle of incidence i at this surface.
4. Refraction at **B** by the application of Snell's law, which connects the angles of incidence i and refraction i' with the refractive indices, n and n', by

$$n' \sin(i') = n \sin(i) \tag{A1.1}$$

to find the angle of refraction i' and angle u' the ray makes with the optical axis (Figure

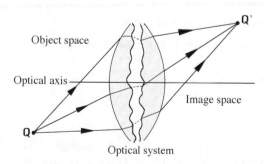

Object space

Optical axis

Image space

Q'

Q

Optical system

Figure A1.1. Ideal imagery.

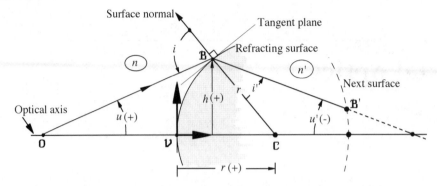

Figure A1.2. Refraction by a surface, showing important variables and the sign convention.

A1.2). These angles specify the direction of the refracted ray. This is called the 'refraction' step. If there is more than one surface in the system, the above steps 2–4 are repeated until the last surface is reached. Each return to step 2 requires the point of intersection with the next surface to be found. Figure A1.2 shows a ray-trace to the point **B'** on the next surface. The process of tracing to the next surface is called the 'transfer' step.

5. Locating the point of intersection with the optical axis or the expected image surface.

The sign convention used for tracing rays is that shown in Figure A1.2. Distances to the left of a surface or below the optical axis are negative and those to the right or above are positive. Angles due to an anticlockwise rotation of the ray from the optical axis are positive, and those due to a clockwise rotation are negative. The origin for axes at each surface is the vertex **V**. The signs enclosed in brackets indicate the signs of the quantities shown in the figure.

The paraxial approximations and paraxial rays

If rays are traced very close to the optical axis, then all the angles shown in Figure A1.2 are small. For small angles x expressed in radians,

$$\tan(x) \approx \sin(x) \approx x \qquad (A1.2)$$

This approximation improves as the size of the angle decreases. When we apply this paraxial approximation to ray-tracing equa-

tions, Snell's law reduces to

$$n'i' = ni \qquad (A1.3)$$

The useful outcome of this paraxial approximation is that, if all the rays within the beam shown in Figure A1.1 are traced as paraxial rays, they are all concurrent at some point in image space. In this sense, paraxial rays are aberration-free rays.

Definition of a paraxial ray

A paraxial ray is a finite ray traced close to the optical axis, in which the angles involved are sufficiently small that replacing the sines and tangents of the angles by the angles themselves (in radians) in ray-trace equations produces a negligible error.

Paraxial ray-trace equations

There are two paraxial ray-trace equations that are used for steps 2–4 in the previous section.

Paraxial refraction equation

This equation is used to determine the new direction of the ray after refraction:

$$n'u' - nu = -hF \qquad (A1.4)$$

where

$$F = C(n' - n) \qquad (A1.5)$$

is the refractive power of the surface, C is the surface curvature ($= 1/r$), and the other variables are shown in Figure A1.2.

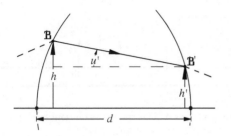

Figure A1.3. Ray-tracing: the transfer step.

Paraxial transfer equation

This equation is used to locate the intersection point or height at the next surface:

$$h' = h + u'd \qquad (A1.6)$$

This equation can be derived with the quantities shown in Figure A1.3.

A paraxial ray-tracing scheme

Since most optical systems consist of more than one surface, equations (A1.4) to (A1.6) are used repeatedly. The following scheme shows how this is done, with a small change in notation. The variables given in the following equations are defined in Figure A1.4.

Step 1: choosing a ray

We assume that the position of the axial point **O**, which is the origin of the ray or where an off-axis ray crosses the axis, is known. Let the distance of this point from the first surface vertex be l_v. We now choose a direction of the ray by selecting a pair of values u_1 and h_1

which satisfy the equation

$$l_v = -h_1/u_1 \qquad (A1.7)$$

Step 2: refraction at the jth surface

Starting at the first surface (i.e. $j = 1$), we use equation (A1.4), i.e.

$$n'_j u'_j - n_j u_j = -h_j F_j \qquad (A1.8)$$

where

$$F_j = C_j(n'_j - n_j) \qquad (A1.9)$$

is the power of the jth surface.

Step 3: transfer to the next (j + 1)th surface

Here we use equation (A1.6), i.e.

$$h_{j+1} = h_j + u'_j d_j \qquad (A1.10)$$

Steps 2 and 3 are repeated at each surface, using the following equivalences:

$$n'_j = n_{j+1} \text{ and } u'_j = u_{j+1} \qquad (A1.11)$$

until the last (kth) surface is reached. At this stage, the axial distance l'_v from the last surface vertex of the point where this ray crosses the axis is given by the equation

$$l'_v = -h_k/u'_k \qquad (A1.12)$$

Image size and magnification

Usually, we need to know the transverse magnification M of the image, which is

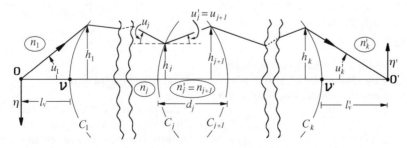

Figure A1.4. The tracing of a paraxial ray through a general system consisting of k surfaces.

defined as

$$M = \frac{\text{image size } (\eta')}{\text{object size } (\eta)} \qquad (A1.13)$$

where the object value (η) and image size (η') are shown in Figure A1.4. The value of this magnification can be found from the above ray-trace and is given by the equation

$$M = \frac{n_1 u_1}{n'_k u'_k} \qquad (A1.14)$$

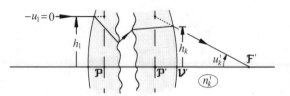

Figure A1.5. Particular ray-traces for determining the positions of the back cardinal points.

Cardinal points and equivalent power

The location of the back cardinal points $\mathbf{P}'$ and $\mathbf{F}'$ can be found from the results of a paraxial ray-trace from object space to image space, initially parallel to the axis (i.e. $u_1 = 0$), as shown in Figure A1.5. Given the initial ray height h_1, final ray height h_k and final angle u'_k, the positions of these points can be found from the equations

$$\mathbf{P'F'} = -h_1/u'_k \qquad (A1.16)$$

$$\mathbf{V'F'} = -h_k/u'_k \qquad (A1.17)$$

The equivalent power F is given by the equation

$$F = n'_k/\mathbf{P'F'} \qquad (A1.18)$$

The position of the back nodal point $\mathbf{N}'$ is given by the equation

$$\mathbf{P'N'} = (n'_k - n_1)/F \qquad (A1.19)$$

The positions of the front cardinal points $\mathbf{P}$, $\mathbf{F}$ and $\mathbf{N}$ can be found by tracing a similar paraxial ray from the image space (i.e. $u'_k = 0$) back through the system into object space. The equivalent power can also be calculated from this ray-trace and, if the equivalent of equation (A1.18) is used, it gives the same numerical value. It can also be found that

$$\mathbf{PN} = \mathbf{P'N'} \qquad (A1.20)$$

The lens equation

If the positions of the cardinal points and the equivalent power of an optical system are known, the position of an image can be found without the above detailed ray-tracing. Instead, it can be found by the direct appli-

Special case of the object at infinity

If the object is at infinity, equation (A1.7) cannot be used to generate a ray because the value of l_v is infinite. In this case, $u_1 = 0$, and we can choose any suitable value of h_1.

Choice of ray

Since paraxial rays are aberration-free rays, all paraxial rays in a beam arising from an object point are concurrent at the image point. To locate the image point, we need in principle to trace only two rays in the beam to find the point of concurrency. However, for an axial object point, one of these rays may be taken as the optical axis. Therefore, for axial objects we need to trace only one ray, and where this ray intersects the optical axis is the image point and the location of the paraxial image plane.

The optical invariant

If two distinct paraxial rays, denoted by A and B, are traced through any optical system, the quantity

$$n_A(u_A h_B - u_B h_A)$$

at any surface and on either side of the surface has the same value throughout the system, and thus its value is invariant. Using the symbol H to denote its value,

$$H = n_A(u_A h_B - u_B h_A) \qquad (A1.15)$$

This quantity is useful in aberration theory, which we discuss in Appendix 2.

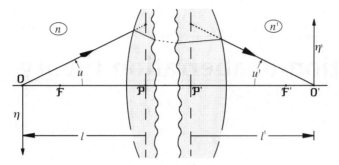

Figure A1.6. The general system and the lens equation.

cation of the lens equation

$$n'/l' - n/l = L' - L = F \qquad (A1.21)$$

where n' and n are the object and image space refractive indices, L is the object vergence ($= n/l$) and L' is the image vergence ($= n'/l'$), the distance l is measured from the front principal plane at **P** and the distance l' is measured from the back principal plane at **P'**. F is the equivalent power of the system, defined by equation (A1.18), and is the power of an equivalent thin lens placed at the principal planes (Figure A1.6).

In this situation, equation (A1.14) for the transverse magnification is still applicable and, using the symbols shown in Figure A1.6, this equation can be written as

$$M = nu/(n'u') \qquad (A1.22)$$

It can also be expressed in terms of the distances l and l' of the object and images from the respective principal planes by the equation

$$M = nl'/(n'l) \qquad (A1.23)$$

Gaussian optics

Sometimes it is useful to assume that rays that are beyond the paraxial region, according to the approximation in equation (A1.2), nevertheless behave as if they are paraxial rays (i.e. are aberration-free). The application of par-axial approximations beyond the paraxial region is called Gaussian optics.

Summary of main symbols

i angle of incidence
u paraxial ray angle
h paraxial ray height
n refractive index
F (equivalent) power of a surface or lens
C surface curvature (reciprocal of radius of curvature)
d separation between adjacent refracting surfaces
l For thin components, this is the distance from the vertex **V** of the component to the axial object point **O**. For thick components, the distance is measured from the front principal plane **P** to the axial object point **O**
L corresponding vergence ($= n/l$)
M transverse magnification
H optical invariant
η object size
F   focal point
N   nodal point
P   principal point
Q   off-axis object point
O   on-axis object point
V   vertex point

A prime (') superscript following the above symbols (except F, C, d, M, and H) means that a quantity occurs after refraction or in image space.

A2

Introduction to aberration theory

Quantification of aberrations

In the absence of aberrations, diffraction and scatter, all rays from any point in object space, that are refracted by an optical system, are focused to one point in the image plane – that is, they are concurrent. The position of this point can be predicted by using the paraxial equations described in Appendix 1. In the presence of aberrations, the rays are not concurrent at the expected image point, but intersect the paraxial image plane in a spread-out pattern.

There are three common ways of quantifying the aberrations of an optical system; namely **wave**, **transverse** and **longitudinal**. Aberrations of a system are often determined by calculating the aberrations of representative rays. For each ray, there is always a wave and a transverse aberration, and sometimes a longitudinal aberration. Figure A2.1 shows a schematic system and typical rays traversing the system. The wave, transverse and longitudinal aberrations of this ray are described as follows.

Rays from an axial point

Figure A2.1a shows a particular real ray **OBB'H** in a beam from the point **O**. This ray should cross the optical axis and the paraxial image plane at the point **O'** but, because of aberrations, it intersects the axis at the point **G** and the paraxial image plane at the point **H**.

The path **OBO'** indicates the route of the corresponding unaberrated ray. The aberration may be specified in terms of any of the following quantities:

Longitudinal
  aberration $\qquad$ $O'G = \delta l'$

Transverse aberration
  $\qquad$ $O'H$

Wave (path length)
  aberration $\qquad$ $[OEE'O'] - [OBO']$
  $\hfill$ (A2.1a)

where the square brackets refer to optical path lengths, which are products of physical path lengths and refractive indices. The wave aberration is the difference in optical path length between that of the pupil ray (the central ray of the beam) and that of any other ray of the beam. In this case, it is assumed that the pupil ray of the beam travels along the optical axis.

Rays from an off-axis point

Figure A2.1b shows a general ray from an off-axis point **Q**. If such a ray does not intersect the optical axis or the pupil ray of the beam, longitudinal aberration is not applicable to the ray. The transverse aberration is **Q'H**. The wave aberration is similar to that given by equation (A2.1a), but now the pupil ray follows the path **QEE'Q'** instead of the optical axis. In summary,

Exit pupil

$\delta l'$ O'

B'

G

H

Entrance pupil

B

E'

B

E

Pupil ray

O

(a)

H

Q'

O'

Y

B'

B

ϕ

E'

r

E

O

Pupil ray

X

O

η

Q

(b)

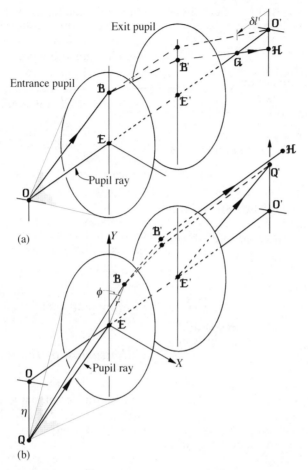

Figure A2.1. Three forms for quantifying the aberrations of a ray: wave, transverse and longitudinal.

Transverse aberration

Q'H

Wave (path length)
 aberration

[QEE'Q'] – [QBQ']
 (A2.1b)

There are other methods of quantifying the level of aberrations of rays and beams that depend upon the particular aberration. For example, the spherical aberration of the eye is often expressed as an equivalent power error.

The wave aberration function

The aberration of a particular ray depends upon the co-ordinates of the point **B**, where the ray passes through the entrance pupil. If we set up a (X, Y) co-ordinate system in the entrance pupil, as shown in Figure A2.1b, we can express the wave aberration as a function of X and Y. The wave aberration for the ray through **B** is also a function of the position η of the object point **Q** in the field. The wave aberration W is thus a function of X, Y, and η and can be expressed as a power series in these variables. For a rotationally symmetric system, it has the form

$$W(\eta;X,Y) = {}_0W_{4,0}(X^2 + Y^2)^2 + {}_1W_{3,1}\eta(X^2 + Y^2)Y + {}_2W_{2,0}\eta^2(X^2 + Y^2) + {}_2W_{2,2}\eta^2Y^2 + {}_3W_{1,1}\eta^3Y + \text{higher order aberrations} \quad (A2.2)$$

The first five terms in this expansion are the

primary aberrations or **third order aberrations**, and are known as

$$_0W_{4,0}(X^2 + Y^2)^2 \quad \text{spherical aberration}$$
$$_1W_{3,1}\eta(X^2 + Y^2)Y \quad \text{coma}$$
$$_2W_{2,0}\eta^2(X^2 + Y^2) \quad \text{field curvature}$$
$$_2W_{2,2}\eta^2Y^2 \quad \text{astigmatism}$$
$$_3W_{1,1}\eta^3Y \quad \text{distortion}$$

It is often more convenient to express this function in terms of polar co-ordinates (r,ϕ) where

$$X = r\sin(\phi) \text{ and } Y = r\cos(\phi) \quad (A2.3)$$

and ϕ is the angle between the line **EB** and the Y axis, as shown in Figure A2.1b. The above polynomial can then be expressed in the form

$$W(\eta;r,\phi) = {_0W_{4,0}}r^4 + {_1W_{3,1}}\eta r^3 \cos(\phi)$$
$$+ {_2W_{2,0}}\eta^2 r^2 + {_2W_{2,2}}\eta^2 r^2 \cos^2(\phi)$$
$$+ {_3W_{1,1}}\eta^3 r \cos(\phi)$$
$$+ \text{ higher order aberrations} \quad (A2.4)$$

The level of the wave aberration need only be as large as a wavelength to have a significant effect on image quality.

Units of aberrations

All the aberrations defined above are distances or differences in distances, and therefore have units of length. Because even very small values can be significant, it is common practice to express wave aberrations in units of the wavelength. For example, a distance of 0.001 mm is equivalent to two wavelengths if the wavelength is 500 nm.

Defocus and wave aberration

The wave aberration polynomial is very useful in studying the effects of a defocus as well as aberrations on an image. If a defocus is present, we can add the following term:

$$_0W_{2,0}r^2$$

to the wave aberration polynomial given by equation (A2.4), and the value of $_0W_{2,0}$ is related to the defocus ΔF by the equation

$$\Delta F = 2{_0W_{2,0}} \quad (A2.5)$$

where ΔF is the change in power required to produce that level of defocus.

Calculation of the wave aberration function

The definition of wave aberration given by equations (A2.1a and b) is ideal for the theoretical analysis of, and deriving explicit equations for, the wave aberration, but only for relatively simple systems. For complex systems, it is easier in practice to determine

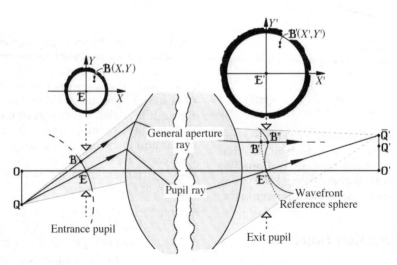

Figure A2.2. The distortion of a wavefront passing through an optical system and the wave aberration [**B'B''**]

the wave aberration by numerically ray-tracing specific rays. Such ray-traces do not give the path **QBQ'** but the path **QBB'H**, so we cannot determine the wave aberration using equation (A2.1a or b). Therefore, in practice, we need a different and more practical definition of wave aberration.

In the ideal optical system, a point source can be thought of as emitting light with spherical wavefronts as shown in Figure A2.2. These wavefronts enter the system through the entrance pupil. If the imagery is perfect, these wavefronts exit the system also with a spherical shape. However, if aberrations are present, the wavefronts are distorted. The wave aberration is a measure of the distortion.

Figure A2.2 shows a distorted or aberrated wavefront leaving the exit pupil, and also shows an undistorted wavefront (the reference sphere). The wave aberration of any ray is the optical distance along the ray between the distorted wavefront and the reference sphere. Arbitrarily, the two wavefronts are defined to coincide at the centre of the exit pupil.

$$W = [QEE'] - [QBB'] \quad (A2.6)$$

As

$$[QEE'] = [QBB'B''],$$

equation (A2.6) reduces to

$$W = [B'B''] \quad (A2.7)$$

Since for any specific optical system the position and shapes of all the surfaces are known, the ray intersection points with each surface can be found by conventional geometrical and trigonometrical rules and the above path differences can be calculated for any specific ray.

The two definitions of wave aberration used (equations (A2.1 and A2.7)) are slightly different, but for low levels of aberrations will lead to very similar results. They will give different results for large levels of aberrations, but in this case, some other equations used in the chapters covering aberrations will also be in error; for example, the relationship between wave, transverse and longitudinal aberrations used in Chapter 15.

Seidel aberrations

There are seven Seidel aberrations, and these are listed in Table A2.1 along with some of their properties. Only five of these are monochromatic aberrations, and these are related to the primary wave aberrations given in equation (A2.2). The Seidel aberrations can be calculated from the paths of the paraxial marginal and paraxial pupil rays.

Seidel aberrations are usually calculated as wave aberrations, although they are occasionally calculated in the transverse or longitudinal aberration forms. Equations for their calculations can be found in texts by Welford (1986) and Smith and Atchison (1997). They are calculated from the system constructional parameters (refractive indices, surface curvatures and shapes and surface separations), and depend upon the beam width and the field-of-view, which in turn are

Table A2.1. The seven Seidel aberrations.

Aberration	Symbol	Imagery point to point	Dependence on* aperture (p)	field (q)
Monochromatic				
Spherical	S_1	no	4	0
Coma	S_2	no	3	1
Astigmatism	S_3	no	2	2
Field curvature	S_4	yes	2	2
Distortion	S_5	yes	1	3
% distortion			0	2
Chromatic				
Longitudinal	C_L	no	2	0
Transverse	C_T	no	1	1

*These values are for wave aberrations, except for distortion expressed as a percentage. For transverse aberrations the p power dependence reduces by 1, and for longitudinal aberrations the p power dependence reduces by 2.

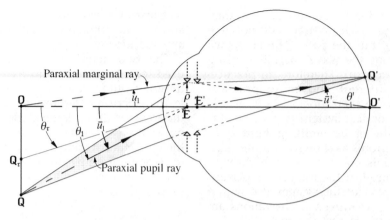

Figure A2.3. Field points and field angles.

defined by the paraxial marginal and paraxial pupil rays. Values are given in Appendix 3 for selected schematic eyes, and are calculated for a beam width limited by the paraxial marginal ray passing through the edge of an 8 mm diameter entrance pupil (that is, through the edge of pupil of radius $\bar{\rho} = 4$ mm), and for a field width specified by the paraxial pupil ray inclined at angle of 5° to the optical axis. Figure A2.3 shows a beam arising from the point **Q**, which is at the edge of the nominal field of view and subtends an angle θ_1 at the entrance pupil at **E**. The pupil ray subtends a paraxial angle $\bar{u}_1$ to the axis, and this paraxial angle is the tangent of the real angle according to

$$\bar{u}_1 = \tan(\theta_1) \qquad (A2.8)$$

Thus, in this case, $\theta_1 = 5°$ and so

$$\bar{u}_1 = \tan(5°) = 0.087488663 \qquad (A2.8a)$$

The combination of beam width and field size is embodied in the optical invariant H, which we introduced in Appendix 1. Using the paraxial marginal and pupil rays, we have

$$H = n(\bar{u}h - u\bar{h}) \qquad (A2.9)$$

where u and h are the marginal ray angle and height at any plane in the system, $\bar{u}$ and $\bar{h}$ are the corresponding pupil ray values, and n is the refractive index on the side of the plane where the above paraxial angles are measured. At the entrance pupil plane,

$$H = n\bar{u}_1\bar{\rho} \qquad (A2.9a)$$

Therefore, for the data in Appendix 3,

$$H = 1 \times 0.0874887 \times 4 = 0.349955 \qquad (A2.10)$$

For a beam with a different width and from a different field point, the aberrations are different and can be found from

New aberration
value = old aberration value
$\times$ (fractional pupil radius)^p
$\times$ (fractional field position τ)^q (A2.11)

where the values of p and q are given in Table A2.1.

The fractional value τ can be used to specify the position of some other field point, say the point $\mathbf{Q}_\tau$ shown in Figure A2.3, and this point is off-axis by an angle $\theta_{\tau'}$ measured at the entrance pupil. The fractional field value τ is defined as

$$\tau = \tan(\theta_\tau)/\tan(\theta_1) \qquad (A2.12)$$

where θ_τ is an off-axis angle point inside or outside the 5° field.

Seidel aberrations and the primary wave aberration co-efficients

The five monochromatic Seidel aberrations are directly related to the wave aberration co-efficients of equations (A2.2) and (A2.4) as follows:

$$S_1 = 8_0W_{4,0}\bar{\rho}^4 \qquad \text{spherical aberration} \qquad (A2.13a)$$

$S_2 = 2_1 W_{3,1} \bar{\rho}^3$ coma   (A2.13b)

$S_3 = 2_2 W_{2,2} \bar{\rho}^2$ astigmatism

(A2.13c)

$S_4 = (4_2 W_{2,0} - 2_2 W_{2,2}) \bar{\rho}^2$ Petzval curvature

(A2.13d)

$S_5 = 2_3 W_{1,1} \bar{\rho}$ distortion   (A2.13e)

The Seidel aberration values can be found from the wave aberration polynomial co-efficients, if the latter are known, as well as from the Seidel formulae given in texts such as Welford (1986) and Smith and Atchison (1997). If the Seidel aberrations are known, the wave aberration co-efficients can be calculated after re-arranging the above equations as

$_0 W_{4,0} = S_1 / (8 \bar{\rho}^4)$ spherical   (A2.14a)

$_1 W_{3,1} = S_2 / (2 \bar{\rho}^3)$ coma   (A2.14b)

$_2 W_{2,0} = (S_3 + S_4) / (4 \bar{\rho}^2)$ field curvature

(A2.14c)

$_2 W_{2,2} = S_3 / (2 \bar{\rho}^2)$ astigmatism

(A2.14d)

$_3 W_{1,1} = S_5 / (2 \bar{\rho})$ distortion   (A2.14e)

Sagittal, tangential and Petzval surfaces

In the Seidel approximation, the sagittal and tangential surfaces are spherical with radii of curvatures given by the following equations (Smith and Atchison, 1997)

$$r_s = - \frac{H^2}{n'(S_3 + S_4)} \text{ sagittal surface} \quad (A2.15a)$$

$$r_t = - \frac{H^2}{n'(3S_3 + S_4)} \text{ tangential surface} \quad (A2.15b)$$

In the absence of astigmatism, i.e. $S_3 = 0$, we can see from the above equations that the two radii of curvatures are the same. The corresponding surface is known as the Petzval surface, and it follows that its radius of curvature, denoted as r_P, is

$$r_P = - \frac{H^2}{n' S_4} \text{ Petzval surface} \quad (A2.15c)$$

The sagittal and tangential image surfaces can

be represented by the corresponding vergences L_s and L_t. This is particularly useful if the image plane is at infinity, because then the image surfaces cease to have any meaning. Using equations in Smith and Atchison (1997), for ray-tracing out of the eye and for the object (instead of the image) at infinity, we can show that the vergences are related to the off-axis angle θ by the equations

$$L_s(\theta) \approx \frac{\theta^2}{2 n_{vit} r_s} \quad (A2.16a)$$

$$L_t(\theta) \approx \frac{\theta^2}{2 n_{vit} r_t} \quad (A2.16b)$$

where θ is the off-axis angle in radians. These vergences are the same as peripheral power errors as used in Chapters 15 and 16.

Wave aberration co-efficients $W_{2,0}$ and $W_{2,2}$

In visual optics, the peripheral power errors $L_s(\theta)$ and $L_t(\theta)$ are more meaningful than the Seidel or wave aberration values. However, if we wish to calculate the point spread or optical transfer functions, we need to know the corresponding wave aberration co-efficients $W_{2,0}$ and $W_{2,2}$. We have

$$W_{2,0} = -L_s(\theta)/2 \quad (A2.17a)$$

$$W_{2,2} = [L_s(\theta) - L_t(\theta)]/2 \quad (A2.17b)$$

or

$$L_s(\theta) = -2W_{2,0} \quad (A2.18a)$$

$$L_t(\theta) = -2(W_{2,0} + W_{2,2}) \quad (A2.18b)$$

Modifications for a curved retina

The use of Seidel aberrations assumes usually that the image surface is flat. Some of the above equations can be modified by taking into account the radius of curvature of the retina. The equivalent of equations (A2.16a and b), for the sagittal and tangential surface vergences, now become

$$L_s(\theta) \approx \frac{\theta^2}{2 n_{vit}} \left[\frac{1}{r_s} - \frac{1}{r_R} \right] \quad (A2.19a)$$

$$L_t(\theta) \approx \frac{\theta^2}{2n_{vit}}\left[\frac{1}{r_t} - \frac{1}{r_R}\right] \tag{A2.19b}$$

where r_R is the radius of curvature of the retina.

In the Seidel approximation, the wave aberration $W_{2,2}$ is independent of the retinal radius, but the co-efficient $W_{2,0}$ changes by an amount $\Delta W_{2,0}$ where

$$\Delta W_{2,0} = \frac{\theta^2}{4n_{vit}r_R} \tag{A2.20}$$

Seidel aberrations of a gradient index medium

Sands (1970) presented a set of equations for determining the Seidel aberrations of gradient index media. To make these equations consistent with the Seidel aberrations of Hopkins (1950) and Welford (1986), Sands' aberration values must be multiplied by a factor of two and the signs changed. The aberrations are broken up into two types: the refractive contribution arising at the surfaces, and the transfer contribution arising from the passage of the rays through the lens from the anterior to the posterior surface.

Refractive contribution

$$\kappa = +2C_1\{2N_1(0) + 0.5C_1 dN_0(0)/dZ\}$$
$$- 2C_2\{2N_1(d) + 0.5C_2 dN_0(d)/dZ\} \tag{A2.21}$$

Spherical aberration (S_1)	κh^4
Coma (S_2)	$\kappa h^3\bar{h}$
Astigmatism (S_3)	$\kappa h^2\bar{h}^2$
Field curvature (S_4)	0
Distortion (S_5)	$\kappa h\bar{h}^3$

where C_1 and C_2 are the front and back surface curvatures of the lens, d is its thickness, $dN_0(Z)/dZ$ is the differential of $N_0(Z)$ with respect to Z, h is the paraxial marginal ray height at the surface, and $\bar{h}$ is the paraxial pupil ray height at the surface.

Transfer contribution

Spherical aberration (S_1)

$$- \{N_0(d)h(d)u^3(d) - N_0(0)h(0)u^3(0)\}$$

$$- \{2\int_0^d[4N_2(Z)h^4(Z) + 2N_1(Z)h^2(Z)u^2(Z)$$

$$- 0.5N_0(Z)u^4(Z)]dZ\}$$

Coma (S_2)

$$- \{N_0(d)h(d)u^2(d)\bar{u}(d) - N_0(0)h(0)u^2(0)\bar{u}(0)\}$$

$$- \{2\int_0^d[4N_2(Z)h^3(Z)\bar{h}(Z)$$

$$+ N_1(Z)h(Z)u(Z)[h(Z)\bar{u}(Z) + \bar{h}(Z)u(Z)]$$

$$- 0.5N_0(Z)u^3(Z)\bar{u}(Z)]dZ\}$$

Astigmatism (S_3)

$$- \{N_0(d)h(d)u(d)\bar{u}^2(d) - N_0(0)h(0)u(0)\bar{u}^2(0)\}$$

$$- \{2\int_0^d[4N_2(Z)h^2(Z)\bar{h}^2(Z)$$

$$+ 2N_1(Z)h(Z)\bar{h}(Z)u(Z)\bar{u}(Z)$$

$$- 0.5N_0(Z)u^2(Z)\bar{u}^2(Z)]dZ\}$$

Distortion (S_5)

$$- \{N_0(d)h(d)\bar{u}^3(d) - N_0(0)h(0)\bar{u}^3(0)\}$$

$$- \{2\int_0^d[4N_2(Z)h(Z)\bar{h}^3(Z)$$

$$+ N_1(Z)\bar{h}(Z)\bar{u}(Z)[h(Z)\bar{u}(Z) + \bar{h}(Z)u(Z)]$$

$$- 0.5N_0(Z)u(Z)\bar{u}^3(Z)]dZ\}$$

Relevance of gradient index expressions to the eye

If a ray passing through the lens of the eye has a shallow trajectory, the angle $u(Z)$ is small. In the expressions above, the effects of the $N_0(Z)$ and $N_1(Z)$ co-efficients are attenuated by the value of u, and so their contributions are also likely to be small. The $N_2(Z)$ co-efficients are likely to be the main gradient index contributors to Seidel aberration of the lens. The equations show that the spherical aberration has the opposite sign to that of the $N_2(Z)$ co-efficients. Thus, if the gradient index medium is to reduce the spherical aberration of the eye, the sign of these co-efficients must be positive.

Summary of main symbols

λ	vacuum wavelength
n'	refractive index of the vitreous humour
$\bar{\rho}$	radius of entrance pupil

r ray height in pupil (say in millimetres)

τ relative field position defined by equation (A2.12)

H optical invariant defined by equation (A2.9)

θ direction of a point in the object field

η distance of object from axis

Seidel aberrations

S_1 spherical aberration
S_2 coma
S_3 astigmatism
S_4 Petzval curvature
S_5 distortion
C_L longitudinal chromatic aberration

C_T transverse chromatic aberration

$W(r)$ wave aberration for ray passing through the pupil at a height r

$_0W_{4,0}$ etc. wave aberration co-efficients

References

Hopkins, H. H. (1950). *The Wave Theory of Aberrations*. Clarendon Press.

Sands, P. J. (1970). Third order aberrations of inhomogeneous lenses. *J. Opt. Soc. Am.*, **60**, 1436–43.

Smith, G. and Atchison, D. A. (1997). In *The Eye and Visual Optical Instruments*, Ch. 33. Cambridge University Press.

Welford, W. T. (1986). *Aberrations of Optical Systems*. Adam Hilger.

A3

Schematic eyes

Introduction

This appendix lists constructional data, Gaussian constants such as the pupil positions and sizes, the positions of the cardinal points, and the Seidel aberrations of several paraxial and finite schematic eyes. The constructional data were taken from references, but Gaussian and aberration values were determined by the authors.

Seidel aberrations were evaluated for the schematic eyes using an 8 mm entrance pupil diameter, a semi-field angle of 5° and a reference wavelength of 589 nm. The optical invariant H has the value 0.349955. The V-value of all ocular media is taken as 50.23, based on equations (17.15) and (17.17).

Units

Distances are in millimetres and are generally measured from the front surface vertex of the cornea.

Powers are expressed in units of dioptres (D or m^{-1}).

Accommodation levels are measured at the anterior corneal surface vertex.

The Seidel aberrations and the primary wave aberration co-efficients are given in units of wavelengths ($\lambda = 589$ nm), except for S_5 and C_T, which are given as percentages.

Paraxial schematic eyes

List of eyes

Gullstrand exact (Gullstrand, 1909)
  relaxed
  accommodated 10.878 D
Le Grand theoretical (Le Grand and El Hage, 1980)
  relaxed
  accommodated 7.053 D
Gullstrand–Emsley simplified (Emsley, 1952)
  relaxed
  accommodated 8.599 D
Bennett–Rabbetts simplified (Rabbetts, 1998)
  relaxed
Emsley reduced (Emsley, 1952).

Relaxed 'exact' schematic eyes

Gullstrand exact or number 1

Medium	n	R	d	Equivalent powers		
				Surface	Component	Whole eye
Air	1.000					
		7.700		48.831		
Cornea	1.376		0.500		43.053	
		6.800		−5.882		
Aqueous	1.336		3.100			
		10.000		5.000		58.636
Lens: Cortex	1.386		0.546			
		7.911		2.528		
Core	1.406		2.419		19.111	
		−5.760		3.472		
Cortex	1.386		0.635			
		−6.000		8.333		
Vitreous	1.336		17.18540			

Le Grand full theoretical eye

Medium	n	R	d	Equivalent powers		
				Surface	Component	Whole eye
Air	1.0000					
		7.800		48.346		
Cornea	1.3771		0.550		42.356	
		6.500		−6.108		
Aqueous	1.3374		3.050			
		10.200		8.098		59.940
Lens	1.4200		4.000		21.779	
		−6.000		14.000		
Vitreous	1.3360		16.59655			

Relaxed simplified schematic eyes

Gullstrand–Emsley

Medium	n	R	d	Equivalent powers		
				Surface	Component	Whole eye
Air	1.000					
		7.800		42.735	42.735	
Cornea	4/3		3.6			60.483
		10.000		8.267		
Lens	1.416		3.6		21.755	
		−6.00		13.778		
Vitreous	4/3		16.69620			

Bennett–Rabbetts

| Medium | n | R | d | Equivalent powers | | |
				Surface	Component	Whole eye
Air	1.000					
		7.800		43.077	43.077	
Cornea	1.336		3.6			
		11.000		7.818		60.000
Lens	1.422		3.7		20.828	
		−6.47515		13.280		
Vitreous	1.336		16.78627			

Reduced eyes

Emsley

| Medium | n | R | d | Equivalent powers | | |
				Surface	Component	Whole eye
Air	1.000					
		5.555̇				60.00
Vitreous	4/3		22.22222			

Accommodated 'exact' schematic eyes

Gullstrand (accommodation distance = −92.00 mm (≈ 10.878 D))

| Medium | n | R | d | Equivalent powers | | |
				Surface	Component	Whole eye
Air	1.000					
		7.700		48.831		
Cornea	1.376		0.500		43.053	
		6.800		−5.882		
Aqueous	1.336		2.700			
		5.333		9.376		70.576
Lens: Cortex	1.386		0.6725			
		2.655		7.533		
Core	1.406		2.6550		33.057	
		−2.655		7.533		
Cortex	1.386		0.6725			
		5.333		9.376		
Vitreous	1.336		17.18540			

Le Grand full theoretical eye (accommodation distance = −141.793 mm (≈ 7.053 D))

Medium	n	R	d	Equivalent powers		
				Surface	Component	Whole eye
Air	1.0000					
		7.800		48.346		
Cornea	1.3771		0.550		42.356	
		6.500		−6.108		
Aqueous	1.3374		2.650			67.677
		6.000		14.933		
Lens	1.4270		4.500		30.700	
		−5.500		16.545		
Vitreous	1.3360		16.49655			

Accommodated simplified schematic eyes

Gullstrand–Emsley (accommodation distance = −116.298 mm (≈ 8.599 D))

Medium	n	R	d	Equivalent powers		
				Surface	Component	Whole eye
Air	1.000					
		7.8		42.735	42.735	
Cornea	4/3		3.2			69.721
		5.0		16.533		
Lens	1.416		4.0		32.295	
		−5.0		16.533		
Vitreous	4/3		16.69621			

Gaussian properties

	Relaxed eyes					Accommodated eyes		
	'Exact'		Simplified		Reduced		'Exact'	Simplified
	Gull. 1	Le Grand	Gull–Ems	B–R	Emsley	Gull.	Le Grand	Gull–Ems
Power (D)	58.636	59.940	60.483	60	60	70.576	67.677	69.721
Eye length	24.385	24.197	23.896	24.086	22.222			
VV′	7.2	7.6	7.2	7.3	*	7.2	7.7	7.2
OV	∞	∞	∞	∞	∞	92.000	141.792	116.298
Accom. level (D)	0	0	0	0	0	10.870	7.053	8.599
Cardinal point positions								
VF	−15.706	−15.089	−14.983	−15.156	−16.667	−12.397	−12.957	−12.561
VF′	24.385	24.197	23.896	24.086	22.222	21.016	21.932	21.252
VP	1.348	1.595	1.550	1.511	0.000	1.772	1.819	1.782
VP′	1.601	1.908	1.851	1.819	0.000	2.086	2.192	2.128
VN	7.078	7.200	7.062	7.111	5.556	6.533	6.784	6.562
VN′	7.331	7.513	7.363	7.419	5.556	6.847	7.156	6.909
PN = P′N′	5.730	5.606	5.511	5.600	5.556	4.761	4.965	4.781
FP = N′F′	17.054	16.683	16.534	16.667	16.667	14.169	14.776	14.343
P′F′ = FN	22.785	22.289	22.045	22.267	22.222	18.930	19.741	19.124
N′R′						17.539	17.041	16.987
F′R′						3.370	2.264	2.644

Continued overleaf

Gaussian properties *continued*

| | Relaxed eyes | | | | Reduced | | Accommodated eyes | |
| | 'Exact' | | Simplified | | | | 'Exact' | | Simplified |
	Gull. 1	Le Grand	Gull–Ems	B–R	Emsley	Gull.	Le Grand	Gull–Ems
Pupils: (NA for 8 mm diameter pupil)								
VE	3.047	3.038	3.052	3.048	0.000	2.668	2.660	2.674
VE′	3.665	3.682	3.687	3.699	0.000	3.212	3.255	3.249
$\overline{M}_{EA}$	1.133	1.131	1.130	1.131	1.000	1.117	1.115	1.114
$\overline{M}_{E'A}$	1.031	1.041	1.036	1.036	1.000	1.051	1.055	1.049
$N\bar{A}$	0	0	0	0	0	0.0423	0.0277	0.0375
$N\bar{A}'$	0.2345	0.240	0.242	0.240	0.240	0.2374	0.2414	0.2710
$\overline{m}$	0.823085	0.813243	0.818128	0.817532	0.750000	0.795850	0.791122	0.796683
E′R′	20.720	20.515	20.209	20.387	22.222	21.173	20.942	20.647

Seidel aberrations

	$S_1/8$	$S_2/2$	$S_3/4$	$S_4/4$	$\%S_5$	$C_L/2$	$\%C_T$
Relaxed eyes							
Gullstrand exact eye (by surface contribution)							
1	23.6327	9.6202	0.4895	1.8447	−0.0800	9.5960	−0.3287
2	−2.0030	−0.7207	−0.0324	−0.1663	0.0060	−0.8665	0.0262
3	0.1577	0.2090	0.0346	0.1404	−0.0195	0.4821	−0.0538
4	0.2057	0.2100	0.0268	0.0675	−0.0081	0.2489	−0.0214
5	5.1871	−1.0374	0.0259	0.0926	0.0020	0.5175	0.0087
6	11.7803	−2.0552	0.0449	0.2340	0.0041	1.2479	0.0183
Total	38.9605	6.2258	0.5893	2.2127	−0.0955	11.2259	−0.3506
Le Grand	39.1445	6.2642	0.5619	2.2578	−0.1012	11.3592	−0.3694
Gullstrand–Emsley	41.2324	5.8719	0.5901	2.2731	−0.0990	11.5061	−0.3603
Bennett–Rabbetts	38.5293	5.8075	0.5819	2.2534	−0.0997	11.4031	−0.3622
Emsley	59.4091	28.8757	1.7543	2.3392	−0.1674	12.1682	−0.4977
Accommodated eyes							
Gullstrand exact eye (by surface contribution)							
1	29.6779	12.4057	0.6482	1.8447	−0.0877	9.8212	−0.3455
2	−2.5355	−0.9513	−0.0446	−0.1663	0.0067	−0.8856	0.0280
3	5.6696	2.8705	0.1817	0.2632	−0.0190	1.2617	−0.0538
4	22.8734	6.7077	0.2458	0.2009	−0.0110	1.0154	−0.0251
5	34.7899	1.8831	0.0127	0.2009	−0.0010	1.0154	−0.0046
6	15.8359	−1.4826	0.0173	0.2632	0.0021	1.3966	0.0110
Total	106.3111	21.4332	1.0613	2.6066	−0.1098	13.6247	−0.3900
Le Grand	53.5239	12.0929	0.8439	2.5104	−0.1126	12.9305	−0.4044
Gullstrand–Emsley	65.9357	14.0976	0.9216	2.5765	−0.1092	13.4028	−0.3921

Finite schematic eyes

List of eyes

Lotmar (1971)
Kooijman (1983)
Navarro *et al.* (1985)
Liou and Brennan (1997)

Further information about these model eyes is given in Chapters 16 and 17.

Lotmar (1971) – same as Le Grand eye except for surface asphericities

Medium	n	R	Q	d	Equivalent powers		
					Surface	Component	Whole eye
Air	1.0000						
		7.8	–0.286*		48.346		
Cornea	1.3771			0.55		42.356	
		6.5	0		–6.108		
Aqueous	1.3374			3.05			59.940
		10.2	0		8.098		
Lens	1.4200			4.00		21.779	
		–6.0	–1.0		14.000		
Vitreous	1.3360			16.59655			
		–12.3					

*Lotmar represented the front surface of the cornea by equation (17.23), and the above value of Q is the value for a figured conicoid fitted to equation (17.25). The conicoid asphericity and figuring co-efficients are:
$Q = -0.2857143$, $f_4 = 0.0$, $f_6 = -2.547626E-06$, $f_8 = -8.104263E-09$, $f_{10} = -6.660308E-11$, $f_{12} = -5.864599E-13$
The termination of the figuring co-efficients at the a_{12} term gives an error of less than 2E-06 at a ray height of $h = 4$ mm.

Kooijman (1983) – same as Le Grand eye except for surface asphericities

Medium	n	R	Q	d	Equivalent powers		
					Surface	Component	Whole eye
Air	1.0000						
		7.8	–0.25		48.346		
Cornea	1.3771			0.50		42.356	
		6.5	–0.25		–6.108		
Aqueous	1.3374			3.05			59.940
		10.2	–3.06		8.098		
Lens	1.4200			4.00		21.779	
		–6.0	–1.0		14.000		
Vitreous	1.3360			16.59655			

Two models of retinal radius were offered; one with a radius of curvature of –10.8 mm and a Q value of 0, and the other with a radius of curvature of –14.1 mm and a Q value of 0.346.

Navarro *et al.* (1985)

Medium	n	R	Q	d	Equivalent powers		
					Surface	Component	Whole eye
Air	1.0000						
		7.72	–0.26		48.705		
Cornea	1.376			0.55		42.882	
		6.5	0		–5.983		
Aqueous	1.3374			$(3.05)d_2$			60.416
		$(10.2)R_3$	$(-3.1316)Q_3$			8.098	
Lens	$(1.42)n_3$			$(4.00)d_3$		21.779	
		$(-6.0)R_4$	$(-1.0)Q_4$			14.000	
Vitreous	1.3360			16.40398			
		–12.0					

The bracketed values are for the relaxed condition.

The model is set any level of accommodation by the following equations:

$$R_3 = 10.2 \quad - 1.75 \quad \ln(A + 1)$$
$$R_4 = -6.0 \quad + 0.2294 \ \ln(A + 1)$$
$$d_2 = 3.05 \quad - 0.05 \quad \ln(A + 1)$$
$$d_3 = 4.0 \quad + 0.1 \quad \ln(A + 1)$$
$$n_3 = 1.42 \quad + 9\times10^{-5} \ (10A + A^2)$$
$$Q_3 = -3.1316 - 0.34 \quad \ln(A + 1)$$
$$Q_4 = -1.0 \quad - 0.125 \quad \ln(A + 1)$$

where A is the accommodation level (dioptres).
For example, at 10 D of accommodation,

Medium	n	R	Q	d	Equivalent powers		
					Surface	Component	Whole eye
Air	1.0000						
		7.72	−0.26		48.705		
Cornea	1.376			0.50		42.882	
		6.5	0		−5.938		
Aqueous	1.3374			2.930110			71.145
		6.00368	−3.94688		16.756		
Lens	1.438			4.23979		34.548	
		−5.44992	−1.29974		18.716		
Vitreous	1.3360			16.28415			
		−12.0					

Liou and Brennan (1997)

Medium	n	R	Q	d	Equivalent powers		
					Surface	Component	Whole eye
Air	1.000						
		7.77	−0.18		48.391		
Cornea	1.376			0.55		42.262	
		6.40	−0.60		−6.250		
Aqueous	1.336			3.16			60.314
		12.40	−0.94		2.581		
Lens	Grad A			1.59	6.283		
		∞	−			22.134	
Lens	Grad P			2.43	9.586		
		−8.10	+0.96		3.950		
Vitreous	1.336			16.23883			

Gradient index details of lens:

	Grad A	Grad P
$N_{0,0} =$	1.368	1.407
$N_{0,1} =$	0.049057	0.000000
$N_{0,2} =$	−0.015427	−0.006605
$N_{1,0} =$	−0.001978	−0.001978

No retinal radius of curvature was provided.
The stop is displaced 0.5 mm from the optical axis to the nasal side.

Gaussian properties

	Lotmar*, Kooijman*	Navarro Relaxed	Navarro Accomm (10 D)	Liou and Brennan
Eye length	24.196552	24.003979	24.003979	23.950014
Power	59.940	60.416	71.145	60.343
Cardinal point positions				
VF	−15.089	−14.969	−12.051	−15.040
VF′	24.197	24.004	21.172	23.950
VP	1.595	1.583	2.005	1.532
VP′	1.908	1.890	2.393	1.810
VN	7.200	7.145	6.727	7.100
VN′	7.513	7.452	7.116	7.378
PN = P′N′	5.606	5.561	4.723	5.568
FP = N′F′	16.683	16.552	14.056	16.572
P′F′ = FN	22.289	22.114	18.779	22.140
F′R′	0.000	0.000	2.832	0.000
Pupils:				
VE	3.038	3.042	2.928	3.098
VE′	3.682	3.682	3.551	3.720
$\overline{M}_{EA}$	1.133	1.133	1.128	1.133
$\overline{M}_{E′A}$	1.041	1.041	1.058	1.035
$\overline{m}$	0.813243	0.814493	0.797668	0.819238

*Same as Le Grand full theoretical eye.

Seidel aberrations

	$S_1/8$	$S_2/2$	$S_3/4$	$S_4/4$	$\%S_5$
Relaxed eyes					
Lotmar (1971)	20.3144	7.1107	0.3392	2.2578	−0.1001
Kooijman (1983)	15.7668	6.2829	0.3648	2.2578	−0.0995
Navarro *et al.* (1985)	13.8628	7.0582	0.3421	2.2775	−0.0991
Liou and Brennan* (1997)	7.3745	1.6754	0.5424	1.8371	−0.2064
Accommodated eyes					
Navarro *et al.* (1985) (10 D)	−26.1827	9.0316	0.4876	2.6315	−0.1019

*The stop is displaced 0.5 mm from the optical axis to the nasal side, but this has been ignored for the analysis.

Summary of symbols

n	refractive index	**R′**	Position of retina (at axial pole)
r	radius of curvature	$\overline{M}_{EA}, \overline{M}_{E′A}$	magnification of entrance pupil
d	surface separations		and exit pupil
E, E′	Entrance and exit pupils	$\overline{m}$	ratio of the paraxial pupil ray
F, F′	Front and back focal points		angles in image and object
P, P′	Front and back principal points		space
N, N′	Front and back nodal points	*NA, NA′*	numerical apertures in object
V, V′	Front and back vertex points		and image spaces

References

Emsley, H. H. (1952). *Visual Optics*, vol. 1, 5th edn, pp. 40–41, 346. Butterworths.

Gullstrand, A. (1909). Appendix II: Procedure of rays in the eye. Imagery – laws of the first order. In *Helmholtz's Handbuch der Physiologischen Optik*, vol. 1, 3rd edn (English translation edited by J. P. Southall, Optical Society of America, 1924).

Helmholtz, H. von (1909). *Handbuch der Physiologischen Optik*, vol. 1, 3rd edn (English translation edited by J. P. Southall, Optical Society of America, 1924).

Kooijman, A. C. (1983). Light distribution on the retina of a wide-angle theoretical eye. *J. Opt. Soc. Am.*, **73**, 1544–50.

Le Grand, Y. and El Hage, S. G. (1980). *Physiological Optics*. Translation and update of Le Grand Y. (1968). *La dioptrique de l'oeil et sa correction*, vol. I of *Optique physiologique*, pp. 65–7. Springer-Verlag.

Liou, H.-L. and Brennan, N. A. (1997). Anatomically accurate, finite model eye for optical modeling. *J. Opt. Soc. Am. A.*, **14**, 1684–95.

Lotmar, W. (1971). Theoretical eye model with aspheric surfaces. *J. Opt. Soc. Am.*, **61**, 1522–9.

Navarro, R., Santamaría, J. and Bescós, J. (1985). Accommodation-dependent model of the human eye with aspherics. *J. Opt. Soc. Am. A.*, **2**, 1273–81.

Rabbetts, R. B. (1998). *Bennett and Rabbetts' Clinical Visual Optics*, 3rd edn, pp. 209–13. Butterworth-Heinemann.

A4

Calculation of PSF and OTF from aberrations of an optical system

The point spread function (PSF)

We show how to calculate the PSF, taking into account diffraction, defocus, aberrations, polychromatic light, the photopic luminous efficiency function $V(\lambda)$ and the Stiles–Crawford effect. Scatter is more difficult to include in these calculations, so we will neglect it.

The PSF can be calculated if the wave aberration in the pupil of the eye is known. From optical image formation theory (see Smith and Atchison, 1997), the PSF is related to the wave aberration via a Fourier transform. The background for the following equations is taken from the above reference.

Rather than express the PSF as a light distribution at the retina, we will express it as the equivalent distribution projected back into object space. The major difference will be that, in the first case spatial co-ordinates will be in linear quantities such as millimetres, and in the second case they will be in angular units. Calculating the point spread function back in object space, taken as air, also avoids the need to use the image space refractive index in the diffraction integral.

Before we present equations for calculating the PSF from the wave aberration in the pupil, we must first distinguish the amplitude PSF from the intensity PSF. The amplitude PSF is the complex amplitude of the light distribution, whereas the intensity PSF is the actual light distribution that we measure with a light meter. When we refer to the PSF, we mean the intensity PSF unless otherwise indicated.

If we denote the amplitude PSF as $g_a(u,v)$, where u and v are the directions in object space, and the PSF as $g(u,v)$, these two quantities are related by the equation

$$g(u,v) = g_a(u,v)g^*_a(u,v) \tag{A4.1}$$

where * refers to the complex conjugate. The amplitude PSF is related to the wave aberration $W(X,Y)$ by the equation

$$g_a(u,v) = C\iint_E P(X,Y)e^{-i2\pi(uX + vY)}dXdY \tag{A4.2}$$

where

$$C \text{ is a constant} = (1/\lambda) \tag{A4.3}$$

E implies integration over the pupil of radius $\bar{\rho}$, (u, v) are related to the actual angles (in radians) θ_x and θ_y in the X and Y directions, respectively, by the equations

$$\theta_x = \lambda u \text{ and } \theta_y = \lambda v \tag{A4.4}$$

(X, Y) are the cartesian co-ordinates in the pupil, and $P(X, Y)$ is the complex amplitude in the pupil known as the **pupil function**, which is mathematically defined as

$$P(X, Y) = A(X,Y)e^{[-ikW(X,Y)]} \tag{A4.5}$$

The constant $k = 2\pi/\lambda$, $A(X, Y)$ is the amplitude transmittance at the point (X, Y) in the pupil, and is included to allow for the Stiles–Crawford effect. $W(X, Y)$ is the wave aberration as an optical path difference, and is expressed in normal units of distance and not wavelength.

Equation (A4.2) is a Fourier transform of

the pupil function $P(X, Y)$, and is zero outside the pupil. However, it would not be a Fourier transform if the object space variables were the real angles θ_x and θ_y, instead of u and v. In other words, the use of u and v and not θ_x and θ_y allows the amplitude point spread function to be expressed as a Fourier transform.

We will regard the Stiles–Crawford effect as rotationally symmetric in the pupil, and can write it as

$$A(X, Y) = e^{[-(\beta/2)(X^2 + Y^2)]} \tag{A4.6}$$

where β is the Stiles–Crawford attenuation factor to base e and the '/2' factor is included because we must use an 'amplitude' Stiles–Crawford effect and not the normal 'intensity' effect (Krakau, 1974). Typical values for β are given in Chapter 13.

The wave aberration function W(X, Y)

The wave aberration function $W(X, Y)$ is described in detail in Appendix 2. It is one way of quantifying the level of aberrations. The function is a polynomial in X and Y, and the different terms represent the different aberrations – e.g. spherical aberration and coma. It can also incorporate defocus and chromatic aberrations.

Defocus

If the eye is defocused by an amount ΔF, e.g. 0.5 D, a defocus term $W_{2,0}(X^2 + Y^2)$ can be added to the wave aberration polynomial, where ΔF and the co-efficient $W_{2,0}$ are related by equation (A2.5), i.e.

$$W_{2,0} = \Delta F / 2 \tag{A4.7}$$

For example, a defocus of +0.5 D gives $W_{2,0} = +0.00025 \text{ mm}^{-1}$.

Chromatic aberration

As discussed in Chapter 17, longitudinal and transverse chromatic aberration arise because of the dispersion of the ocular media. The dispersion leads to a chromatic change in power $\Delta F(\lambda)$ given by the equation

$$\Delta F(\lambda) = F(\lambda) - F(\bar{\lambda}) \tag{A4.8}$$

where $F(\lambda)$ is the power at the wavelength λ and $\bar{\lambda}$ is the reference wavelength for zero chromatic aberration. Equations for $F(\lambda)$ are given in Chapter 17.

For on-axis and off-axis point spread functions, longitudinal chromatic aberration is taken into account with a wave aberration term $W_{2,0}(\lambda)(X^2 + Y^2)$. The co-efficient is related to the chromatic change in power $\Delta F(\lambda)$ by the equation

$$W_{2,0}(\lambda) = \Delta F(\lambda) / 2 \tag{A4.9}$$

For off-axis point spread functions, transverse chromatic aberration is taken into account with a wave aberration term $W_{1,1}(\lambda)Y$ or $W_{1,1}(\lambda)X$. The co-efficient is related to the chromatic change in power $\Delta F(\lambda)$ by the equation

$$W_{1,1}(\lambda) = \bar{\theta}\mathbf{EN}\Delta F(\lambda) / n(\lambda) \tag{A4.10}$$

where $\bar{\theta}$ is the angular distance off-axis, $\mathbf{EN}$ is the distance from the entrance pupil to the front nodal point, and $n(\lambda)$ is the refractive index of the vitreous medium. Transverse chromatic aberration leads to a PSF having a transverse shift that is wavelength dependent.

Polychromatic sources

For polychromatic light sources, the PSF is calculated at a number of wavelengths. The chromatic aberrations are included in the wave aberration function. Each point spread function is weighted by both the relative sensitivity of the eye $V(\lambda)$ (Chapter 11) and the relative radiance of the source $S(\lambda)$. The polychromatic point spread function is formed by adding the weighted individual point spread functions, but only after these have been expressed in terms of the real angles θ_x and θ_y, instead of u and v. That is,

$$g(\theta_x, \theta_y) = \Sigma_\lambda V(\lambda) S(\lambda) g(\theta_x, \theta_y)_\lambda \tag{A4.11}$$

Computation checks

For any computation of the point spread function via equation (A4.2), it is good practice to have independent checks of the final result. The following three conditions can be used:

1. If the system is free of aberration:

$$g(0, 0) = |g_a(0, 0)|^2 = |C\iint_E P(X, Y)dXdY|^2$$
$$= \{(\pi/\lambda)\{1 - \exp[-(\beta/2)\bar{\rho}^2]\}/(\beta/2)\}^2$$

$$(A4.12)$$

If no Stiles–Crawford apodization is present, i.e. $\beta = 0$,

$$g(0, 0) = [(\pi/\lambda)\bar{\rho}^2]^2 \qquad (A4.12a)$$

2. Volume under PSF = effective flux passing through pupil

$$= \pi(1 - \exp(-\beta\bar{\rho}^2)]/\beta \qquad (A4.13)$$

If no Stiles–Crawford apodization is present, i.e. $\beta = 0$,

$$\text{Volume} = \pi\bar{\rho}^2 \qquad (A4.13a)$$

3. For an off-axis calculation on a rotationally symmetric system and a single wavelength, the peak of the point spread function should occur at the angle in equation (A4.10), i.e.

$$\theta_{peak} = \bar{\theta} \qquad (A4.14)$$

The optical transfer function (OTF)

A sinusoidal pattern with a real spatial frequency σ and an orientation ψ is shown in Figure A4.1. The spatial frequency components in the X and Y directions are

$$\sigma_x = \sigma \cos(\psi) \text{ and } \sigma_y = \sigma \sin(\psi) \qquad (A4.15)$$

The two dimensional OTF, which we write as $G(\sigma_x, \sigma_y)$, is the Fourier transform of the PSF

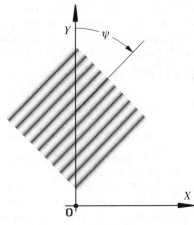

Figure A4.1. Sinusoidal pattern of grating inclined at an angle ψ.

$g(\theta_x, \theta_y)$, that is

$$G(\sigma_x, \sigma_y) = \int\int_{-\infty}^{+\infty+\infty} g(\theta_x, \theta_y)e^{-i2\pi(\theta_x\sigma_x + \theta_y\sigma_y)}d\theta_x d\theta_y$$

$$(A4.16)$$

However, calculation of the OTF by this direct relationship is not necessarily the best approach, because the PSF has no bounds and the integral should therefore be carried out over an infinite range. In practice we must use finite bounds but, depending upon how much of the PSF is outside these bounds, there will be errors in the final results. A better alternative is to use a Fourier transform identity (Bracewell, 1986), that states that the Fourier transform of the product of the transforms of

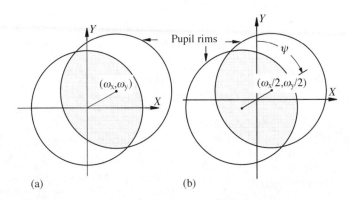

Figure A4.2. The sheared pupils used to calculate the OTF from equations (A4.17) and (A4.18).

two functions is the convolution of two functions. In this case, equation (A4.16) reduces to a convolution of the pupil function $P(X, Y)$ with its complex conjugate, as follows:

$$G(\omega_x, \omega_y) = \iint_c P(X, Y)P^*(X - \omega_x, Y - \omega_y)dXdY$$

(A4.17)

where

$$\omega_x = \sigma_x \lambda \text{ and } \omega_y = \sigma_y \lambda \qquad (A4.17a)$$

replace σ_x and σ_y in G and the integrand.

Since the pupil function $P(X, Y)$ is zero outside the pupil, the limits of integration reduce to the region 'c' common to the two sheared pupils shown shaded in Figure A4.2a, and we do not have to write the integral limits from $-\infty$ to $+\infty$. A useful alternative and equivalent form of this integral is

$$G(\omega_x, \omega_y) = \iint_c P(X + \omega_x/2, Y + \omega_y/2)P^*(X - \omega_x/2, Y - \omega_y/2)dXdY \qquad (A4.18)$$

with the region of integration now being that shown in Figure A4.2b.

Macdonald (1971) has described such a method for the routine calculation of the OTF based upon the above auto-correlation integral, but with the amplitude function $A(X, Y) = 1$.

It is common practice to normalize the OTF so that $G(0, 0) = 1$.

Summary of main symbols

$g(\theta_x, \theta_y)$	Point spread function (PSF)
θ_x, θ_y	angles in X and Y directions
X, Y	cartesian co-ordinates in the actual pupil
β	Stiles–Crawford parameter to base e
$G(\sigma_x, \sigma_y)$	optical transfer function (OTF)
σ	spatial frequency (c/rad)
σ_x, σ_y	components of σ in the X and Y directions
ω_x, ω_y	corresponding modified spatial frequencies, related to (σ_x, σ_y) by equation (A4.17a)

References

Bracewell, R. (1986). *The Fourier Transform and its Applications*, revised edn, p. 112. McGraw-Hill.

Krakau, C. E. T. (1974). On the Stiles–Crawford phenomenon and resolution power. *Acta Ophthal.*, **52**, 581–3.

Macdonald, J. (1971). The calculation of the optical transfer function. *Optica Acta*, 18, 269–90.

Smith, G. and Atchison, D. A. (1997). Image quality criteria. In *The Eye and Visual Optical Instruments*. Cambridge University Press pp. 647–72.

Index